D0847354

SHELTON STATE LIBRARY

Discarded

SSCC

RT
85
.H87
1991

Husted, Gladys L.

Ethical decision
making in nursing

33626000350648

DATE DUE

ETHICAL DECISION MAKING IN NURSING

Discarded
SSCC

ETHICAL DECISION MAKING IN NURSING

Gladys L. Husted, R.N., Ph.D.

Associate Professor
Duquesne University School of Nursing
Pittsburgh, Pennsylvania

James H. Husted

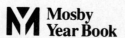 Mosby
Year Book

St. Louis Baltimore Boston Chicago London Philadelphia Sydney Toronto

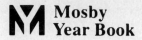

Mosby
Year Book

Dedicated to Publishing Excellence

Editor: Linda L. Duncan
Project Manager: Annette Hall

Copyright © 1991 by Mosby–Year Book, Inc.
A Mosby imprint of Mosby–Year Book, Inc.

All rights reserved. No part of this publication may be
reproduced, stored in a retrieval system, or transmitted, in
any form or by any means, electronic, mechanical,
photocopying, recording, or otherwise, without prior written
permission from the publisher.

Printed in the United States of America

Mosby–Year Book, Inc.
11830 Westline Industrial Drive
St. Louis, MO 63146

Library of Congress Cataloging in Publication Data

Husted, Gladys L.
    Ethical decision making in nursing / Gladys L. Husted, James H.
  Husted. — 1st ed.
        p.   cm.
    Includes bibliographical references and index.
    ISBN 0-8016-3382-6
    1. Nursing ethics.   I. Husted, James H.   II. Title.
    [DNLM: 1. Decision Making—nurses' instruction.   2. Ethics,
  Nursing.   3. Models, Theoretical.   WY 85 H872e]
  RT85.H87   1991
  174′.2 – dc20
  DNLM/DLC
  for Library of Congress   90–13682
                                                                  CIP

GW/DC/DC   9   8   7   6   5   4   3   2   1

ACKNOWLEDGMENTS

We wish to acknowledge our indebtedness to the following people:

Linda Duncan, who had the courage to entertain a new idea.

Joanna May, whose editorial comments and suggestions on the structure of the book were invaluable.

Annette Hall, who made the task of plucking the thorns from the final product enjoyable.

M. Carroll Miller, a friend and colleague, for her critiques of early drafts of each chapter and for her constant encouragement and support.

Tabitha A. Husted, our daughter, who gave us the gifts of time, love, encouragement, and support.

The graduate nursing students of N. 761 who served as a crucible for refining the dominant ideas in this book.

The Arkangels for their enthusiasm and friendship.

And finally to **Charlie** — Charlie to whom this book is dedicated.

PREFACE

The past thirty or forty years have seen an ethical revolution in biomedicine. The hope of one traditional ethical outlook gaining general assent has given way to modern bioethics. Bioethics, as we shall see, is an ethical system appropriate to a wide range of cultural outlooks but dependent on none of them.

Nurses today practice in a "melting pot" society. No nurse can hope to find his or her beliefs shared by everyone in the biomedical setting. Everyone wants to act in ways believed to be ethically right. Whatever your ethical beliefs, however, you, as a nurse, will be faced with the necessity of taking actions that you consider wrong.

This is not a reason for you to ignore questions of right and wrong. It is, in fact, a very important reason for you to understand your ethical beliefs. You are at a very great disadvantage if you do not understand why you consider one action right and another action wrong. You will be unable to interact on an equal footing with your colleagues. You will not be able to objectively and effectively defend the actions you take. You will have no objective means of moral self-defense.

Bioethics is, by conscious design, an ethic appropriate to people practicing a profession as professionals. It is a set of standards of behavior, requiring contextual understanding, through which biomedical professionals can choose and justify their ethical decisions and actions.

APPROACH

A person cannot learn anything well without experiencing it. A nurse learns best about bioethics in the biomedical situation. The approach of this book is to guide the nurse's experience—to suggest what she should look for.

In mastering bioethics you, as a nurse, will learn *why* you hold the ethical positions of your profession. You may learn that some of your prior ethical beliefs are inappropriate to the biomedical context. You may have to give up those beliefs. You could, conceivably, learn that you cannot accept some of the ethical standards of nursing. In learning the reasons why the bioethical standards are appropriate to nursing, you will become better able to meet the ethical demands of nursing.

ETHICS AS PURPOSIVE

Bioethics is purposive through and through. The decision-making standards presented here are the commonly accepted ideals of the biomedical professions, not the invention or creation of the authors. The bioethical literature is filled with discussions of the bioethical standards. This book attempts to draw out the implications of these standards and discuss their contextual application.

The bioethical standards not only serve as guides to bioethical decision making and action, they, themselves, *are* ethical decisions. They are decisions reached by thousands of biomedical professionals through decades of experience—the experience of that which is successful and right and that which is unsuccessful and wrong.

One bioethical standard is the decision that every patient has a right to be treated according to his unique character structure.

Another is the decision that every patient has a right to decide and act on his own values.

Yet another is the decision that every patient, under ordinary circumstances, has a right to expect complete and objective information.

Still another is the decision that every patient has a right to self-ownership.

The decision that every patient has a right to expect whatever benefit is possible in the health care setting, and to expect no harm, is another bioethical standard.

The standard that every patient has a right to expect that the agreements between himself and health care professionals will be kept is also a universally held bioethical decision.

The bioethical standards are tools of justification. They are generally accepted; but not always consistently applied. This text subjects the applications of these standards to stringent examination and analysis.

REALISM AND PURPOSE

In this book we take the position that a nurse's ethical motivations ought to be focused on the purposes of nursing. We argue that the purpose of a nurse's ethical actions is set by the mutual expectations of the nurse and her patient when they enter into the agreement that establishes their relationship as nurse and patient.

Bioethics, when it is consistent, is centered entirely on the welfare of the bioethical professional's patient. It is, therefore, of necessity a form of ethical realism.

Ethical realism is the theory that every ethical truth arises from the situations in which it is true. It is an ethic appropriate — and faithful — to the ethical context. As an ethical system for professionals, bioethics takes ethical realism for granted. There is no possibility of objective justification and no possibility of a nurse acting as an independent bioethical agent without this ethical realism.

With ethical realism absolute infallibility is impossible. You, the nurse, cannot hold infallibility as a rational standard. However, you can, and must, hold justifiability as your standard. No one, not even you yourself, can rationally expect more than that you did the best you could have done under a particular set of circumstances.

Bioethics is not only realistic; it is also a purposive ethic.

A professional ethic must allow you to:

1. Have some basis for believing that your decisions and actions are appropriate to the profession of nursing.
2. Contrast your ethical position with other positions in such a way that you can judge whether yours is superior.
3. Be able to justify your decisions and actions.

This is only possible if your actions are guided by an objective purpose.

In the context of a purposive ethic, reason (thinking) must be an element of the decision-making process.

A professional ethic that does not put reason at its center is no different from that of the "man in the street." If it were no different from the ethical system of the man in the street, it would not, in any relevant sense, be a professional ethic.

SCOPE OF THE DISCUSSION

This book covers every type of bioethical dilemma from bedwetting to euthanasia. It demonstrates the relevance of the contemporary bioethical standards to these (and by extension to all) bioethical dilemmas. It rigorously examines how the contemporary bioethical standards must be defined and understood in order to be used in ethical decision making.

This approach brings the reader into the center of the bioethical environment. The ethical decision-making process presented throughout the book should enable a person entering a nursing career to more quickly be at home in the profession.

Although we recognize that the nurse should not break the law, we do not address legal issues in this text. The ethical is something in and of itself, and it is logically prior to the legal.

History shows that atrocious ethical actions can be enacted into law. Whatever the law on abortion, half the population will consider it immoral. If a distinction between the legal and the ethical is not made, no law will ever be changed. If, in your practice, you take an entirely legalistic approach to ethical issues, then you are failing to take ethical issues seriously. If you fail to take ethical issues seriously, then quite obviously you will never master ethical decision making.

OVERVIEW

We begin Part One by discussing just enough of the history and nature of ethics to set the context of what is to follow. Then we discuss:

- The crucial necessity of justification.
- The function of the nurse/patient agreement in the ethical interaction of nurse and patient.
- The appropriateness of the traditional ethical theories to the biomedical setting.
- The radical importance of the context in ethical decision making and action.
- The occurrence of conflicts among the bioethical standards.

In Part Two we discuss:

- The elements of autonomy as resolutions to conflicts among the bioethical standards.
- The elements of autonomy as keys to the context.
- The function of introspection in ethical decision making.
- The bioethical context as an interweaving of the individual contexts of autonomous agents.

In Part Three the dilemmas are resolved* according to the theoretical

---

*The reader will notice that, beginning with Chapter 3, certain paragraphs are numbered. The numbers refer to the dilemma described in the paragraph. Part Three contains the resolutions of the dilemmas found in Parts One and Two double-numbered by chapter. This will enable the reader to quickly refer back to the particular dilemma in either of the first two parts.

HUSTED'S FORMAL ETHICAL DECISION MAKING MODEL

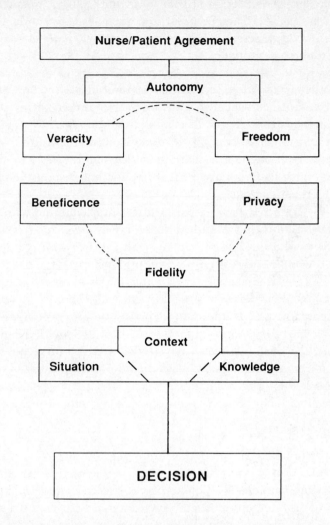

bases developed throughout Parts One and Two. The reader cannot expect to understand the logic behind the resolutions without understanding the theoretical bases on which the dilemmas were resolved.

The book sets out an ethical decision-making model based on a contextual application of the bioethical standards. The model is structured to help nurses make contextually appropriate (justifiable) ethical decisions.

In one way or another all of a nurse's ethical decisions involve the terms of an implicit agreement that she makes with her patient. Husted's model is derived from this agreement. It is based upon six noncontroversial but crucial points.

Husted's Formal Ethical Decision-Making Model

1. In order to grasp the terms of the nurse/patient agreement the nurse needs to be aware of her patient's unique nature (autonomy). Every patient is a unique personality. To interact with a patient is to interact with that unique personality.

   When a nurse acts as a researcher, an educator, or an administrator, she will not be aware of the unique characteristics of any individual patient. She must, however, always be aware of the unique characteristics of patients *as patients*. If a nursing action is to be justifiable, it must, directly or indirectly, be an action oriented toward patients. A nurse who fails to recognize the unique character of her patient fails to honor the nurse/patient agreement. She fails her responsibility to take justifiable ethical actions.

2. In order to interact with a patient a nurse must interact with his freedom. Every action that a patient takes arises from his freedom. The precondition of a nurse's interacting with the freedom of a patient is that she recognize and respect his freedom. A nurse who fails to respect her patient's freedom is not interacting *with her patient*. She, therefore, fails to honor the agreement she has made with him.

3. In order for a person to interact according to an agreement he must understand the terms of the agreement. This understanding cannot exist unless the relationship between the parties is based on a rational trust, and rational trust cannot exist unless the relationship is based on veracity. Except in rare circumstances a nurse who does not communicate and interact with her patient on the basis of objective truth violates the agreement she has made with him.

4. A situation where interaction takes place by agreement, yet one party to the agreement has been coerced, is an impossible situation. If any party to the interaction is coerced, there is no agreement. If an interaction occurs through agreement, then no one is coerced into this interaction. No party to an interaction based on an agreement agrees to be forced. No one *can* agree to be forced. Wherever there is interaction based on agreement, there is the implicit presumption of the self-ownership (privacy) of the parties to the agreement. Any agreement is invalid if it, implicitly or explicitly, denies the self-ownership of one of the parties to the agreement. It, in effect, leaves one party to the agreement out of the agreement.

5. Wherever there is an agreement, there is a final purpose of the agreement. An agreement without a final purpose would be unintelligible. It would be an agreement to do nothing, and, therefore, no agreement at all. Whatever the nature of this final purpose the exchange of values that the agreement calls for is beneficent action. Every agreement, by

its nature, calls for beneficient action. A nurse who fails to act beneficently toward her patient fails to fulfill the agreement she has with him.

6. Wherever there is an agreement there must be fidelity to the agreement.
   An agreement that will not be honored is a contradiction in terms. No
   nurse can ever justify an ethical decision or action that violates the
   implicit agreement she has with her patient.

All these considerations form the ethical context of the interaction between
nurse and patient. The ethical effectiveness of this interaction depends upon
the nurse's acquisition of optimal awareness—the widest possible context of
knowledge—and on her bringing about, as nearly as possible, ideal conditions for what she and her patient intend. This book is designed to help you
acquire that optimal awareness.

Your ethical decision ought to be based on the context of the ethical
situation. It ought to be the product of your actual context of knowledge.

Your ethical decision ought to be the realization of your fidelity to the
agreement.

Your realization of fidelity to the agreement is an expression of beneficence.

Ideally this expression of beneficence results in an enhancement of your
self-ownership and the self-ownership of your patient.

Fidelity to the agreement involves veracity on the part of the parties to the
agreement.

Fidelity to the agreement presupposes an essentially free interaction between nurse and patient.

All of this presupposes some understanding, on the part of each party, of
the autonomy of the other.

All of this is facilitated by an increase in a nurse's actual context of
knowledge. This book is designed to bring about that increase.

* * *

We predominantly use the pronoun "she" to designate the nurse. This is,
we hope, justified by the fact that over 90 percent of nurses are women. On
the other hand, we almost invariably use the pronoun "he" to designate the
patient. This is not because the majority of patients are men, but simply for
the reader's ease of understanding.

Gladys L. Husted
James H. Husted

CONTENTS

ETHICAL DECISION MAKING IN NURSING

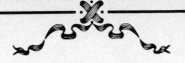

PART ONE

ELEMENTS OF THE ETHICAL DECISION-MAKING MODEL

CHAPTER
1

A Critical History of Ethics

Every field of study has a purpose. Human beings need to navigate the seas, someone creates astronomy. Curious about living things, someone creates biology. Someone creates mathematics for the purpose of computation. Someone creates medicine from a desire to heal. Every science and every art arises from need or from curiosity. This is as true of ethics as it is of any other field of study.

In observing human lives one often perceives tragedy. People bring about the conditions of their own unhappiness. At the end of their lives they may look back with regret. When they observe what they have become, they may find consolation in misery.

Socrates, the founder of ethics, was not the first person ever to think about these very basic human problems. He was probably the first to think about them rigorously and systematically. He proposed a systematic examination of human life as the way to a solution. This began that part of philosophy that is ethics. It was a study of the *good life* (Aristotle cited in McKeon, 1941). Ethics examines good and evil in terms of the demands of successful living.

In an ethical context that which is contrary to human welfare is the "evil." That which tends to promote human welfare is the "good." In an ethical context a "successful" life is a life that one experiences as worth living.

The demands of successful living are the natural principles of ethics. For instance, successful living requires the virtue of courage (Plato cited in Jowett, 1937). Therefore courage is one of the natural principles of ethics.

In a derivative way ethics, also, involves a study of the interactions of ethical agents. This study is made in terms of right and wrong. The study deals with the conditions under which one agent has, or has not, the right to expect to benefit from the action of another.

In an interpersonal context ethics is the study of what brings good or evil into human life through human interaction. It looks to the nature of agreements and the proper behavior of ethical agents when an agreement is lacking. It is concerned with the nature of the goals that agents ought to pursue together. It examines the decisions and choices agents ought to make in regard to these goals.

In an interpersonal ethical context the "wrong" is that which involves deception or coercion. The "right" is that which is based on objective agreement.

Ethics examines the processes of decision making and the ways in which agents reach, or fail to reach, their goals.

For all these reasons ethics has traditionally been called "the practical science". The ability to engage in processes of ethical analysis is known as *practical reason.*"[Since] ethics is fundamentally a practical discipline [it is] concerned with what we should do and how we should live..." (Churchill, 1989, p. 28).

THE BIRTH OF ETHICS

In order for a new science to be discovered certain conditions are necessary:

1. The science must yield very abstract and general knowledge. There can be no science of crab apple trees. The discovery rf how the speed of hair growth can be predicted would not constitute a science. These subjects are too narrow. Science is concerned with very broad areas of human interest.
2. There must be a purpose for the discovery. If it fulfills no need, it cannot be a science. There is no *scientific* way to harness flying horses. There is no possibility of anyone needing to harness a flying horse.
3. It must be possible to make the discovery. There must be something out in the world to be discovered. There can be no scientific way to study the effects of time travel. So far, at least, there are no effects of time travel.

In addition to these conditions the discoverer must possess certain qualities. A discoverer must:

1. Love the pursuit of knowledge.
2. Have a tireless curiousity concerning the subject matter.
3. Possess genius.

Most of us must content ourselves with possessing the first two qualities. Therefore very few of us will ever discover a new science. But we can share the adventure of discovery.

The founder of ethics possessed all three qualities in abundance. He is, perhaps, the most famous philosopher who ever lived. The adventure of his discovery has been immortalized in the *Dialogues of Plato*. It all began in ancient Greece about 450 B.C.

Inspired by the belief that "The unexamined life is not worth living," Socrates was the first philosopher to turn his attention to the affairs of human life. Socrates, the son of a stone mason and a midwife, saw himself as following his mother's profession. With this difference: Where his mother assisted at the birth of children, he assisted at the birth of ideas. This he did through a method which he called *dialectic*. This method involves disciplined conversation. Socrates would begin by posing a question. When a member of his audience offered an answer, he would question the answer. Through this method (which has come to be known as the maieutic method, the method of midwifery) Socrates led his audience to make ethical inductions. That is to say, by reflecting on concrete facts they were led to wide-ranging ethical generalizations.

Socrates was convinced that no virtue and no ethical action is possible without knowledge. He also believed that no ethical knowledge is possible without an understanding of the meaning of ethical terms. To have a knowledge of virtuous action one must first know what virtue is. To gain an understanding of actions as just or unjust one must understand the essential nature of justice. To know the requirements of happiness one must first know the defining properties of happiness (Plato cited in Jowett, 1937).

These conversations often led the people of Athens into areas where they had no desire to go. Their ethical beliefs consisted entirely of social mores and conventions. To engage them in Practical Reasoning Socrates had to call their beliefs into question. To have one's beliefs called into question is a painful experience. To call one's own beliefs into question is a very unpopular activity. But no ethical reasoning is possible without it.

As is well known, Socrates' curiosity cost him his life. He was executed by the state for teaching heresy and "corrupting the youth of Athens." Then, as now, many people would rather kill, or die, before engaging in Practical Reasoning.

BIOETHICS

Bioethics—ethics as it relates to the health care professions—came into existence as an independent discipline about 1970. "During this same period medicine has shifted from a near exclusive focus on disease toward a primary concern with the sick person. . . . In these last decades, then, the vocabulary of the moral—of right and wrong—has been added to the vocabulary of scientific medicine—of fact and content" (Cassell, 1984, p. 35).

The development of bioethics has, probably, been more like Socrates' method of dialectic than anything in ethics in 2500 years. Many factors— social, cultural, legal—have set the direction of this development.

The fundamental background of bioethics, which forms its essential nature is:

1. The nature and needs of humans as living, thinking beings.
2. The purpose and function of the health care system in a human society.
3. An increased cultural awareness of human beings' essential moral status.

All this forms the nature of the biomedical context. The needs and conditions of people who enter this context do not allow for the purposeless and the arbitrary. The interpersonal relationships of health care professionals and patients give added dimension to this context. The values, which the biomedical sciences offer those who can profit from them, are intimate, complex, and vitally important.

At the same time the threat to a patient's values is very real. The relationship between the biomedical professional and patient is extraordinarily intimate.

Biomedical professionals possess an undesirable degree of power over patients. They may be tempted to take actions that can be justified only through rationalization. Patients are vulnerable.

Bioethics arose in this context. It is becoming more and more reality-oriented, well-reasoned, and centered on the individual. Two influences upon this trend have been especially important: (1) The fact that humans often serve as the subjects of medical research, and (2) The growing threat of medical malpractice lawsuits.

The Influence of Research

People often serve in medical research. The possibility of exploitation and harm is greater here than in any other aspect of biomedicine. Children, for example, participate in research from which they will gain no benefit. This places an intense ethical responsibility on researchers.

Organ transplants are now possible. The techniques of cloning and genetic engineering are being perfected. The application of modern medical knowledge and technology gives rise to the most difficult ethical dilemmas in human experience. Everyone who participates faces these dilemmas.

In general the role of people in research demands acute awareness of ethical parameters. The application of complex technologies to patients is often hard to justify ethically. Many times this knowledge and technology complicate otherwise ordinary health care contexts. This calls for very abstract and complex processes of ethical analysis. It is impossible to deal with these issues ethically without intense analysis.

Thomas Aquinas never tired of saying "A small mistake in the beginning makes for a large mistake at the end." So it is in ethics. It is an inexcusable mistake to attempt to resolve these complex dilemmas by means of hunches or rules of thumb. It is no less a mistake to attempt to resolve simple dilemmas in this way.

When to tell a patient the truth and when not to cannot be dealt with on the basis of moral rules. It might well be impossible to justify telling a heart attack victim that his wife has been killed. Issues of confidentiality and promise keeping cannot be decided by urges and hunches.

- A psychiatric patient tells a nurse he plans to harm someone. She has pledged confidentiality. Is she bound by this pledge?
- Is a nurse in restraining a senile patient practicing unjustifiable paternalism?
- A physician orders a potentially lethal dose of digoxin. A nurse notices this. She cannot contact the physician. Rather than not giving the drug, the nurse gives the normal dose. Should one "blow the whistle" on the physician? On the nurse? On both? On neither?

Unanalyzed rules or guidelines can lead health care professionals into very unjustifiable actions.

The right choice in a bioethical context—to do the right thing at the right time, for the right reason, and in the right proportion (if possible!)—can be extraordinarily difficult. Under the best of circumstances ethical certainty is very hard to attain. To deal with the choices she must make, a nurse must develop a sensitivity to what is happening.

Nursing is an interpersonal art. A nurse never acts strictly alone and for herself. Right action demands that she respect her patient's viewpoint. She must be able to tolerate ethical outlooks that differ from her own. Her patient's viewpoint must outweigh the rules she is accustomed to or her own ethical hunches (President's Commission, 1982). Someone who cannot accept these limitations on her actions should not become a nurse.

Bioethics is, or, one day, may become one of the life sciences. For this to come about it must be optimally appropriate to living and thinking beings (Bourke, 1983).

The Influence of Medical Malpractice Suits

Today's ethical problems may become tomorrow's legal problems. We live in a secular and pluralistic society. In such a society it is necessary to build bridges of ethical understanding between people from diverse backgrounds. These bridges are made possible by a secular moral code.

Without such bridges a nurse may find herself confronted by an attorney. Attorneys are skilled and professional adversaries. The attorney's whole interest will lie in invalidating the nurse's reasoning and decision. She needs more than "the - way - I - was - brought - up" in order to defend herself. Or she may have to justify her decisions and actions to a jury of twelve women and men from very diverse backgrounds. Platitudes of duty or ethical intuition or idealistic political inspiration may well prove an inadequate defense.

She may need an attorney for her legal defense. But she has a responsibility for knowing the ethical implications of her actions. And this responsibility is entirely her own.

> If one attempts to chart the conceptual and value commitments of individuals in approaching and resolving biomedical problems . . . one will find a world view that is secular, though not anti-religious . . . the peaceable context of a neutral secular understanding provides the circumstance, within which religious views and special secular traditions can be embraced and pursued in security. A general secular bioethics must function as the logic of a pluralism, as the means for the peaceable negotiation of moral intuitions.
>
> Secular bioethics as the provision of a neutral framework to address moral problems in biomedicine is a peaceable solution to the problems of delivery of health care, when physicians, nurses, patients, and individuals generally hold a diversity of moral views. If one is not to . . . impose by force or coercion . . . a particular secular tradition, then one will need to content oneself with a general moral framework that lacks such moorings. (Englehardt, 1986, pp 11-12)

Ethical decisions are sometimes made from a predetermined ethical commitment. These out-of-context decisions can lead a health care professional into conflict with patients, with peers, and with the legal system.

Patients entering the health care setting are aware of their rights. The days of "the physician knows best" or "the nurse knows best" are no more. Medical malpractice suits have made it obvious that unexamined ethical assumptions may not justify ethical decisions.

One beneficial result has come of this change. It has turned the ethical code of health care professionals back to the biomedical contexts in which their decisions are made (Zaner, 1988). This return to reality may prove to be one of medicine's most significant contributions to ethics and, therefore, to human happiness.

ETHICS IN CONTEXT

An ethical decision-making model is a systematic arrangement of principles to motivate and guide ethical actions. These principles also serve to explain and justify an agent's actions. Ethical action takes two forms:

1. In the primary sense ethical actions are the actions an agent takes in the pursuit of vital and fundamental goals. These are the actions that inspired the study of ethics.

2. Actions involving the rights of others are also ethical actions. The actions that a nurse takes in her role as nurse always have an ethical aspect. In her role as nurse a nurse acts as agent for her patient. This is a complex ethical relationship.

An implicit or explicit agreement arises from every human relationship. The agreement that arises between the nurse and patient is one instance of this. The principles or elements by which a nurse makes a decision ought to be derived from the actual dynamics of this agreement. Elements of this agreement are formed by the values a patient seeks to attain, maintain, or regain in the relationship. On the nurse's part, they are the values which a nurse agrees to help her patient regain.

THE NURSE/PATIENT AGREEMENT

A patient, in becoming a patient, has a specific purpose. A nurse, in becoming a nurse, also has a specific purpose. These purposes interface. They interface by design. The condition of a patient determines the role of a nurse.

A nurse, in being a nurse, becomes the agent of her patient. A nurse does for her patient what he would do for himself had he not lost his power of agency (President's Commission, 1982).

The interrelationship between them is formed by the nature of a nurse and the nature of a patient. In the interaction of nurse and patient their roles form an implicit agreement between them. They agree, in effect, that, since the patient is a patient, the nurse will be a nurse. The entire area of a nurse's justifiable ethical action lies within these parameters.

A bridge builder cannot excuse the failure to take reasoned and competent actions on the ground of "doing his duty." Nor will "duty" justify mindless and incompetent actions on the part of a nurse. The pursuit of a grand social vision will not justify the collapse of a bridge or an individual patient's unnecessary suffering or loss.

THE STRUCTURE OF AN ETHICAL CODE ILLUSTRATED

In the natural course of a human's life he or she will, of necessity, adopt an ethical code. The code adopted may be Plato's (the pursuit of an unknowable Final Good), Immanuel Kant's (Deontology—action according to the demands of duty), John Stuart Mill's (Utilitarianism—"the greatest good of the greatest number" as the highest ethical goal), Uncle Dick's or Aunt Jane's, or the voice of inner urges. But a person cannot evade the need to find some way of ordering his or her life.

The source of an ethical code is similar in some ways to a travel agent. In order to examine that which is unfamiliar, the inner structure of an ethical code, we can have recourse to that which is more familiar, the itinerary of a vacation.

A vacation involves

The time of departure—precisely when one will leave to go on vacation; the time of arrival—when one can expect to reach one's destination; the time when one will leave the vacation spot to return home; the location where one is going to spend one's vacation and the attractions and facilities that are found there; where one will stay—the accommodation one can expect and how accessible everything will be; the means of transportation to and from one's vacation spot; the cost of one's vacation; the luggage one should take.

Would any sensible person put his entire vacation into the hands of a travel agent? Would he let the agent decide when he will leave; where he will go; how long he will stay; when he will return home; where he will stay; how he will get there; and even the cost of his vacation?

The choice among vacation spots would be made according to the agent's evaluations.

The traveler's desires would play no part in the planning of his vacation.

No sensible person would agree to this arrangement. Yet, incredibly, many otherwise thinking people will make this arrangement with an ethicist. One whom they have chosen at random. They choose a random ethicist to plan the purpose and course of their entire life.

In our culture, at this time, two broad theories of ethics are dominant.

Deontology

Deontology makes "right" and "wrong" the central ethical concepts. Ethical action consists in doing one's duty. To do one's duty is right. To shirk one's duty is wrong. The ethical agent has a duty to do what is right and to refrain from doing what is wrong. Beyond this nothing is ethically relevant. The results of an action may be desired or deplored. But they have no ethical relevance (Arras and Hunt cited in Arras & Rhoden, 1989).

> [According to a deontological ethic] one is not morally responsible for the results of his actions, or for any consequences whatever; his duty is to moral law, an unempirical, nonfactual principle which must be freely obeyed by the rational will as his sole responsibility. (Sahakian, 1974, p. 107)

The notion of duty as central to ethics arose with the Stoic philosophers about 300 B.C. But its most powerful impetus was given by the German philosopher Immanuel Kant (1724-1804).

The concept of duty is unrelated to life and everyday concerns. Kant's duty-ethic was a reaction to the social-subjectivism of David Hume (1711-1776) ("X is right" means society approves X; "X is wrong" means society disapproves of X). In turn, all Kantian-type ethics were attacked by the

English philosopher G.E. Moore (1873-1958). Moore described the attempt to get an "ought" (a duty) from an "is" (a fact relevant to human existence) as a fallacious mode of thinking. He named this the naturalistic fallacy (Schilpp, 1968).

"Ought" and "right" are both defined by a duty ethic in terms of duty. This makes a duty ethic viciously circular. The "right" is that which one "ought" to do (has a duty to do). Because one "ought" to do that which is "right" (that which one has a duty to do). And this for no reason other than that the "right" is that which one "ought" to do (Hospers, 1967).

No deontologist has ever found the reason for duty in the demands of human life. The Stoics located it in a Platonist "World-Soul." The duties of people, the revolutions of the sun, the wetness of water are all part of the same thing—the laws that govern nature.

There is a logical drawback to this. It proves that which is doubtful (that people have duties) in terms of that which is even more doubtful (the existence of Plato's "World-Soul"). It is like proving that Jane will be in town at noon (a doubtful possibility) by declaring that Martians will "beam" her to town at noon (a much more doubtful possibility).

Kant held that the concept of "duty" is an innate idea. One is born knowing that he must do his duty (Kant in Paton, 1964). This notion is also highly doubtful. In order to know that the demands of duty lay upon him the newborn would need to know of the relationships existing between himself and the world. In order to know this he would need to know of the nature of the world. He would need to know this before he knew that there is a world. And this is impossible.

Historically, notions of "the right" have been in flux. Every neighboring culture and every succeeding age has its own view of the right. Every era and culture is entirely convinced that its view of the right is part of the make-up of the natural world.

Deontology demands that actions be taken without regard to consequences. A nurse cannot justify taking an action without concern for the consequences. She should always be able to justify her decisions.

> Deontololgical ethics maintains that, if one acts from a genuine sense of moral duty, then one's action is morally approvable irrespective of its actual consequences . . . [But] the deliberate ignoring of forseeable consequences of one's actions is an abandonment of the primary function of Practical Reasoning . . . [This is in opposition to the] virtuous capacity of the good person to look forward to the most likely results of a given decision or voluntary act. (Bourke, 1983, p. 10)

Could a nurse justify causing harm to a patient by saying "I was doing my duty"? This would not suffice legally. It surely does not suffice ethically—not if "ethically" is understood in any practical or rational sense.

Deontology is not an ethical system. It is the absence of an ethical system. Consider this: The original deontologists preached the rightness of duty in action. They saw that a certain state of mind must, necessarily, follow these actions. The permanent possession of this state of mind was the *purpose* of deontology.

The Stoics called this state of mind *apatheia*, which means indifference (a modern name for *apatheia* is *"burnout"*). *Apatheia* demands indifference to pain or pleasure, health or illness, happiness or misery. The father of modern deontology, Immanuel Kant, sings the praises of apathy in the *Preface to The Metaphysical Elements of Ethics* in a section entitled "Virtue Necessarily Presupposses Apathy (Considered as Strength)" (Kant in Paton, 1964).

Indifference is an undesirable quality in a nurse. It is the opposite of what a nurse's state of mind ought to be. But one cannot, consistently, practice deontology without it.

Nevertheless many ethicists regard "duty" and "morality" as equivalent terms. They claim that "ethics" and "deontology" are identical. If this is true, then the only task of ethics is to list a person's duties, and every ethical action is simply an act of obedience.

A nurse cannot escape taking the role of ethical agent. One option open to her is to answer the demands of her innate and prerational sense of duty. To do this she must be aware of having an innate and prerational sense of duty. But no one can ever be certain that *any* idea is innate.

Utilitarianism

The central ethical concepts of utilitarianism are "good" and "evil." Utilitarianism finds its basis in the doctrine of psychological hedonism. Hedonism is the doctrine that ethical agents ought to be motivated solely by pleasure and pain. David Hume's famous aphorism, "Reason is, and rightly ought to be, the slave of the passions [emotions]," would serve as a motto for hedonism.

Utilitarianism was first formulated in terms of psychological hedonism, which means that determinism was the first inspiration of utilitarianism.

Determinism is the doctrine that every human action is a response to a prior action. This prior action originates outside of the person who is (apparently) acting. The determinist holds that deciding and choosing are illusions. Determinists have described the feeling of being able to control one's thoughts and actions as a kind of dream. Psychological hedonism is a form of determinism. It holds that one acts only to seek pleasure and to avoid pain. It holds that one *cannot* act otherwise. This tendency it describes as being inborn (Hospers, 1972).

The utilitarians claimed that people cannot escape viewing pleasure as "the good." Their next stop was to argue for the necessity of:

...the principle which approves or disapproves of every action whatsoever according to the tendency which it appears to have to augment or diminish the happiness of the party whose interest is in question. ... (Bentham, 1879/1962)

Then they went on to argue, in effect, that the good of two persons is a greater good than the good of one. The greatest possible good, then, would be the good of everyone, or, the good of the greatest possible number. This good they declared ought to be the goal of every ethical agent.

Early opponents were quick to point out flaws in this reasoning. Thomas Carlyle (1795-1881) called utilitarianism a "pig philosophy." He noted that, in every conceivable way, a symphony by Beethoven was a greater good than the victory of a pig wrestler. In fact Beethoven's creativity, from every point of view, seems a greater good than the good of a large number of pig wrestlers (Trail, 1896).

In response to this the utilitarians amended their standard to read "The greatest (or highest) good of the greatest number." This reasoning ignores several relevant facts:

1. Let us grant that a person, through psychological necessity, holds his own pleasure to be an end in itself. This fact, in itself, gives him no reason, logical or otherwise, to concern himself with the good of others. A person might hold his good to be of value to him not because it is *a* good but because it is *his* good. There is no logical flaw in this attitude, and any claim that it is ethically flawed begs the question. A person cannot know whether something is right or wrong before he knows what it means for something to be right or wrong. (This was the point of Socrates' insistence on the importance of definitions.)

   There is no rational reason for an agent to believe that *his* good is freely interchangeable with the good of other agents. His good might be uniquely valued by him. He might hold that, if it is computed along with the good of another, it loses its ethical relevance.

   Let us imagine someone for whom this is not the case:
   Joe is very excited about going to a rock concert. Sally tells him that she is also going. Now Joe is no longer excited. If Sally is going it does not matter to Joe whether he goes or not as long as someone goes. Joe regards values as interchangeable.

   Psychologically this does not make sense. But it is utilitarianism's view of human nature.

2. It is difficult to see how a nurse could justify her actions by reference to "the greatest good for the greatest number." Her primary responsibility is to her individual patient. Her patient, in turn, has a right to choose his own goals and the consequences he seeks. He has a

right to choose highly individualistic goals based solely on his own desires.

Utilitarianism not only directs us to consider the results of an action when making moral judgments but also holds that we should look only to results. Considerations of an agent's intentions, feelings, or convictions are seen as irrelevant to the question "What is the right thing to do?" (Arras & Hunt cited in Arras & Rhoden, 1989, p. 8)

A nurse in pursuit of "the greatest good of the greatest number" would have no time to attend to her individual patients. Nor would they have any right to expect individualized nursing treatment from her. Being a nurse would not allow her to take ethical action. It would be a wall between her and the possibility of ethical action.

3. Utilitarianism collapses into deontology (Veatch, 1985). This has finally been recognized even by utilitarians. To avoid this flaw, a distinction is drawn between "rule" and "act" utilitarianism. Rule utilitarians claim that an agent has a duty to obey certain rules. These are the rules best adapted to bring about the greatest good for the greatest number. Act utilitarians declare that the value of an action is determined by its goal. This simply means that an agent has a duty to aim for a specific goal. He has a duty to act to bring about the greatest good for the greatest number.

Utilitarians cannot escape deontology.

4. Utilitarianism is also an ethical theory peculiar in this:

Justice is the most highly honored interpersonal virtue of our society. It is the goal of our entire legal system. And utilitarianism is a prescription for injustice.

"One such limitation [of utilitarianism as an ethical theory] is violation of personal autonomy . . . its inherent potential for discrimination, the possibility that what is perceived as "good" for the majority may be bad for the minority." (Franklin, 1988)

In fact it's somewhat worse than that:

Utilitarianism . . . has fallen into bad odor, and particularly when it comes to a defense of individual rights and personal liberties . . . suppose . . . the general welfare of the community, or the greatest happiness of the greatest number, might conceivably be furthered or increased by the sacrifice of the liberty, or the well-being, or even the life of a single individual. . . . [Would not this sacrifice be] . . . the moral consequence of anyone's adhering strictly to Utilitarian principles. (Veatch, 1985, pp. 30-31)

Nevertheless, utilitarianism is today's dominant ethical trend. Many nursing ethics texts recommend it as a tool for ethical decision making. It is an alternative theory which a nurse might want to consider. But:

> Utilitarianism requires an agent to do that action which brings about the greatest balance of good over evil in the universe as a whole ... to maximize the good of all humans ... to consider all of the available alternatives and perform that act which will maximize the good of all affected parties. (McConnell, 1982, p. 14)

This is what utilitarianism is. Does it not seem unreasonable to expect a nurse to know:

1. What action will bring about the greatest balance of good over evil in the universe as a whole?
2. What the nature of "the greatest balance of good over evil in the universe as a whole" would be?
3. How she might "maximize the good of all humans"?
4. The precise number of "all of the available alternatives"?
5. Precisely that "act which will maximize the good of all affected parties"?

Suppose that, by some miracle, the nurse could know all this. How could utilitarianism be justified in a health care system that places a high value on the individual's rights and autonomy?

The utilitarian's ethical advice consists in emotionally charged, high flying, and empty phrases. It is a fatally impractical approach to the Practical Science. If an agent accepts the necessity of doing the impossible, he will become a fanatic. Or he will do nothing.

REFERENCES

Arras, J., & Rhoden, N. (Eds.). (1989). *Ethical issues in modern medicine* (3rd ed.). Mountain View, CA: Mayfield Publishing.

Bentham, J. (1962). *The works of Jeremy Bentham.* (J. Bowring, Ed.). New York: Russell & Russell (Original work published 1879).

Bourke, V. (1983, May). *The teleological and deontological dichotomy.* Paper presented at Duquesne University First Annual Ethics Conference, Pittsburgh, PA.

Cassell, E.J. (1984). Life as a work of art. *Hastings Center Report, 14*(4), 35-37.

Churchill, L.R. (1989). Reviving a distinctive medical ethic. *Hastings Center Report, 19*(3), 28-30.

Engelhardt, H.T., Jr. (1986). *The foundations of bioethics.* New York: Oxford University Press.

Franklin, C. (1988). Commentary on case study. *Hastings Center Report, 18*(6), 35-36.

Hospers, J. (1967). *An introduction to philosophical analysis* (2nd ed). Englewood Cliffs, NJ: Prentice Hall.

Hospers, J. (1972). *Human conduct.* New York: Harcourt Brace Jovanovich, Inc.

Jowett, M.A. (Trans.) (1937). *The dialogues of Plato*. New York: Random House.

Kant, I. (1964). *Groundwork for the metaphysics of morals* (J.H. Paton, (Trans.) New York: Harper & Row. (Original work published 1785.)

McConnell, T.C. (1982). *Moral issues in health care*. Monterey, CA: Wadsworth Health Science Division.

McKeon, R. (Ed.). (1941). The basic works of Aristotle. New York: Random House.

President's Commission for the Study of Ethical Problems in Medical Biomedical and Behavioral Research. (1982). *Making health care decisions: The ethical and legal implications of informed consent in the patient-practitioner relationship*, (Vol. I). Washington, D.C.: U.S. Government Printing Office.

Sahakian, W.S. (1974). *Ethics: An introduction to theories and problems*. New York: Barnes & Noble.

Schilpp, P.A. (Ed.). (1968). *The philosophy of G. E. Moore* (Vol. II). LaSalle, IL: Open Court.

Trail, H.N. (Ed.). (1896). *The centenary edition of Carlyle's work*. New York: Oxford Press.

Veatch, H.B. (1985). *Human rights: Fact or fancy?* Baton Rouge, LA: Louisiana State University Press.

Zaner, R. (1988). *Ethics and the clinical encounter*. Englewood Cliffs, NJ: Prentice Hall.

The First Step of Bioethical Decision Making

The philosopher Lao Tzu (dates unknown) has told us that "The longest journey begins with the first step." This is so obvious that we can see it for ourselves. We can hardly avoid seeing it. But it is so obvious that, without Lao Tzu, we might never have noticed the importance of it.

It is also obvious that the first step of a journey can be taken in confusion. If it is taken in confusion, it might be in the wrong direction. If it is taken in the wrong direction, at the end of his journey, a traveler may find himself very far from his destination.

This is true of any journey one makes. A series of "actions taken in the pursuit of vital and fundamental goals" may be regarded as an ethical journey. The possibility of an undesired destination, then, is especially true of an ethical journey.

THE APPROPRIATE AND THE JUSTIFIABLE

Some ethical decisions are appropriate. The agent who makes them makes them for a reason. There is a likelihood that they will accomplish that reasoned purpose. And, while accomplishing this purpose, they will injure neither the agent nor anyone else. Often they are made on the basis of hunches and intuitions. They may, nevertheless, be appropriate to the context in which they are made. But nothing is learned from them. No principles are drawn. They are not repeatable. The agent really did not know *why* he did what he did.

Some ethical decisions are justifiable. They are appropriate to the contexts in which they are made. They accomplish the purposes of the agent. They injure no one. That they will bring about some benefit and avoid bringing about harm is forseeable by the agent who makes them. The acting agent can see the connections between his decision, the actions he takes, and the results of his decision. He knows why he made this decision. If it were necessary, he could explain and justify his motives to an objective judge. Before he took his ethical action, he explained and justified his motives to himself. Thereby he made a justifiable decision.

Any ethical decision that is justifiable must be appropriate to the context in which it was made. Otherwise it would not be justifiable. One cannot, in any logical sense, justify an inappropriate ethical decision. That an ethical decision is justifiable *presupposes* that it is appropriate.

But an (apparently) appropriate ethical decision is not necessarily justifiable:

- The agent may not be able to explain his motivations. He may not be clearly aware of his motivations.
- He may be unable to give a description that explains all the connections between his motivations and his decision.
- He may be unable to give a description explaining all the predictable connections between his decision and the accomplishment of his purpose.

He may not have a clear and coherent knowledge of why his decisions are appropriate. So, while these decisions are justifiable in principle, *he* cannot justify them.

Ethical decisions made under these conditions are not justifiable. In a very strong sense, they are not even appropriate because under these conditions it is objectively inappropriate to make ethical decisions. The agent's intention may be flawless. But he cannot foresee the consequences of his actions.

Such situations are too confused for justifiable decisions to be made. An ethical situation may involve the most fundamental purposes of the people involved. It may impinge upon a whole network of purposes. It may tie into the sources of their self-images. It may have results extending far into their futures.

The complexity of the elements of a situation do not allow for such decisions to be appropriate.

Mr. Dietrich is hospitalized.

All his desires and all his intentions have been interrupted.

As with every human being the processes of thought, choice, decision, and action are natural to Mr. Dietrich. But now he cannot translate thought into action.

Mr. Dietrich's life-style and his life itself are threatened.

His power of agency is nullified; all his purposeful and goal-directed actions are frustrated.

To seek values and to arrange these values into a more perfect life is natural to all humans. But Mr. Dietrich can only seek to rid himself of a severe disvalue.

Mr. Dietrich expects beneficence from his nurse. He cannot know, and probably would not believe, that his nurse would make an ethical decision involving him without her knowing, objectively, *why* she made that decision. To do so would be a failure of beneficence. Mr. Dietrich, like every patient, assumes beneficence on the part of his nurse.

Mr. Dietrich is in the final stages of cancer. He probably will not live out the week. His physician has ordered physical therapy for him. Mr. Dietrich does not want to go to therapy. His nurse assumes that the physician has some reason for the therapy and decides that she will not question his decision.

Can the nurse justify her decision? She has no reason to believe that it was an appropriate decision for the physician to make. In fact it seems obvious that it is an inappropriate decision.

Mr. Dietrich would have no reason to imagine that his nurse has no clear awareness of the relationship between the decision to make him endure the pain of therapy and the purposes appropriate to his context.

There is no *ethical* justification for Mr. Dietrich's nurse to remain unaware. Yet, as we have seen in Chapter 1, all too often ethical decisions suffer this sort of defect. We all know this. But we do not like to think about it. All the same, a nurse has an ethical responsibility to think about it.

Generally, experience will, more or less, teach a nurse what is to be done. But no one can function well without an awareness of what he is doing, and why he is doing it. In addition, the nurse's role is difficult. Her environment is filled with distractions.

Even under conditions that make justifiable ethical decisions impossible, a nurse can make appropriate ethical decisions. But not with perfect assurance, not with serenity, and not consistently.

Justifiable ethical decision making is not impossible. It is not even difficult in most situations. But it is impossible solely on the basis of hunches and intuitions.

PREPARING FOR THE ETHICAL JOURNEY

If a nurse can develop the ability to objectively justify her ethical decisions, she has, by that very fact, developed the ability to make appropriate decisions. But it seems impossible that she could develop an ability to consistently make appropriate decisions if she does not possess the ability to justify her decisions.

In order for her to develop the ability to make justifiable decisions, she must have a sound ethical orientation toward her role as nurse. If she has this orientation to her profession, she can begin any ethical journey with calm assurance.

To get the direction of the first step precisely right the initial preparations are very important. For that which we call the "first step" is pivotal in the ethical decision making of any professional. In order to be certain of its discovery, several conditions of the search are desirable:

1. The work-a-day world should not be considered. The work-a-day world is, to borrow a phrase from William James, "a blooming, buzzing confusion." The ethical aspects of a situation are usually so snarled up in logistic and administrative concerns and the demands of "hands on" care that the ethical aspects are obscured.

2. The authentically ethical aspects of a situation should be clearly perceived. It will also be desirable to be able to fill in the details of the health care setting. These details, held in the mind's eye, will keep one in the context of one's profession. But, being only in the mind's eye, they will not interfere with ethical analysis and discovery.

3. The essential qualities of the ethical situation should be visualized. For instance, it is a common thing to know that bioethics calls for a patient's right to privacy to be respected. A patient's "right to privacy" can be a fuzzy abstraction. Its outline may become visible only in extreme situations.

   A disoriented patient is being transferred on a gurney. He throws off his covers. The situation almost beckons to the nurse to replace them. However, very few situations are as simple as this.

   A cloudy understanding of a patient's right to privacy is better than no ethical understanding at all. But it is better, and far more useful, if a nurse understands that her patient has a right to be protected against undesired or undesirable interaction of *any* sort. This is what "privacy" is.

   Knowing that there is a word "privacy" is not the same as knowing what the word means — out in the world.

   The essential qualities of a situation are those qualities that can, properly, guide the nurse's ethical actions. They are like landmarks on a trip, guiding the traveler to his destination.

4. The ethical aspects of a situation should be isolated. It is better to be able to draw general conclusions to apply to every similar situation. Without these general conclusions a nurse has to face similar situations, one by one, without understanding.

5. One's decisions should be based on stable and permanent values, not on changing and impermanent ones. It is better, therefore, to see where these stable and permanent values are than to identify transitory ones.

6. It is important to make decisions that have a beneficial momentum into the future. It is of little importance to make decisions whose benefits cease the moment the actions are taken. Ethical actions do not have to occur in disjointed series. They can be taken in an ongoing integrated sequence.

In regard to this an ethical decision maker is very much like a pool player. An unskilled pool player merely attempts to put a ball into a pocket. An unskilled decision maker decides on what she believes to be the best decision and acts on it.

A skilled pool player "sets up" her shots. She tries to put a ball into a pocket and, at the same time, to leave her cueball in such a position that it will be easy to make her next shot. A skilled decision maker makes decisions purposefully. A skilled nurse makes her decisions based on the purposes of her patient and on what is necessary to accomplish them. A skilled decision maker does not find it necessary to exert intense mental effort in order to make arrhythmic ethical decisions. She masters the process of bioethical decision making as a skill.

THE NATURE OF ETHICAL ASPECTS

Before justifiable and effective ethical decisions can be made, one must be able to perceive the purely ethical aspects of a situation. This is often quite difficult. There are nonethical aspects to every situation. Otherwise the situation would not be a situation. This is the difference between a situation in the world and a hypothesis held in the mind. There is no such thing in the "extra-mental" world as a situation that is nothing but an ethical situation.

Take the sparsest situation imaginable. Imagine two people meeting and beginning to interact in the middle of a waste land. Not even in this situation is every aspect an ethical aspect. One person plans to follow the north star and walk out of the wasteland. The other intends to build a fire and lay down debris spelling out "Help" in the hope that a passing airplane will sight him.

Each person has come from different conditions of life. Each has different motivations. Each has different ways of going about things. And each will return to different conditions of life. Each has a unique set of abilities and a unique set of strengths and weaknesses. The way each has chosen to escape the wasteland is not an ethical aspect of the situation. Neither is the background from which each has come, nor the conditions of life to which each hopes to return. Their state of health is not an ethical aspect and neither is their knowledge or lack of knowledge. Taken in itself, their way of approaching problems is not an ethical aspect of the situation. It becomes an ethical aspect only in relation to the situation they actually face. Every ethical aspect of a situation arises in relation to aspects which are not, in themselves, ethical.

The nonethical aspects of a situation determine what can be done. The ethical aspects, in relation to a purpose, determine what ought to be done.

Jane sees her daughter, Josephine, drowning. Jane cannot swim. There is a life preserver at hand. This establishes what Jane can do but not what Jane ought to do. Jane's desire to save Josephine determines what she ought to do.

Ethics has to do with "actions taken in the pursuit of vital and fundamental goals." The rescue of her daughter is, at that time, Jane's only vital and fundamental goal. This desire and the fact that she can attain her goal are the ethical aspects of the situation. Jane's purposes bring the ethical aspects of the situation into being.

Suppose, when this event occurred, Jane had not been present, and Josephine saved her own life by grabbing onto a log that came floating by. In doing this she achieved a vital and fundamental goal. She saved her life. The floating log is, obviously, not an ethical aspect of this situation. The *action* of Jane's daughter is its only ethical aspect. Only those aspects of a situation that arise by virtue of human purposes are ethical aspects of the situation.

To put it another way, the ethical aspects of a situation are determined by what is important in the situation. What is important in any situation is determined by the purposes of the agents who can act in it. That something is important, of necessity, implies that it is important in relation to a purpose.

This is not to say that what one ought to do in any situation is simply relative to one's desires. To go from "I want X" to "Therefore it is good (or right) that I do Y" is neither ethical nor rational. Justifiability is radically important to ethical decision making. To be the source of justifiable actions one's desires must be justifiable in terms of their long-term consequences.

One's decision that pleasure is one of one's vital and fundamental goals is an ethical decision. In itself it is a perfectly justifiable ethical decision. But if one decides that one of the ways he will pursue pleasure is by becoming addicted to crack, this decision defeats the first decision on which it was based. For, eventually, the crack will destroy one's capacity to enjoy food, music, sex, travel . . . everything. Not by law or convention, but by physiological necessity, the decision to become addicted to crack is an immoral decision. It is logically on a par with one's decision to jump off a roof to enjoy the experience of flying.

Without a motivating desire nothing is important. But desire itself is important. Therefore desire must always be subject to reason. For desire has no means of self-defense. Reason—and only reason—has the resources necessary to defend itself and to defend an agent's capacity to desire.

Desires are formulated into purposes. There are three types of purpose which determine the ethical aspects of a situation:

- *A purpose set by an individual agent's desire.*
  Desire motivates an agent's action toward every goal. Desire is the principal basis of every human purpose.
- *A purpose set by the recognition of rights.*
  By recognizing the rights of others one sets uncoerced cooperation as the standard of purposive interaction.
- *A purpose projected and acted upon among individuals through explicit agreements, promises, etc.*
  This purpose must always be motivated by desire and, ethically, must recognize the rights of everyone involved.

THE FIRST STEP

The most important ethical quality of any nurse is the quality of beneficence. Beneficence motivates a nurse to act effectively as the agent of her patient.

In order for a nurse to practice beneficence, she must be able to act with understanding. If a nurse is to do nothing that will bring about evil and everything possible that will bring about good—if she is to practice beneficence—she must know why she is doing what she is doing. To have ethical understanding it is necessary to gain understanding. To gain understanding is the first step of ethical action.

There are two ways to gain understanding.

Trial and Error

Since no two human beings are utterly different, every nurse can feel a certain empathy with human hopes and fears. Thus she has the basic resources necessary to learn through experience. She can master ethical action through trial and error.

But this is the slowest possible way. While she is learning in this way she may make many blunders. She may do many things which, eventually, will bring about harm. She may fail to do many things which would have brought about much good. She may never learn what principles are right for ethical action always and in every similar situation. She may never master the art of applying these principles well in specific cases. Many ethical agents never do.

Reliable Authority

The only other possibility is for a nurse to learn the requirements of right action from a reliable authority on the subject. Which leaves her with the problem of discovering an authority who is *reliable*.

1. *Certain authorities advise a nurse to adopt formalistic standards.* These are standards that are to be applied indiscriminately without regard to consequences.

    But if a nurse is to act beneficently, she will be able to justify only those actions that bring about an extreme preponderance of benefit over harm. Actions taken ritualistically without concern for the nature of their effects are not actions that are intended to avoid evil and bring about good. Actions can be taken without a prior and specific process of ethical analysis. However, these actions, properly speaking, do not have an ethical motivation.

    Animals without the power of reason never reach the level of the ethical—nor even the level of the beneficent. This is true whether they lack the power of reason by nature or by choice. If the actions they take avoid evil and bring about good, this is not by design but by accident.

    So, for the purposes of a nurse, authorities who offer formalistic rules are not reliable.

2. *Other authorities would advise a nurse to hold the convenience of others as her standard of ethical judgment.* This standard is, at best, the standard of etiquette. Taken beyond the level of etiquette it ignores the fact that a nurse is a nurse. It seems apparent that this is inappropriate if a nurse has a specific role. This standard would make it impossible for a nurse to fill her role as a nurse.

Jake, recovering from open heart surgery, is attached to a number of confining apparatuses. This is making Jake increasingly agitated from inactivity. Jake's family has asked his nurse not to get him out of bed until they arrive. This would be very pleasant and convenient for both Jake and his family. However, his agitation is causing a fluctuation in his vital signs. Proper nursing practice requires Jake's nurse to set aside convenience as a standard of judgment. Rational bioethical decision making requires precisely the same thing.

If the standard of convenience were appropriate, robots would make ideal nurses because robots are specifically designed for convenience.

The nurse is not a robot, and there is little reason to leap to the conclusion that the betrayal of her knowledge and the sacrifice of her mind is her answer to the problem of ethical decision making. In order to practice her profession ethically, a nurse must be able to do good while she avoids doing evil. She must be free to use her judgment in the practice of her profession. In fact, this exercise of judgment is the first demand of beneficence.

So there is still a need to find an authority who possesses reliable information.

THE NURSE'S ETHICAL AUTHORITY

That which is good or evil is good or evil in relation to some purpose. A purpose is attained through that which is good. A purpose is frustrated by that which is evil.

A nurse must be concerned with the appropriateness of her purposes and the forseeable effects of her ethical actions. A formalistic standard is explicitly unconcerned with purposes and with effects.

The purposes fitting a convenience standard are too unstable and transitory to be of any fundamental benefit. There is, very often, a crucial difference between the purpose that yields the greatest benefit — the purpose on which one should act and the first purpose that springs into one's mind. A convenience standard provides no way of differentiating between these two.

THE FINAL AUTHORITY

It is her patient who provides a nurse's reason for being a nurse.

It is her patient who enables a nurse to discover what it is to be a nurse.

To be a nurse is to do for a patient what the patient would do for himself if he were able. To be a nurse is to be the agent of one's patient. This relationship is codified in an informal agreement between nurse and patient. In light of this agreement there is only one authority to whom a nurse can turn for ethical advice: her patient.

Any bioethical system that does not make the patient, through the agreement, the final authority in ethical decision making drives a wedge between nurse and patient. It alienates the nurse and her patient, and it alienates the nurse from her role as nurse.

Directly or indirectly every nurse has patients. Some nurses are engaged in research. The purpose of the research is the benefit of patients. Others are engaged in education. The ultimate purpose of the educator is the benefit of patients. Still others are engaged in administration. Again, their ultimate purpose is the benefit of patients.

All these purposes are concretized in the implicit agreement between nurse and patient. Every ethical decision that a nurse makes as nurse must hold the patient as its central focus. Otherwise her action misses its mark.

Patients came before nurses. Without patients there would be no such thing as nurses. Without hospitals nurses would find somewhere else to care for patients. Without physicians or medicine nurses would do what they could—as nurses sometimes must do. Without educators nurses would act according to their best judgment. Without administrators nurses would act without administration.

But without patients the profession of nursing would disappear.

A simple examination of the nature of nursing makes the first step of justifiable ethical action obvious. In order to make a bioethical decision a nurse, whatever her specific function might be, must first refer to her agreement with her patient. In matters pertaining to her professional ethical decision making, the patient *is* the nurse's final authority.

Who would have a better knowledge of the patient's side of the agreement than the patient himself?

The purposes of the patient and of the nurse, as a nurse, are codified in the agreement. The ethical status of any decision, choice, or action is a function of the relation of that decision, choice, or action to these purposes. The agreement, then, is the first step of a nurse's ethical journey—and its standard. The agreement cannot be understood without the patient. It cannot even be formed without the patient.

SUMMARY

Reference to the nurse/patient agreement is the first step in the nurse's ethical decision-making process. The nurse/patient agreement is the court of last resort for a nurse in justifying her decisions. The more effectively the nurse meets the ethical agreement the more real she is as an ethical agent and as a nurse. On the other hand it is possible for a nurse to fulfill the agreement so ineffectively that she will hardly be a nurse or an ethical agent at all.

CHAPTER

3

The Nurse/Patient Agreement

In the early 1970s, along with bioethics, general agreement on certain bioethical standards came into being. Before this bioethical standards had not been generally or explicitly recognized despite their importance to biomedical professionals. They are part of the professional obligation of nurses and of every biomedical professional. They are preconditions of any agreement between nurse and patient.

THE FIRST STEP OF ETHICAL INTERACTION

Imagine two people engaged together in some behavior: They are playing volleyball, carrying a plank, going out to dinner, robbing a jewelry store, holding hands at the movies, taking a rocket to the moon. There are three possible sources of their behavior.

- *Their behavior is directed by coercion.* One person is forcing another to "interact." Or both are being forced by a third person.
- *Their behavior is directed by deception.* One person is aware of what he or she is doing while the other has been deceived into cooperating. Or both have been deceived by a third person.
- *Neither is forced. Neither is deceived.* They are acting together by agreement. The terms of their agreement are understood by both.

Only the third source of their interaction, only that which is directed by objective agreement, can be justifiable ethical interaction. Force or deception violates the rights of the person who is forced or deceived. There is no way to justify violating a person's rights. "Rights" is *the* fundamental interpersonal ethical concept.

The recognition of rights is the first step of the ethical interaction between nurse and patient—that their interaction shall arise "through voluntary consent, objectively gained."

Because agreement is the first step of the nurse/patient interaction, certain bioethical standards must be in place. These standards form the nature of the nurse/patient agreement. Likewise, they are implied by the terms of the agreement. The contemporary bioethical standards that we will discuss are:

- Autonomy
- Freedom
- Veracity
- Privacy
- Beneficence
- Fidelity

An objective agreement is any agreement in which both parties to the agreement are aware of the reason for the agreement, the terms of the agreement, and the intentions of the other party to the agreement.

These bioethical standards are *presupposed* by any objective agreement between nurse and patient. It is important to understand how these standards function in the nurse/patient agreement.

AUTONOMY[1]

An autonomous agent is one with the right and power to take actions according to personal desire and without obtaining permission. One cannot make an agreement without being an autonomous agent.

Two students in the same class might both possess autonomy and never agree to interact. But no one can make an agreement to interact unless that person has the right and power to take autonomous actions. If one of the students is, for instance, a convict, he cannot take autonomous actions. He cannot make any significant ethical agreement to interact with an autonomous agent.

The making of an agreement to interact and the consequent interaction are autonomous actions only possible to autonomous agents. Autonomy is an individual's "moral property." It is his or her right to be unique and to be treated according to that uniqueness. Every agent is an autonomous agent. There cannot be such a thing as a nonautonomous agent. Every action is an autonomous action. A nonautonomous action is a logical impossibility.

Joe, a patient with cardiovascular disease, is given to high living and carousing around. His nurse, Anne, is prim, proper, and upright. The same facts hold true of Mark and his nurse, Amy. Anne devotes a great deal of time to trying to reform Joe. Joe devotes a great deal of effort in trying to corrupt Anne. Mark and Amy, for the most part, accept each other as they are. Amy and Mark respect each other's autonomy and Joe and Anne do not. Amy and Mark have a better understanding and a firmer agreement than do Anne and Joe. If nothing else Amy and Mark have more time and energy to devote to the nurse/patient relationship than do Anne and Joe.

Without the recognition of another's autonomy there is no basis for noncoercion and respect for the other's rights. Using this definition, "coercive" actions taken toward stones, trees, machines, or animals cannot be regarded as evil. These things possess no autonomy. Autonomy is a property arising from an agent's capacity to reason and to take purposive action. It is the ability, and the consequent right, to take self-determined, independent, and long-range action.

FREEDOM[2]

One can possess freedom without making an agreement, but one cannot make an agreement without possessing freedom.

Susan is walking down the street. Suddenly she is struck by the attractiveness of the dresses in a department store window. She stops to admire them. So far Susan is passive. The dresses are, so to speak, coming out and influencing Susan. Susan is taking no external action in relation to them. In the context of this experience she is a patient.

Susan decides to buy a dress. She enters the department store, and she chooses one. She makes an agreement with a clerk. Susan pays the clerk the price of the dress and acquires it.

In these experiences Susan is active. She is an agent taking action toward a goal.

Susan might very well have decided not to buy a dress. This would also have been an action and an exercise of her freedom. But it would have been an exercise of her freedom not involving any agreement or any other person.

Suppose Susan was unable to decide which dress to buy. Her subsequent actions, including her agreement with the clerk, would never have occurred. She would have been passive throughout the whole event. Without the right and power to make voluntary choices there can be no "meeting of the minds." Without a "meeting of the minds" there can be no agreement.

Without agreement there can be no ethical interaction. Freedom is presupposed in any attempt to take ethical interaction.

✂ **DILEMMA 3-1**   Ralph has suffered a myocardial infarction. He is now out of the coronary care unit and seems to be doing well. His physician has given him instructions to stop smoking, increase his activity, and discontinue the work he has been doing while in the hospital. His nurse, Joyce, declares war on his cigarette smoking. Ralph will not stop smoking. If Joyce were willing to recognize Ralph's right to take independent action, she might be able to persuade him to increase his activity and to, at least, cut down on the work he is doing in the hospital. But Ralph resents her interference with his right to take free action, and Joyce is able to accomplish nothing.

When one person refuses to respect the rights of another a "meeting of the minds" between them is impossible. The conflict between them leaves no room for an agreement. In the absence of an agreement there is no basis between them for trust and ethical interaction.

VERACITY

It is logically impossible to have confidence in an agreement if one cannot have confidence in the truthfulness of the people making the agreement. An agreement in which no one has any confidence is really no agreement at all.

Ricky's nurse is going off her shift. Ricky, a seven-year-old patient, is frightened and crying. He asks his nurse if she will come back the next day. She replies that she will. The nurse is off the next day. She does not return. Thereafter Ricky lacks all trust in the truthfulness of health care personnel.

It is easy to see that one can tell the truth without entering into an agreement. The sun is bright. Paul reports to Marcy that the sun is bright. Paul has stated the truth. But no agreement has been entered into between Paul and Marcy.

On the other hand, no one can enter into an agreement unless the parties to the agreement are truthful. Harry and Sid agree to share the driving on a trip to Fort Lauderdale. Harry does not know how to drive. Harry and Sid have not really entered into an agreement.

One can tell the truth without entering into an agreement. But one does not enter into an agreement unless one tells the truth.

PRIVACY[3]

Privacy is the right of an individual to be free of undesired interactions or relationships. One can be a private person and never make agreements. Making an agreement may involve giving up a part of one's privacy. But the practical benefits of making agreements would not be possible to one who did not possess this right. Many of the benefits of long-term planning, whether or not this involves agreements with others, would be lost to one who lacked the right to privacy.

A patient voluntarily gives up a part of his privacy to a health care professional. This much is obvious. There is, however, no reason for a health care professional to assume that her patient gives up *all* right to privacy.

Privacy, as a standard, is the health care professional's obligation to protect her patient from undesirable interactions. The whole world does not have the right of access to a patient's private affairs. This is implied by the patient's right to autonomy. No one has a right to violate a patient's rights.

Confidentiality

A very important part of the standard of privacy is a nurse's obligation to maintain confidentiality regarding her patient's affairs. For her to reveal details of his condition or situation to inappropriate others would be to force him into an undesired relationship with these others.

Each party to an agreement has the right to divulge personal information only to those to whom he wants it divulged.

In the particular circumstances of the patient he is unable to protect himself from unwanted intrusions by others. This responsibility falls on the health care professional. It is one of her functions as agent of her patient.

Privacy and confidentiality are intricately bound up with trust. Trust is an essential part of their agreement.

No agreement is possible without trust.

BENEFICENCE

It is a scandal of modern medicine that a nurse's ability to exercise beneficence is severely circumscribed.

> In February 1985, [the] New Jersey appellate court ruled that a hospital had the right to dismiss a nurse who refused, for "moral, medical and philosophic" reasons, to administer kidney dialysis treatments to a terminally ill double amputee. . . . Mrs. Warthen [the nurse] asked to be replaced, arguing that she could not submit the man to dialysis because he was dying and the procedure was causing additional complications. She . . . was fired. . . . The three judge appellate panel agreed with the hospital. . . . (Humphry & Wickett, 1986, p. 122)

Mrs. Warthen was motivated to take her position by her understanding of beneficence. Most health care professionals would agree that her stand was beneficent. No doubt the hospital where Mrs. Warthen worked held the value of beneficence in high esteem. But the value of their beneficence was not very influential here.

Health care professionals sometimes appeal to a concern for beneficence in order to violate a patient's autonomy.

✂ **DILEMMA 3-2**   Harold has a gangrenous leg. Harold's physician wants to perform an amputation in order to save Harold's life. Harold refuses the surgery. Harold's physician tells himself: "No one could possibly want this." He gets a court order declaring Harold incompetent. The court order permits him to perform the surgery. Harold's physician tells himself that he has acted benevolently. At the same time he has violated Harold's autonomy.

This pseudo-beneficence often seems to get lost in the case of terminally ill and suffering patients.

✂ **DILEMMA 3-3**   Martha has bone cancer. She is suffering excruciating pain. Treatment has been unsuccessful. She is dying. Heroic measures are used in order to keep her alive. A nurse's suggestion that Martha be allowed to die is met with outrage from her colleagues. The only benefit the nurse's colleagues can envision is Martha's sacrifice to "ethical" ideals essentially irrelevant to Martha's situation. If ethical ideals do demand this, it is unfortunate because this idea certainly debases the concept of benevolence.

Beneficence is an intention "to help or at least to do no harm" (Hippocrates cited in Jones, 1923). It is conceivable (but not very conceivable) that a person could act beneficently without making agreements. (for example, on a desert island there is no one toward whom one could feel benevolence). Under most circumstances, it is inconceivable that people without benevolence would make agreements. What possible purpose could be served by making an agreement with someone who had no intention "to help or at least to do no harm"?

FIDELITY

For a nurse fidelity is commitment to the obligation she has accepted as a nurse. Fidelity is commitment to a promise. For a nurse this is the promise to honor her agreement with her patient.

A nurse has an obligation to attend to her patient in the sense of providing care for him. She also has an obligation to attend to him in the sense of listening to him and counseling him. At the very least she has an obligation to protect him from preventable harm (Mappes cited in Arras & Rhoden, 1989).

A patient whose well being is threatened by a nurse has a right to "blow the whistle" on the nurse. The nurse is violating their agreement.

A nurse, on the other hand, has no agreement with a physician or hospital that particular things will be done for the benefit of patients. Therefore she has no primary right to blow the whistle on a physician or hospital. But a patient has this right. And a patient has a right to expect a nurse, as his agent, to blow the whistle when this is appropriate.

Any person, including a nurse, has a right to speak out to protect any other person, including a patient, from harm. This is an aspect of beneficence.

When a nurse blows the whistle to protect a patient, she relies on something more central to their agreement than mere benevolence. Whistle blowing is an aspect of fidelity.

For a patient the demands of fidelity are quite different from those of the nurse. This is because the roles of nurse and patient are very different. A nurse's role, by definition, is much more active than a patient's.

This certainly does not mean that a patient has no moral obligation to exercise fidelity. If a nurse is to be the agent of a patient, the patient must cooperate in the exercise of this agency (Pellegrino and Thomasma, 1988). Fidelity on the part of a patient is simply a recognition of the reality of the nurse. It is the avoidance of behavior that makes contradictory demands on her.

- After surgery a patient expects a nurse to protect him from pneumonia. But he refuses to cough and practice deep breathing postoperatively.
- A patient expects a nurse to help him become more mobile after a stroke. But he refuses to go to physical therapy.
- A patient expects a nurse to protect him from injury. But he refuses to get assistance before getting out of bed.

If a patient does not honor the terms implied by his agreement with the nurse, he violates this agreement. Worse still, he violates his own purposes.

Fidelity means fidelity to an agreement. So, of course, it is not possible to practice fidelity without making agreements. It is also not possible to keep agreements without practicing fidelity. An agreement made without the anticipation of fidelity is a logical impossibility.

However, in expecting fidelity from her patient, a nurse must always bear in mind the incapacities that his condition forces upon him. When she does not receive the cooperation of a patient, she must remember her commitment to her profession. Even when things cannot be done well, she must do the best she can. This is her obligation to her profession—and to herself.

MOTIVATIONS

Between a nurse and a patient there emerges a most intimate ethical relationship. This relationship is formed on the side of the patient by the desire to regain a state of agency. The loss of agency is a frightening experience. It can involve, to a degree, the loss of the patient's self-image. It can be a very painful experience. It makes a patient dependent on others.

On the nurse's side the relationship is formed by her response to the patient. Ideally it will not be formed by any value the dependency of a patient has for a nurse but by the nurse's emotional intolerance of her patient's misfortune. This is the attitude that led most nurses into nursing. The precise emotional attitude that a tragic play or a movie concerning a person acting against adversity hopes to arouse is the ideal emotional attitude of a nurse toward her patient.

At the same time it is to be hoped that a nurse will be strong enough not to wallow in her emotions and allow them to inhibit her actions. She must not allow herself to be "burned-out" by her emotions. And she must not allow herself to resent the patient for being disabled. It would not do for both to be disabled.

The nurse/patient relationship involves implied expectations and obligations accepted and agreed to by each. In every case the expectations and obligations arise somewhat differently. These differences are determined by a number of contextual factors. Chief among these are the conditions of the patient and the way in which the character structures of nurse and patient mesh or fail to mesh in their interaction.

Their relationship sets the parameters of their interaction.

IS THERE A NURSE/PATIENT AGREEMENT?

The question arises as to whether the nurse/patient relationship is based on an actual agreement between them.

For a moment let us entertain the idea that there is no form of agreement between nurse and patient.

If there is no form of agreement between them, there can be no fidelity between them. There is no fidelity between two people who pass each other on the street, simply because there is no common purpose between them. No agreement on a common purpose is possible where there is no common purpose. Therefore, there is simply no objective basis for fidelity between them. Since they have no plans to interact, there is no reason for an agreement between them.

Fidelity is, essentially, fidelity to the terms of an agreement. Without the terms of an agreement there is nothing to establish the parameters of fidelity. A nurse would have no basis for a stable commitment to her patient. A patient would have no objective reason to feel confident under the care of his nurse.

Without an agreement between them nurse and patient would have no explicit understanding of their roles. A patient could not begin to understand the functioning and the fidelity of a nurse unless an agreement existed between them.

To the extent that there is no explicit understanding of the nurse/patient roles, there is no foundation for their interaction. There is no way for them to structure their interaction. What action could a nurse take if she had no idea what the response of a patient would be? What actions could a patient expect a nurse to take if he had no certain knowledge that she was acting in her capacity as nurse?

Without a prior agreement a nurse could not be certain that her patient regarded himself as her patient. Without this agreement a patient could not be sure that the nurse regarded herself as his nurse.

But these problems do not arise between nurse and patient. They do not arise simply because there *is* an agreement between them.

This agreement makes it possible for each to function. It also makes it necessary for each to apply ethical reasoning to his and her actions. Because of this agreement, as Levine (1989) observed, "All nursing actions are moral statements."

JUSTIFICATION AND THE AGREEMENT

It is logically impossible for a nurse to be able to justify her thinking and yet be blameworthy for her actions. If she has done the best she can, given the context of her knowledge, this is all that can be asked of her.

It is also impossible for a nurse to be praiseworthy for her actions while she is unable to justify the thinking that produced those actions. If the good results that came from her actions were accidental, there is nothing in this for which she can be praised. Both intention and effect are relevant to the quality of an ethical action.

An agent justifies his actions by describing how these actions accomplish an ethical purpose. Where there is an agreement, the purpose that justifies his actions is the subject of the agreement. Along with the purpose there may also be an agreement on the actions that may or may not be taken.

For a decision or action to be justified, then, four conditions are necessary:

1. The goal of the decision or action must be this predetermined purpose.
2. There must be reason to believe that this decision or action will tend to bring about the accomplishment of its purpose.
3. It must not be an action prohibited by the agreement.
4. It must not be an action that would interfere with actions specified in the agreement.

In a health care setting the bioethical agreement is an instrument by which both nurse and patient can maximize the benefits of their relationship.

The relationship takes the form of contractual agreement. The role of the nurse becomes one of "contracted clinician" (Brock cited in Barry, 1982).

An implied contract comes into existence when any person seeks the advice and help of another human and that other person accepts the appeal [in return for some acceptable consideration]. Whether the details are verbalized or not, the sick person and the health worker enter into a contract with one another. Implicitly they accept mutual obligations and rights. (Francoeur, 1983, p. 72)

The nurse enters into an implied but formal agreement with those who come under her care. Without this agreement there could be no expectations and no ethical obligations. Right actions, on the part of the nurse, and of the patient, are actions according to the rights of the other. The rights of each is determined by the terms of the agreement.

Without the agreement there would be no ethical criteria on which to base ethical judgments. Each party to the agreement has ethical responsibilities according to the terms of the agreement and only according to these terms.

The nature and the terms of the agreement between nurse and patient are usually not made explicit for the participants. However, the terms of this contract are generally known and accepted.

A LOSS OF DIRECTION

Actions that are outside of the nurse/patient agreement often fail to enhance the ethical interrelationship between nurse and patient. They often bring discord into that relationship. Marie, a nurse at County General, frequently experiences ethical conflict in her interactions with her patients.

Sometimes she allows her patient to talk her into negotiating personal problems with the patient's family. Other times, when her patient does not give her the information she needs to care for him adequately, she fails to insist that he be candid with her. There are times when she allows a patient to act toward her with controlling behavior and treat her as if she were a servant. She may allow a patient to hold her responsible for his health while he refuses to cooperate in his regimen of care.

All these activities are outside of the nurse/patient agreement. Sometimes Marie submits to performing them. Sometimes she volunteers.

There are times when any of these behaviors are appropriate and even necessary. But, if they are allowed to blur the outlines of the nurse/patient context, they undermine the interaction between Marie and her patient. When Marie neglects her role as professional, her ethical interaction with her patient deteriorates.

Sometimes Marie makes unreasonable demands on her patient. She may lay her personal problems on him. Or she may take the emotional effects of a bad day out on him. She may decide to place the desires of someone else above her patient's desire.

These interactions replace the nurse/patient agreement as Marie's guide to ethical interactions. As the nurse/patient agreement loses its power to direct Marie's interactions, her ethical relationship with her patient comes apart.

In any kind of relationship all interactions that can be understood and described are formed by an agreement. When it becomes evident that the protection afforded by the agreement is lost, the relationship suffers. One or both parties to the agreement feel bewildered and betrayed. He or she may not know why.

The agreement between nurse and patient is an implicit agreement formed by mutual expectations. Being an implicit agreement, it must be protected. Sometimes, even through apparently good intentions, it can be undermined.

Interactions outside of the nurse/patient agreement may have a detrimental effect on a patient's recovery and long-term well being. They are primary contributors to nurse burn-out. By engaging in interactions outside of the nurse/patient agreement, Marie and her patient lose a clear awareness of what nursing is all about. This awareness is a *significant* value.

PURPOSES AND "PRACTICAL REASON"

Ethical realities are common experiences for all persons. They are not something accepted by mere convention. Nor are they something brought into being by legislation. Everyone has desires and purposes. Everyone faces the need to think before he or she takes actions. These factors cannot exist without bringing the need for ethical thought — for "practical reason" — into existence.

That purpose and value are ethical phenomena pertaining to all people, that all people possess rights, and that all people possess ethical agency are not matters on which one decides. They are ethical realities always already there for one to discover.

Ethical realities are human realities, not because people have the power to choose them, but because they are part of human nature and part of the human situation. The supreme interpersonal reality is the network of agreements that makes human interaction possible.

If the desire behind an agreement is a rational, noncoercive, and non–self-destructive desire, then the agreement is the final "court of appeal" concerning interpersonal actions.

NOTES

1   Certain terms used in the book are redefined for the sake of maximum usefulness. Autonomy is one of these terms. In the bioethical literature the terms *autonomy* and *freedom* are very frequently confused and/or equated. Generally speaking "autonomy" is very similar in meaning to "freedom." In this text, we have defined the autonomy of a person as the uniqueness (unique character structure) of that person. Our reason and justification for this is as follows:

"Autonomy" means independent and self-governing. A person's independence and self-governance, however, is captured in the concept of a person's "freedom." Every person is, by nature, free; and every person has a right to freedom. A person's right to freedom is that person's right to self-governance and independent action.

The *way* a person exercises his or her self-governance and right to take independent action is not determined by the mere fact that the person *is* independent and self-governing. It is determined by that person's unique desires and values — his or her unique character structure. A nurse understands her patient better if she makes herself aware of the ways in which he is unique than she does if she simply makes herself aware of his independence and right to self-governance alone.

For the technical sense in which terms are used in this text, the reader is referred to the Glossary.

2   This issue of freedom is usually discussed in the literature under the term *voluntarism.* However, voluntarism is a technical philosophical term that does not encompass the bioethical standard. Therefore we will refer to this standard as "freedom."

Voluntarism, briefly, is the ethical theory that the will, rather than the intellect, is the faculty by which people make ethical decisions. It is the theory that the will is the basic factor in human experience, and therefore ought to come before reason, duty, or any other source of ethical guidance. Voluntarism is, quite obviously, neither appropriate to the context of a nurse nor to that of a patient.

3   Privacy is another term that we use in a technical sense. The dictionary defines "privacy" as "the condition of being secluded or isolated from the view of, or from contact with, others; concealment; secrecy." But behind this definition there is the fact of the patient's self-ownership. If a person enjoys self-ownership, then he or she has a right to privacy (in the dictionary sense). If a person does not enjoy self-ownership, then there is no possible basis for that person's right to privacy.

A nurse's awareness of her patient's self-ownership provides a much better standard of ethical behavior than her, much narrower, awareness of his right to privacy.

REFERENCES

Arras, J., & Rhoden, N. (1989). *Ethical issues in modern medicine* (3rd ed.). Mountain View, CA: Mayfield Publication Co.

Barry, V. (1982). *Moral aspects of health care.* Belmont, CA: Wadsworth.

Francoeur, R.T. (1983). *Biomedical ethics: A guide to decision making.* New York: John Wiley & Sons.

Humphry, D., & Wickett, A. (1986). *The right to die: Understanding euthanasia.* New York: Harper and Row.

Jones, W.H.S. (trans.). (1923). *Hippocrates.* Cambridge, Mass.: Harvard University Press.

Levine, M.E., (1989). The ethics of nursing rhetoric. *Image, 21*(1), 46.

Pellegrino, E.D., & Thomasma, D.C. (1988). *The restoration of beneficence in health care.* New York: Oxford University Press.

CHAPTER

4

Contemporary Ethical Standards

In any society or culture[1] autonomous individuals can misunderstand each other. Even when they do understand each other, it is possible for them to disagree. In our pluralistic society the failure of people to understand each other is very common. The health care system, in common with every other segment of society, has found it necessary to find ways to create understanding and agreement. When individuals interact, they often begin without any ground of understanding. This is true even of people whose backgrounds are identical. Some common ground must be created or found.

The function of bioethics, in our society, is to make agreement possible (Engelhardt, 1986). Nurses and patients meet as strangers. They may come from diverse backgrounds. They may come from different subcultures. Their ways of looking at and approaching the world may be quite different.

There is no situation in which creating harmony is always an easy task. It is especially difficult in a nursing situation. A patient is in unfamiliar surroundings. He must contend with pain and inactivity. He faces the threat to his values[2] posed by disability. A nurse must deal with responsibility and strain. Because nursing is not always recognized as a profession, the nurse is sometimes held in low esteem by other professionals. She must establish and maintain several delicate balances. Among these is the balance between her rights and autonomy and the demands and obligations she faces as a nurse.

Yet, with all the responsibility and strain, nursing provides unique opportunities for personal fulfillment. Without giving up her rights or her autonomy, a nurse can provide great benefits for herself and her patient.

One of the greatest benefits a nurse can provide to a patient is free and open communication with him. Without this she does not deal with her patient as a fellow human. This means that she does not treat herself as fully human.

One of the greatest benefits a nurse can gain for herself is communication with her patient. This keeps her aware of the importance of her art. It is a central part of this art to be able to deal with her patient as a fellow human being.

CONTEMPORARY BIOETHICAL STANDARDS

Bioethical standards serve to make it possible for nurse and patient to deal with each other on a human level. They tend to create respect for her patient in a nurse. This heightens a nurse's self-respect. The standards make it appropriate for a patient to respect his nurse. Bioethical standards make it possible for strangers to achieve understanding. If they are not always successful in bringing about agreement, they can be successful in bringing about toleration. They make it possible for nurse and patient to agree on and respect each other's rights.

Contemporary bioethical standards make possible what much of traditional ethics would make impossible. They make it possible for nurse and patient to interact on the basis of shared goals.

The major contemporary bioethical standards are:

• Autonomy
• Freedom
• Veracity
• Privacy
• Beneficience
• Fidelity

A few preliminary observations concerning the bioethical standards are in order.

Principles

In the literature contemporary bioethical standards are usually referred to as principles. In common usage the term "principle" is used to mean "a basic truth or law" (*American Heritage Dictionary*, 1985). Principles are basic or necessary truths.

For instance, a society whose every member attempted to survive by theft would not survive. As the things that were stolen were consumed, there would be less and less to steal. Finally there would be nothing to steal and no way for the members of the society to survive. Thus the evil of theft is an ethical principle enforced by the nature of reality. It is a necessary truth.

On the other hand, the members of a society can perceive the benefits to be gained, for instance, by respecting each other's privacy.[3] They may agree among themselves to do this. This does not make respect for privacy a necessary and permanent truth. The failure to respect privacy will probably cause dissension and discord, but it will not necessarily destroy the society as theft would.

It is possible to imagine a society in which there was no concept of privacy. Whatever disadvantages this might have, the society would not be destroyed by this lack. It is virtually impossible to imagine a society that holds no prohibitions on theft. The continuous existence of this society would be impossible. The members of every society can depend upon the inappropriateness of theft as a cultural norm. They can trust that theft will be regarded as unusual and criminal. They cannot have the same trust in respect for their privacy. Principles are not subject to change. They are permanent—part of the nature of things. Standards are chosen. They are not permanent; they can be discarded at will. The destructive nature of theft is a principle. It is the way things are. Respect for privacy is a standard. It is the product of an agreement.

It is unreasonable to expect that any ethical standard upon which a society agrees will gain permanent acceptance. Ethical standards, unlike ethical principles, are notoriously impermanent.

Standards are "a measure for comparison of quantitative or qualitative value" (American Heritage Dictionary, 1985). Thus as a culture's values change, its standards change. The phrase "contemporary standards" does not involve an internal contradiction; the phrase "contemporary principles" does. If something is a principle, it is not contemporary. If it is contemporary, it is not a principle. Thus we will refer to autonomy, freedom, veracity, privacy, beneficience, and fidelity as "standards," not "principles." Although, no doubt, it would be a great blessing if these standards were principles.

Justice

Justice, in terms of the allocation of scarce resources, the distribution of health care, and so on will not be dealt with here. In our contemporary culture, the allocation of resources, the "right" to health care, and issues of this type are treated as political issues. And although every political issue has an ethical foundation, not one has a *bioethical* foundation.

"Justice," in the contemporary biomedical milieu, is an undefined term. There are two major outlooks on the nature of justice: (1) that justice is the fairest or most equal distribution of values, and (2) that justice is the unimpeded exchange of values between (or among) autonomous individuals.

In the nature of things an undefined term does not designate either a principle or a standard. It designates a problem. Therefore "justice" is not included among the contemporary bioethical standards listed on p. 40.

STANDARDS AND THE NURSE/PATIENT AGREEMENT

The health care setting always functions against the background of the culture within which it exists. Ethical ideas governing the health care setting, historically, have reflected the ethical ideas of the culture itself. Sometimes the inhumane ideas of right and wrong that a culture holds find frightful expression in the health care system. But the health care system generally functions on a more realistic and more humane level than that of the overall culture.

The invention of anesthesia was greeted with cries of dismay from a segment of society that feared a violation of ethical principles. The Bible condemned the daughters of Eve to bear children in pain and travail. Anesthesia was seen, rightly, as a way for women to escape this. But cultural institutions changed, and the use of anesthesia survived.

In the biomedical setting the nature of an individual, and of the human condition, becomes evident. The relevance and irrelevance of a culture's ethical beliefs are revealed in this setting, much as the skeletal structure of a patient is revealed by x-rays.

The health care system has arisen by virtue of specific human desires and needs. It serves a definite purpose. These needs, desires, and purposes determine the role of everyone in the health care system. They determine the nature of the role filled by nurses.

These human needs, desires, and purposes, in relation to the role of the nurse, cause an implied agreement to arise between nurse and patient. A patient agrees to be a patient.[4] A nurse, in turn agrees to be a nurse.

A nurse in a health care setting knows why she is there. A patient knows, or comes to know, why he is there. His nurse also knows why he is there. He is there to regain his power to take actions toward his goals.

One's power of agency is his power or capacity to initiate and carry out actions directed toward goals. A patient comes into the health care setting in order to overcome a physical or psychological disability. He is there to regain his power of agency. But no patient regards agency as his final purpose. His final purposes are the goals toward which he directs purposeful action. Agency is a value in that it enables an agent to realize purposes beyond itself. A patient is in the health care setting so that he will be able to return to the football field or the concert stage or the factory floor. He is there in order to return to his family.

Unless the patient or his nurse is comatose, both understand this. This understanding is the *motive* of their agreement. It determines the nature of their agreement.

   Given the volitional and rational nature of the parties to the agreement, the contemporary bioethical standards seem perfectly appropriate to it.

AUTONOMY

Autonomy involves, but is not limited to, the right of an agent to take individual actions. Individual actions are actions directed toward goals that are exclusively the agent's own. Autonomy is a right that an agent possesses by virtue of the fact that he has the power and the desire to take actions. "To respect autonomy is to respect the individual's right of self governance according to a plan that is chosen and followed by the individual" (Fowler & Levine-Ariff, 1987, p. 40). As a bioethical standard, respect for autonomy is the necessity placed on health care professionals of accepting the uniqueness of a patient.

   Every contemporary bioethical standard is derived from the standard of autonomy. If the standard of autonomy cannot be defended, then no bioethical standard can be defended. In the context of contemporary bioethical standards, autonomy is the ultimate standard of the rightness or wrongness of a nurse's ethical decisions. If a nurse is to be able to justify her actions, it is imperative that she be able to defend the standard of her decisions.

   Autonomy has to do with the uniqueness of the individual. It is his right to be what he is.

   Recognition of the right to autonomy involves a willingness not to interfere with actions toward goals that are not one's own. It involves recognition of the fact that a patient's purposes cannot be abridged on the grounds that the patient or his purposes are different from some societal norm. A nurse has no right to attempt to frustrate a patient's purposes no matter how much they differ from or clash with her own. Nor does any health care professional have a right to enforce on a patient an obligation which the patient has to himself.

   Peter has carcinoma of the lung. The attending physician decides that chemotherapy is the treatment of choice. The physician does not consult with Peter. He is convinced that Peter has an obligation to himself to undergo the treatment.

   Despite efforts to respect autonomy, it is almost impossible to remove a sense of coercion when the patient is weak, helpless, and at the mercy of others. Furthermore . . . physicians are strongly influenced by their personal values and unconscious motivations. . . . (Orlowski & Kanoti, 1986, p. 48)

   The notion of an obligation which a patient has to himself is ethically unintelligible. Health care professionals are not enforcers. An agent's autonomy is recognized through the recognition of his freedom to decide for himself.

Nurses, also, are influenced by "personal values and unconscious motivations." A patient does not make a choice or decision in a vacuum. However, it is the health care professional's responsibility to remove as much coercion or undue influence as possible.

Every ethical agent possesses an autonomy equal to every other—and nothing more. An agent possesses the right to his autonomy (1) by virtue of the fact that he is a (rational, volitional) human being, and (2) to whatever extent he is capable of making individual choices and decisions, or taking individual actions.

A patient contracts with a health care professional in order that he can regain his autonomy. A patient contracts with a nurse for the specific purpose of retaining whatever degree of autonomy he can. A patient cannot lose his right to make autonomous decisions by becoming a patient.

Respect for the autonomy of another is identical with respect for the person of another. It is respect for an individual whose essential nature is the same as one's own.

> To respect persons *simpliciter* is to respect another individual as someone who shares the same human destiny as oneself. To respect self-determined choice is to respect choice as one way that an individual may autonomously realize his or her destiny. . . . (Fry cited in Fowler, 1987, p. 41)

If humans, by nature, possess autonomy then all humans— every being of this nature—possess autonomy.

If one individual, by nature, possesses a right to attack the autonomy of other individuals, then everyone possesses this right. If everyone possesses the right to attack the autonomy of others, then no one possesses a right to autonomy. But if no one possesses a right to autonomy, then no one possesses the autonomous right to attack the autonomy of others.

In a logical and an ethical sense, one who violates the autonomy of another acts according to a line of reasoning that forms a vicious circle.

Paternalism

The most common way of violating a patient's autonomy is "paternalism." Paternalism occurs when the health care professional (1) relates to an adult patient as if the patient were a child, or (2) assumes the authority of a parent in relating to a child.

It is the practice of relating to a patient in such a way that the patient has no choice or responsibility in the decision-making process.

> Paternalism may be defined as the refusal to acquiesce in a person's wishes, choices and actions for that person's own benefit. Both individual and communal beneficience may drive paternalism, but paternalism should be limited

and constrained by respect for persons and their autonomy. (Childress, 1984, p. 31)

Paternalism occurs when an adult is treated like a child. It occurs when a professional treats a patient, in effect, as one would treat a child. It occurs when a professional relates to a patient without respect for the patient's rights and moral dignity. "Paternalism is the interference with a person's liberty of action justified by reasons referring exclusively to the welfare, good, happiness, needs, interest, or values of the person being coerced" (Dworkin, 1972, p. 65).

In Chapter 1 we established that no sensible person would turn the entire planning of his vacation over to a travel agent. Likewise no sensible person would turn the whole process of his hospital stay and health care over to another.

The Propriety of Limited Interventions

There are times, however, when a health care professional *must* act for a patient. These would include times when a patient is, for instance, unconscious or suffering a grand mal seizure. Even in these unusual circumstances, however, a patient has tacitly agreed beforehand to a limited intervention. He has done this by the act of entering the health care system. He has agreed to let health care professionals act as his agent when he is unable to exercise agency on his own.

A health care professional, in acting for a patient in an emergency situation, does not wrongfully take away her patient's autonomy. She does nothing wrong *if* she remembers that a biomedical situation is not a permanent emergency.

Provisions for emergency situations are built into the normal procedures of the health care setting. A patient's consent is not needed for emergency care if there is an immediate threat to the patient's life and health. This does not involve nor imply the loss of a patient's autonomy. In entering a health care setting a patient agrees to these provisions. But taking on the responsibility for fulfilling an agreement is not the same as giving up one's autonomy.

Sometimes a health care professional is tempted to override a patient's autonomy. She might decide to exercise her own independent judgment involving the course of the patient's treatment even when limited intervention is involved. In such a circumstance she might do well to ask herself this question:

"What argument would you accept for someone taking control of your autonomy in a situation where you had not agreed to this?"

If there is no argument that you, the reader, would accept, there is no argument you can offer.

FREEDOM

An agent possesses freedom in two senses:

1. In what might be called an existential sense, every agent possesses freedom in that he is capable of taking independent actions.
2. In an ethical sense, every agent possesses freedom since there is nothing in human nature to justify one agent's right to interfere with the autonomous action of another. Whatever rights an individual possesses, he possesses by virtue of his human nature.

Every ethical agent possesses a human nature. Therefore every ethical agent possesses identical rights. That one human is more human than another and, by this fact, possessed of "superior" rights is an absurdity. It is the same type of absurdity the pigs in George Orwell's *Animal Farm* were guilty of when they declared that "Some animals are more equal than others."

Every ethical agent possesses freedom equal to that of every other ethical agent — and nothing more. An agent's existential freedom is enormously increased by his possession of rights. But it is limited by the fact that others also possess rights. No agent has the ethical freedom to violate the rights of others.

Autonomy accrues to a patient by virtue of the fact that he has the power to pursue goals peculiar to his own unique desires. Freedom accrues to a patient by virtue of the fact that reasoning agents can plan and take actions directed toward future goals.

An agent's freedom is his right to determine for himself the meaning and importance of a context. It is also freedom to (1) form purposes; (2) act; (3) bring about change; and (4) pursue his goals.

It is freedom to act with practical reason.

Freedom is the doctrine that nothing should be done to a patient without the patient's consent. It is a direct implication of the standard of autonomy. Autonomy permits a patient to be what he is. Freedom permits him to act for that which he perceives as his own benefit. Under the standard of freedom one may not interfere with a patient's purposes. One may not compel a patient to act, or to submit to the actions of others, against his will.

Freedom is established by the very same line of reasoning as autonomy. To violate the standard of freedom is to violate the nature of an agent. It is particularly incongruous in a biomedical setting. The whole purpose of a biomedical setting is to enable a patient to *regain* agency, not to assist him in losing it. To work for a patient's agency and, at the same time, to violate it reveals a "contradiction" in one's actions. The nurse/patient agreement does not call for a patient to deliver whatever power of agency he retains to a health care professional. A person's right to freedom is his right to the privacy of his will.

The Interactions of Autonomy and Freedom

Suppose someone wrote a biography of Paul McCartney. Someone else wrote a biography of John Lennon. A third biographer wrote the Life of George Harrison, and a fourth, the Life of Ringo Starr. Suppose, further, that each biography discussed the life of its subject without ever mentioning the existence of the other three. These biographies would miss that which was of historic significance in the life of the Beatles. None would be a complete or even a relevant account of the life of its subject.

The case is very much the same with autonomy and freedom. Neither can be understood without the other. They are intrinsically intertwined.

That an agent is autonomous, that he possesses desires, values, and purposes peculiar to himself, is the sole reason he requires a right to freedom. If he did not possess autonomy, his purposes might be best served by his being in a harness.

At the same time—that an agent has a right to freedom means that he has a right to autonomy. Freedom is freedom to be autonomous.

Informed Consent

> The principle of autonomy is the moral basis for the legal doctrine of informed consent, which includes the right of informed refusal. (Smith and Veatch, 1987, p. 7)

The idea that one may not engage in the "unauthorized touching" of another dates back at least to the eighteenth century. This was decided in *Slater vs. Baker and Stapleton* (1767). This decision made it clear that a person has a right to know what is to be done to his body so that he can "get himself prepared."

This decision did not consider a patient's right to informed *consent*. It recognized only his right to be told what course of treatment he is to undergo.

Between 1767 and 1905 the situation was unchanged. However, in 1905, a case was heard that began what we know today as informed consent. In *Mohe vs. Williams*, the patient won the decision because he had consented to surgery on one ear and the physician operated on both. Shortly thereafter, in 1914, in the case of *Schloendorff vs. The Society of New York Hospital*, the patient again won. In this case the patient had consented to abdominal examination, but the physician had performed abdominal surgery instead. Judge Cardoza ruled that every adult person of sound mind has the right to determine what shall be done with his own body. Surgery had been performed without the patient's consent. This decision established the legal recognition of a patient's right to be informed as to what is going to be done and the right to give or withhold consent. It did not address his right to be informed about the risks involved in the course of his treatment.

The right to give an informed consent in regard to clinical practice was not explicated until 1957 in the case of *Salgo v. Leland Stanford, Jr., University Board of Trustees*. The decision established a patient's right to informed consent, including his right to be advised of the risks involved in the proposed treatment. In this case, the Calfornia Supreme Court ruled in favor of a patient who had not been told the risks involved before an aortography. The patient had become permanently paralyzed. Responding to this decision, individual states began passing laws formalizing the patient's right to informed consent.

The right to informed consent involving research occurred somewhat later, primarily as a result of the trials of German physicians convicted of experimenting on prisoners of war. This led the way for the specific criteria of informed consent that were formalized in the Nuremberg Code. Informed consent was later recognized in the Declaration of Helsinki by the Eighteenth World Medical assembly in 1964 and revised in 1975.

These rulings have to do with the physician's responsibility and do not address the role of the nurse. It is generally agreed that a nurse does not have the primary responsibility for getting informed consent. However, if she realizes that the patient is not informed (not aware of what is going to happen), legally she must act (Rocereto & Maleskin, 1982). Yet no ruling has ever been made as to precisely what she is to do and how she is to do it when the patient is uninformed.

A landmark case involving the role of the nurse in informed consent occurred in Idaho in 1977. Jolene Tuma, a nursing instructor, went to the bedside of a terminally ill woman to start chemotherapy. The woman asked about alternative treatment and was told by Ms. Tuma about several, including laetrile, a controversial drug not approved by the Federal Food and Drug Administration. The patient stopped chemotherapy for a short time but later resumed it. She died shortly thereafter. The patient's son was very upset, and the physician brought charges against the nurse. Ms. Tuma was fired. Her license was also revoked on the ground that her actions "disrupted the physician-patient relationship."

Ms. Tuma took her case through the courts, and in 1979 the Idaho Supreme Court ruled that she could not be found guilty of unprofessional conduct because the Idaho Nurse Practice Act neither "defines unprofessional conduct nor sets guidelines for providing warnings." However, the court did not address the right of a nurse to inform patients. This remains in question to this day.

If the nurse believes that the patient is not properly informed, her first course of action should be to consult the physician and ask him to give the patient the relevant information. If the physician refuses, she must decide what further steps she wants to take. The patient has an absolute moral and legal right to be informed. He has a right to receive full and accurate information.

Yet, paradoxically, a nurse has no firmly established legal right to inform her patient.

The role of the nurse in informed consent is yet to be decided. If the law continues to evolve in the direction of patient autonomy, the nurse will gain a more active function. If the nurse does not gain a more active function, then autonomy as a bioethical standard will be eroded — or destroyed.

VERACITY

Long ago people began to communicate with each other on an abstract level. Early on some genius of our species noted that, if people are going to communicate and interact on this level, truth telling is of the highest importance. Without truth telling there could not be trust among humans. And without trust there could not be communication and interaction.

This was perfectly illustrated in an experiment with newborn cats. The room in which they were kept was covered with linoleum. The linoleum had a block pattern. Half the room in which they were kept was covered with ¼-inch blocks, the other half with 1-inch blocks. The kittens, who began life on the larger blocks, avoided the half of the room with the smaller blocks. From their perspective it appeared that that half of the room was lower and moving onto it would involve a fall (Vander Zander, 1978).

Their perspective deceived them. They were unaware of the truth. So the "truth" on which they acted was the truth that a fall might injure them. This was the truth with the greater survival value.

It is just such a truth that if people do not communicate with each other (for the most part) truthfully, they will suffer through their interaction and communication. Their only recourse would be to give up communication and interaction.

All the contemporary bioethical standards, in one way or another, involve veracity. The standard of veracity requires that a nurse accept (tell herself) the truth concerning the unique nature of her patient. Freedom to choose implies the possession of true ideas. True ideas are the basis of every real choice.

The relation between veracity and privacy is a peculiar one. The standard of privacy protects a patient from having to "volunteer" truth when truth would be detrimental to him. In this way privacy protects the value of truth.

Beneficence is a type of promise keeping. Beneficent actions are the means by which the nurse's promise is kept.

Fidelity is promise keeping itself. It is the form which truth takes in the nurse/patient agreement.

PRIVACY

The right to privacy is an expression of the right to autonomy. In the health care setting, it is the right of a patient to be protected against any form of intrusive contact from others.

> [O]n logical grounds if we concede the existence of individual human rights of any kind, then it is . . . self evident that there must be a "right to privacy" for without it there would be no private individuals to have or exercise those rights. (Thompson, 1979, p. 59)

One does not lose his right to privacy when he becomes a patient in the health care system. Entering the health care system does not mean going on display. This has been recognized since the time of Hippocrates:

> ...whatsoever I shall see or hear in the course of my profession, as well as outside my profession in my intercourse with men, if it be what should not be published abroad, I will never divulge, holding such things to be holy secrets.

It has been reaffirmed in the Nightingale pledge:

> I will . . . hold in confidence all personal matters committed to my keeping, and family affairs coming to my knowledge in the practice of my calling.

Confidentiality

A patient's right to privacy includes a right to confidentiality. Confidentiality extends a patient's self-ownership over to an ownership of his knowledge. Privacy protects his self-ownership. Confidentiality protects his knowledge from being used against his self-ownership. According to the standard of privacy a nurse is ethically obliged not to reveal what a patient tells her in confidence. She is also obliged not to divulge information of a private nature, for example, health records, where this is unwarranted.

Balancing this obligation with the need to inform others, for example, of the presence of contagious disease, can be a delicate matter indeed. At present the laws governing confidentiality are in a state of logical chaos. If a psychiatrist has reason to believe that a patient poses a threat to someone's life, the law demands that he reveal this. If a physician has reason to believe that an AIDS patient is going to attempt to spread his disease as widely as he can, the physician has been legally forbidden to reveal his patient's plans. Thus it has been unlawful for a physician not to attempt to prevent a murder committed with a pistol, while at that same time it has been illegal for a physician to attempt to prevent a murder[5] committed by means of infection with a fatal disease.

It seems reasonable to suggest that when the laws are finally solidified, these discrepancies will no longer exist. But in matters of privacy and confidentiality, the need for a delicate balance seldom exists. A patient's privacy rarely threatens an innocent person.

There is an unambiguous need for a health care professional to protect her patient against the professional herself.

> Damage is done to patients . . . more often as the result of a careless or boastful revelation than from the evil designs or the demands of others outside one's profession." (Cass and Curran in Gorovitz et al., 1983, p. 83)

The patient's right to privacy is one right that a health care professional ought to be especially careful to protect. A violation of this right, as Thompson (1979) points out, involves the unsupportable implication that the patient has no human rights. But the worth and dignity of a health care professional rests in the fact that she deals with people who do possess rights and human dignity.

Demeaning the status of the patient involves demeaning the status of the health care professional herself. Protecting the privacy of a patient is precisely a recognition of his worth and human dignity. Protecting the worth and dignity of the patient is a professional's tribute to her own worth and dignity.

BENEFICENCE

> As to diseases, make a habit of two things—to help, or at least to do no harm. (Hippocrates [460-377 B.C.], EPIDEMICS, BOOK I SEC XI)

This standard counsels a nurse to relate to a patient in a way that will always be beneficial for the patient. It implies that a nurse should scrupulously avoid interacting with a patient in any way that might cause unnecessary and avoidable harm.

> Beneficence is traditionally seen as residing at the foundation of health care and refers specifically to the principle that the goal of actions in relation to patients ought to be to promote health, to relieve from unnecessary pain and suffering and to prolong life. (Beauchamp & Childress, 1983, p. 148)

Beneficence is a quality of actions. It characterizes actions that are motivated by benevolence. Benevolence is a state of mind. It is a consistent attitude of good will toward another (or toward oneself). Beneficence is the practice of acting on the promptings of good will.

Patients do not always find beneficence in a health care setting. The situation is far from perfect today, but it is infinitely better than it once was. The conditions of a hundred years ago led Florence Nightingale to declare:

> It may seem a strange principle to enunciate as the very first requirement in a hospital, that it should do the sick no harm.

Beneficence is, of necessity, an integral part of the nurse/patient agreement. "The bonds of beneficence that tie individuals in special roles . . . are in part contractual. By this I do not mean to suggest an explicit contract but a web of usually implicit understandings" (Engelhardt, 1986, p. 75).

A beneficent nurse acts with empathy for her patient—and without resentment or malice.

Still and all a patient on entering a hospital makes a commitment to let the hospital function as a hospital. A patient has an inalienable right to decline treatment. "To force a patient to undergo treatment against his or her wishes . . . constitutes both a violation of autonomy, and the infliction of harm. In cases such as these, the autonomous patient determines what constitutes unwarranted suffering" (Fowler & Levine-Ariff, 1987, p. 193). Conflicts can arise concerning the demands of beneficence and the natural function of a health care setting. These are, in fact, the most common bioethical conflicts.

FIDELITY

The evolution and traditions of nursing have produced certain cultural expectations concerning the nature of nursing. These also form a bridge of expectations between nurse and patient. When a patient enters the health care system, these expectations form an implicit agreement between them. The terms of the agreement are precisely those expectations as each is aware of them.

A nurse in relating to her patient tacitly promises to live up to her patient's reasonable expectations. Behind this act of making a promise is an implicit commitment to keep it. Thus fidelity is fundamental to the nurse/patient agreement.

> It is widely recognized that acting morally includes the keeping of promises . . . . If people did not generally have an obligation to keep promises, then the very act of making a promise would be meaningless. (Veatch & Fry, 1987, p. 138)

Many of a nurse's ethical dilemmas concern disagreement or confusion over the details of various promises. Dilemmas also arise over which promises make moral commitments between nurse and patient possible.

It is central to the nurse/patient agreement that the nurse is in the health care setting for the benefit of the patient. In recalling this and holding to the agreement the nurse fulfills the promises she has made to the patient. These are also the promises that make moral commitment between nurse and physician possible. Both are there for the benefit of the patient. All that is necessary is that they not interfere with each other's functioning, that they cooperate when appropriate, and that they fulfill their individual functions in a competent manner. The necessity for fidelity is already contained in the standard of autonomy. Fidelity is a way the nurse recognizes the autonomy of her patient—and her own autonomy.

> While nurses may encounter situations in which they are unable to keep a promise made to a patient . . . the breaking of a promise that has been made in

good faith requires special justification that a reasonable person would understand and accept. (Aroskar cited in Fowler, 1987, p. 81)

SUMMARY

Contemporary bioethical standards are all derived, directly or indirectly, from the standard of autonomy. Within the world no two people appear exactly alike. But their values and purposes, their moral beliefs, and their moral characters differ much more than their appearances. Within the human community conflict is inevitable unless the members of the human community rise to a human level. In the biomedical setting bioethical standards allow us to do just this.

NOTES

1 By "culture" is meant a group of people living in the same geographic location and sharing similar traditions, beliefs, and customs.

2 The concept *value* is often used to refer to those traditions or aspects of a culture to which the citizens of the culture are expected to give some form of allegiance. This implicitly denies the importance or even the possibility of individual values.

Social or collective values have no relevance for bioethics and, arguably, for ethics in general. The values with which a nurse deals are her personal and individual values as nurse and those of her patient.

By "values" we are referring to the objects of actions that are motivated by autonomous desires. The disability of a patient diminshes his power of acting. This, necessarily, diminishes his ability to act toward the objects of his desire. In this sense disability poses a threat to his values.

3 "Privacy," for reasons explained on page 38, is used to denote the fact of a person's self-ownership. However, it is used here in its dictionary meaning—the condition of being isolated from contact with others.

4 Very few patients want to be in the hospital. But "wanting to be in the hospital" is not equivalent to "agreeing to be a patient." The general position of a patient is that he does not want to be in the hospital, but while he is there, he agrees to be a patient.

By the same token nurses, in general, want to restore their patients to a state of health and get them out of the hospital. This does not mean that a nurse does not agree to be a nurse. To help her patient to get out of the hospital is a nurse's proper function.

5 Whether the act of intentionally causing the death of another by infecting the person with AIDS is illegal has not yet been firmly established in law. Yet, if one person intentionally brought about the death of another, for example, by injecting him with the hepatitis virus, it seems certain that this would be considered murder. For ethics the traditional definition of murder is "the act of unjustifiably causing the death of another" (Veatch, 1985, *inter alia*). The act of intentionally infecting another with the AIDS virus fits this definition perfectly.

REFERENCES

American heritage dictionary. (1985). (2nd college ed.) Boston, MA: Houghton Mifflin.

Beauchamp, T. & Childress, J. (1983). *Principles of biomedical ethics.* (2nd ed.) New York: Oxford University Press.

Childress, J.F. (1984). Ensuring care, respect, and fairness for the elderly. *Hastings Center Report, 14*(5), 27-31.

Dworkin, G. (1972). Paternalism. *The Monist, 56,* 64-68.

Engelhardt, H.T., Jr. (1986). *The foundations of bioethics.* New York: Oxford English Press.

Fowler, M.D.M., & Levine-Ariff, J. (1987). *Ethics at the bedside.* Philadelphia, PA: J.B. Lippincott.

Gorovitz, S., et al. (1983). *Moral problems in medicine.* Englewood Cliffs, NJ: Prentice Hall.

Orlowski, J.P. and Kanoti, G.A. (Eds.). (1986). Ethical moments in critical care medicine. *Critical Care Clinics, 2*(1), 1-186.

Rocereto, L., and Maleskin, C. (1982). *Legal dimensions of nursing practice: A practical guide.* New York: Springer Publishing.

Smith, D.H. and Veatch, R.M. (Eds.). (1987). *Guidelines on the termination of life-sustaining treatment and the care of the dying: A report by the Hastings Center.* Bloomington, IN: Indiana University Press.

Thompson, I.E. (1979). The nature of confidentiality. *Journal of Medical Ethics, 5,* 58-61.

Vander Zanden, J.W.V. (1978). *Human development.* New York: Alfred A. Knopf.

Veatch, H.B. (1985). *Human rights: Fact or fancy?* Baton Rouge, LA: Louisiana State University Press.

Veatch, R.M., & Fry, S.T. (1987). *Case studies in nursing ethics.* Philadelphia, PA: J.B. Lippincott.

CHAPTER

5

Theories and Standards

Every patient entering the health care system expects to derive some benefit. He hopes to regain his competence to perform his normal functions and to live his life as he chooses. He wishes to enter again into the pursuit of his happiness. At the very least he expects to come out better able to live than when he went into the health care system. Each of the contemporary bioethical standards is, by accident or design, appropriate to these purposes:

1. The *standard of autonomy* enables a patient to maintain his way of understanding himself and his world. (In a psychiatric setting objectivity will replace autonomy as a goal. Objectivity—an awareness of the facts of the external world—is a necessary precondition of autonomy. An autonomous being is autonomous in his relation to the external world.)

Sara is a timorous 82-year-old lady. Leah, her nurse, relates to her in a manner that implies that it is all right to be a timorous 82-year-old lady. When Sara leaves the hospital, she will have a sense of her autonomy as strong as, or stronger than, when she entered.

2. The *standard of freedom* supports a patient's right to function as an independent being. It is the freedom to make the ethical decisions that affect his life.

Billy is a curious 6-year-old boy. Leah talks to Billy. She explains things to him. She asks his opinion. She allows him to make appropriate choices.

Billy leaves the hospital as independent and self-confident as he was when he entered—or more so. In relation to his sense of freedom Billy's hospital stay has had a positive impact.

3. The purpose of *the standard of veracity* is to enable a patient to function as a reasoning being. In order to function as a reasoning being he must have access to the truth of his situation.

Jeff has been put on a low-salt, low-fat diet. Leah takes the time to explain to Jeff why he ought to stay on the diet. She motivates Jeff to stay on his diet by appealing to his understanding (his reason). She does not depend on an emotional motivation which, in a few weeks, would probably fade away.

4. The *standard of privacy* demands recognition of a patient's self-ownership. It is meant to protect him against the possible harm that might be caused by a breach of his privacy. Leah is careful not to say anything about any of her patients that might place them at a disadvantage when they leave the health care system.
5. The *standard of beneficence* protects a patient's reasonable expectation that he will derive some benefit from the health care system. It is also a recognition of his right not to be harmed.
   Leah's final goal is the same as her patients. It is to see them leave the health care system and reenter their lives.
6. The purpose of the *standard of fidelity*—faithfulness to the nurse/patient agreement—is, very simply, to enable everyone to know what he or she is doing. Fidelity establishes a predictable universe for the nurse and for her patient.
   Very early on Leah overcame the tendency to find whimsical justifications for convenient behaviors. She keeps her actions in harmony with her agreement.

The bioethical standards are designed to enable a patient to bring his values into a biomedical setting, retain them while he is there, and have them intact when he leaves.

The existence of these standards cannot be understood, in any objective sense, apart from the patient's purposes and attitudes. The bioethical standards make sense only in the context of the ethical code that circumstances force on a patient. A patient is passive. His entire ethical purpose is to become an agent—to act—to, once again, take charge of his life.

ACTION AND PASSION

In an ethical context a behavior motivated by purpose is an action.[1] The purpose of the acting agent must be a long-range purpose. Something more is necessary. The action must be motivated by the desire of the agent who acts.

ETHICAL ACTION AND DESIRE

Aristotle gives an example of ethical action by his famous discussion of a ship in a storm:

A cargo ship is sailing between two ports carrying a valuable cargo. Suddenly a storm arises and threatens to capsize the ship. The captain orders his crew to throw the cargo overboard in order to save the ship. Aristotle points out that the captain's behavior was voluntary. He could have tried to save the cargo and put the ship in danger of capsizing. Still, his behavior was a passion and not an action. He did what he chose to do, but not what he desired to do (Aristotle cited in McKeon, 1941).

If the sea captain had made a free choice to throw the cargo overboard, motivated only by his desire, his action would be ethically unjustifiable. But, as it is, he was compelled by circumstances to jettison the cargo. The values that might be gained in contrast to the values that might be lost left him no other rational choice. Under the circumstances it was reasonable and justifiable.

Nurses sometimes face similar situations. A nurse may face a conflict between the physician's orders and her ethical outlook.

✖ **DILEMMA 5-1**   Dr. Burton routinely does a hysterectomy on any patient with endometriosis if the patient is past child-bearing years. Nancy, the operating room nurse, believes that the decision to operate ought to be individualized case by case. There is a conflict between Nancy's belief and her behavior. Under these circumstances she is unable to function as an ethical agent.

✖ **DILEMMA 5-2**   The situation is sometimes similar when there is a clash between the legal and the ethical demands of a situation. Sally has a terminal patient, Fred, who is in extreme pain. Fred begs Sally to give him another dose of his pain medication. He has been given 20 mg of morphine two hours ago. The order reads morphine 20 mg every two hours. Sally disagrees with the physician. She believes that this amount of medication may result in Fred's death. Sally believes that to hasten a patient's death is never ethically justifiable. In this situation Sally must choose between a passion (a behavior which is contrary to her desire) and an action (a behavior in harmony with her desire). She believes the passion (giving Fred the morphine) is unethical because it is contrary to her ethical principle. Her alternative course of action (not giving Fred the morphine), however, is illegal because it is contrary to the physician's order. Sally is caught in a conflict between an action and a passion. (Bernal, Hoover, & Aroskar, 1987)

Aristotle also discusses other aspects of the action/passion distinction. According to Aristotle:

- A person ought to guide his actions through the exercise of his powers of reason. "The [proper] function of man is an activity of [his mind] in accordance with reason" (Aristotle cited in McKeon, 1941).

- A good ship's captain is one who has mastered whatever actions are necessary to the safe and successful sailing of a ship. In the same way a good person is one who has mastered whatever actions are appropriate to the type of being he is — a reasoning organism.
- The ultimate good of a person is happiness. Human happiness is produced by living according to one's highest potential — one's reason.

THE BIOMEDICAL CONTEXT AND ITS ETHIC

It might be argued (and we would argue) that Aristotle's description is the blueprint of any ethic appropriate to a rational individual. It is always the implicit ethic of any person who voluntarily becomes a patient. Everyone who becomes a patient first becomes an ethical individualist. If a nurse did not recognize this, there would be no possible ground for understanding or agreement between herself and her patient. If a nurse not only recognizes but concurs with this, there is a ground for more than mere understanding and agreement. There is the necessary and sufficient ground for an alliance — for that which the French very poignantly call "a self-seeking of two."

A patient, in entering into a health care setting, does precisely what reason demands. When a patient enters a health care setting, it is both his mind and body that enter. Both his mind and his body ought to be dealt with by a health care professional.

CONFLICTS AMONG ACTIONS

An agent becomes aware of an object that he evaluates as desirable. Motivated by his desire for the object, he acts to acquire it. For instance: A child spies his rattle and crawls over to play with it. A patient desires to regain the advantages of the values he has lost through sickness or accident, and he contracts with a nurse who agrees to act as his agent. A nurse knows that suffering can sometimes be defeated and death can sometimes be prevented, and she devotes her career to these goals. An ethical agent, in the conduct of his life, develops the ability to analyze and justify the goals he works for and the actions he takes.

All these behaviors are actions. Actions are peculiar in this: If two conflicting actions are attempted at the same time, each will weaken or cancel the other. If a person attempts to jump up and sit down simultaneously, he will accomplish nothing. If he attempts to go to sleep and stay awake at the same time, whichever occurs will be completely out of his control. If he desires to skip class but believes he should not, whatever physical action he takes will be weakened.

Desiring and believing are types of action. Conflicting desires or beliefs tend to cancel effective ethical action.

NURSES AND ETHICAL ACTION

Every person who enters the profession of nursing encounters discussions of a nurse's need for some level of ethical sophistication. Virtually every theorist writing for nurses recommends, as standards of bioethical action:

1. Recognition of a patient's autonomy: No theorist ever *explicitly* counsels a nurse to ignore her patient's uniqueness— although many of the actions they recommend would, necessarily, involve violating a patient's autonomy.
2. Respect for a patient's right to make free and informed decisions and to take autonomous action (*freedom*): No theorist leads a nurse to believe that she has a right to interfere with the desires and actions of her patients . . . in ordinary circumstances.
3. The need for *veracity* in the nurse's dealings with a patient: Theorists counsel the nurse to make veracity an integral part of her interactions with her patients.
4. Respect for a patient's right to self-ownership (*privacy*): This standard implies respect for a patient's right to privacy. It is unlikely that any theorist would counsel a nurse to expose her patient to possible harm through her violation of his right to privacy.
5. Interactions between nurse and patient that will "do good, or at least do no harm" (*beneficence*): No theorist would knowingly recommend that a nurse ignore the requirements of her patient's well-being or accept that which will cause him avoidable harm.
6. A nurse's obligation to keep faith with her agreement with her patient (*fidelity*): No theorist advises a nurse to betray the understanding that arises between nurse and patient.

At the same time every theorist recommends deontology and/or utilitarianism. All advise a nurse to be guided in her professional practice by one or both of these two leading ethical theories. All recommend that, under certain circumstances, a nurse submit dutifully to the demands of tradition or authority and/or to strive to attain the greatest happiness of the greatest number.

THE NATURE OF THE ETHICAL THEORIES

Deontology, in addition to whatever internal merits it may possess, is humanity's oldest ethical theory. By this very fact it demands some form of consideration on the part of a nurse.

Utilitarianism is the most widely accepted ethical theory of contemporary times. It cannot be ignored.

Ideally a nurse will retain an awareness of all the standards in her ethical decision making. She may attempt to combine these standards with attention to duty and to the greatest good for the greatest number. If her effort produces effective ethical action, this will be very unusual. The effective result of these ethical actions would not be unusual because of some innate ethical defect on the part of nurses. It would be unusual simply because in biomedical situations the combination of these bioethical standards and the two all-pervasive ethical theories is internally problematic. There are severe drawbacks in any attempt to harmonize the contemporary bioethical standards and the traditional ethical theories. Every combination, inevitably, produces a conflict between action and passion. A nurse ought to be aware of these drawbacks.

Deontology is "the theory that . . . actions in conformance with . . . formal rules of conduct, are obligatory regardless of their result" (Angeles, 1981, p. 60).

Utilitarianism is the theory that "one should so act as to promote the greatest happiness (pleasure) of the greatest number of people" (Angeles, 1981, p. 307).

Let us examine how well these theories interface with the contemporary bioethical standards.

THE CONFLICT BETWEEN THEORIES AND STANDARDS
Deontology

Many people regard "deontology" and "ethics" as nearly synonymous terms. Ethics, for these people, is simply the study of how a person recognizes and performs his duty.

A deontological theory of ethics is "one which holds that at least some acts are morally obligatory regardless of their consequences for human weal or woe" (Edwards, 1972, p. 343). It would be a mistake to begin with a confused understanding of deontology. To begin with this mistake and to erect flawed patterns of thought and action on it must lead to ethical chaos. Internal contradictions would assert themselves, and more and more actions would come into conflict.

To understand something, a person must isolate it from everything that it is not. So, in order to understand it, let us examine what deontology is not:

1. Deontology is not a theory designed to promote happiness or well-being. There is no purpose to the moral rules that deontology proposes beyond the rules themselves.
2. It is not, in itself, fidelity to an agreement. Ethical agents enter into agreements freely and by choice. A duty is not something an ethical agent deliberates on and chooses. When an ethical agent chooses to accept deontology, he abandons all further choice.

3. It is not a responsibility arising from a person's actions. A person has a duty before he engages in actions. In fact, duty, according to the deontologist, is an agent's only moral responsibility.
4. It is not an orientation toward human values. It is entirely indifferent to human values.
5. It is not an expression of benevolence. The consequences of actions prompted by duty are ethically irrelevant.
6. It is not a way for a nurse to ensure the benefit of her patient. The issue of beneficiary cannot be primary in a deontological context. It can become primary only through the deontological context being abandoned.
7. It is not a way of preventing harm from coming to patients. Harm is as unimportant as benefit.
8. It is not a logically unflawed theory.

The rules of deontology always take the form of a categorical (as opposed to a hypothetical) imperative. The deontologist does not begin by reasoning that *if* he desires a certain result, *then* he must take certain actions (a hypothetical imperative). He begins with the belief that *there is* a particular rule which he must follow regardless of his desires or any forseeable results (a categorical imperative). No circumstance, however extreme, can excuse a deontologist from the performance of his duty. He has no control over the nature of his duty.

By the nature of duty anything, under the right circumstances, can be a duty. Thus it is within the logic of duty that an ethical agent might have a duty not to do his duty. When taken to its logical extreme, the coherence of deontology collapses. Deontology, by its nature, provides its own euthanasia.

Let us examine how deontology interfaces, or fails to interface, with the contemporary bioethical standards.

Deontology and Autonomy. The only possible relevance of the patient's autonomy or uniqueness, for a nurse, is in the effects her various decisions and actions might have on him. From the standpoint of deontology, the effect of a nurse's decisions and actions on her patient is irrelevant to the moral quality of those decisions and actions. If a nurse-deontologist is unconcerned with the effects of her decisions and actions on her patient, she will be equally indifferent to his uniqueness.

DILEMMA 5-3   Zelda believes that she has a duty to give cardiac patients detailed information on the pathology involved in their condition. Mr. Wu and Mr. Goldfarb are two cardiac patients assigned to her. Mr. Wu is very much interested in having this information. But to Mr. Goldfarb it is terrifying. He is greatly depressed by her recitation.

Had Zelda respected the uniqueness of Mr. Goldfarb, she would have given him only that information which would have been of benefit to him and which would have caused him no unnecessary stress. She would have been motivated by beneficence rather than by her sense of duty. This would have necessitated a betrayal of deontology. It is not difficult to see that her fidelity to duty was a betrayal of the best interests of Mr. Goldfarb. But, insofar as duty is Zelda's ethical standard, there is no significant ethical difference between Zelda's relationship to Mr. Goldfarb and her relationship to Mr. Wu.

Deontology is entirely concerned with an agent's actions. It is unconcerned with consequences. It is also indifferent to the agent's intentions. The deontologist can have only one intention—he must intend to do his duty. In principle deontology *demands* indifference to individual autonomy. The recognition of autonomy would require that a nurse make choices appropriate to the uniqueness of her patient. Yet, in deontology the demands of duty are imperative—they do not allow for choices to be made on the part of a nurse. Autonomous differences among patients call for a nurse to analyze each situation. A deontologist who analyzed contextual differences and made choices based on her analysis would have, perhaps unknowingly, abandoned deontology.

To practice deontology a person must divide ethical situations into a limited number of types. One type of situation may demand that the truth be told. Another type may require that the truth be withheld. There is the situation in which a nurse has a duty to obey the law. If she practices in different states, she may have, according to deontology, an *ethical* duty to obey contrary laws. In a situation involving abortion one nurse may feel she has a duty not to assist. In a situation involving euthanasia another nurse may feel that she has a duty to respect the wishes of her patient.

These clearly defined types of ethical situations are necessary in order that the appropriate rule can be applied. It is not possible for a nurse to learn an unlimited number of rules—one for every situation as it arises.

Respect for a patient's autonomy calls for actions to be modified to fit the situation. A deontology that would allow for actions to be modified would no longer be a deontology. Deontology demands absolute adherence to the rule. There is no room for nuances.

Ethical analysis, for a deontologist, can consist in nothing but an attempt to find plausible explanations for his actions. These explanations are rationalizations. They have nothing at all to do with the reason why he took the action.

DILEMMA 5-4 During the performance of a laparotomy for the removal of an ovarian cancer, Dr. Richmond discovers the presence of pre-cancerous gonads in Amelia, his seventeen-year-old patient. This is a condition (testicular feminization) which occurs once in every 50,000 females. Most women who have the condition are not gratified to discover it. Dr. Richmond feels he has a duty to reveal this detail of her condition to Amelia because "she has a right to know it."

It might be argued that this is contrary to a beneficent concern for his patient. This information does Amelia no good whatever and a significant degree of harm. She undergoes severe psychological distress and a gender identity crisis.

Respect for Amelia's autonomy would have inspired in Dr Richmond a desire to mitigate Amelia's suffering, a state of "benevolent forgetfulness" (adapted from Minogue & Taraszewski, 1988).

But if duty has the central place in the decision making of an ethical agent, then the individual patients in the nurse's care have a secondary importance. And, insofar as the individual patient is unimportant, his autonomy is, perhaps even more so, unimportant.

Deontology and Freedom. The standard of freedom supports the pursuit of individual decisions, choices, and actions. Individual choices and actions are in opposition to the pursuit of duty. If duty is the standard of right and wrong, then no biomedical professional should ever support a patient's individual decisions, choices, and actions. To do so would very powerfully tend to corrupt the moral character of her patient.

A nurse who made a practice of frustrating her patient's choices and actions would not be regarded as an effective nurse. The actions of a nurse who denied her patient's right to freedom would not be approved, even by the most authoritarian segments of contemporary society. Yet, if deontology is a valid theory, either a nurse must frustrate her patient's right to free choice and action or she must cooperate in the process by which her patient fails the demands of duty and gradually embraces an antideontological evil.

Deontology is not identical to the neglect of decision and choice. But there is no deontology without this neglect. A person's duty is not revealed through decision and choice but through something deontologists call an "inner life of reason." According to Immanuel Kant, the father of modern deontology, a person's awareness of his duty is an innate idea. A person is *born* knowing what his duties are.

A person does not decide on the course of action that is his duty. His duty is always already there. The decision is always already made. If he embraces deontology, then the choice of duty is the only choice possible. If he chooses his purposes, values, or the course of his life according to a standard other than duty, he has detached himself from deontology.

According to deontology for a nurse to encourage her patient's neglect of duty would be to destroy his moral character. An alternative possibility is for the nurse to pursue her duty while permitting a patient to pursue his own ethical vision. There is a very unfortunate drawback to this. It would effectively bar any possibility of ethical understanding or communication between nurse and patient. Her duty and his freedom and well-being would be in constant conflict. She might need, at any time, for the sake of duty, to take an action that would interfere with her patient's freedom.

�֍ **DILEMMA 5-5**   Mr. Morris' son has a brief layover before flying back to Europe. Mr. Morris has not seen his son for three months. If he does not get to see him now, he will not see him for another three months.

Mr. Morris is scheduled for an arteriogram. The hospital's optimum functioning requires that he be taken for the test at his appointed time. His nurse has a duty to see that the hospital continues to function at its optimum level. She has a duty to keep the schedule. No decision is involved. If she did make a decision, it could only be a decision to shirk her duty.

A duty-ethic is not concerned with the practical and the impractical. None the less the need for a nurse to make choices of this type is not unusual. Effective ethical decision making would certainly require a nurse to choose beforehand between deontology and the bioethical standard of her patient's freedom. The effective pursuit of duty demands a choice of duty, and apathy toward all other considerations—such as her patient's freedom.

In its classic sense *apathy* ("apatheia") refers to tranquility and freedom from the disturbance of emotion. Emotion and human feeling are obstacles to the practice of deontology. For a nurse apathy, in the sense of tranquility, can be attained only if she first attains "apathy" in its modern sense. In its modern sense apathy is "lack of emotion or feeling; lack of interest in things; indifference" (*American Heritage Dictionary*, 1985). An ethical agent can act without concern for consequences only if she develops apathy toward consequences. In fact, a lack of concern for consequences *is* apathy toward consequences.

A nurse *must*, if she is to practice a consistent deontology, develop apathy toward her patients. If justifiable ethical action requires a nurse's allegiance to duty, then justifiable ethical action requires that a nurse develop apathy as her constant emotional state.

✖ **DILEMMA 5-6**   Mrs. Narda, 32-year-old mother of three, is in the final stages of cancer. Her husband died several years ago. She has been promised that a certain experimental treatment will prolong her life. She believes that she has a duty to become a part of the project for the sake of her children.

Jane, her nurse, is a sincere deontologist. Jane knows that this treatment will add no useful time onto Mrs. Narda's life. The treatment will be very painful. The experience of their mother's deteriorating condition and her suffering will very likely have a negative impact on the children. Nothing, except duty, can be served by this course of action.

Only apathy can give Jane the resolve, over the next several months, to encourage Mrs. Narda to continue following this course of treatment. If Jane acted on Mrs. Narda'a right to free action and to give an *informed* consent, Jane's apathy would be no virtue. Jane would then encourage Mrs. Narda to evade her duty and choose for herself. As a consistent deontologist Jane could not do this.

In a biomedical setting a biomedical professional's practice of deontology is incompatible with her patient's right to free and informed action. Deontology does not allow for integrity nor benevolence. It does not allow for fidelity toward the nurse's professional agreement with her patient.

A consistent deontology demands a profound indifference toward a nurse's patients.

Deontology and Veracity. In the history of the race the value of truth became obvious. Truth is an instrument by which human interaction is made possible. In the nurse/patient relationship it makes communication and trust possible. This trust is a source of pride for a nurse and of courage and strength for a patient.

Truth is always spoken in a context. It usually has predictable consequences. It can help to accomplish human purposes.

But, for a deontologist, truth is none of these things. Truth is not a value through which human purposes are attained. It is, simply, one more burden a deontologist must bear.

✖ DILEMMA 5-7   Robin, a 16-year-old, is dying from lupus erythematosus. She is very fearful. Toward the end she screams, over and over, "Don't let me die!"

Robin's parents are called to the hospital, but before they arrive Robin dies. They ask Robin's nurse if their daughter's death was peaceful. Robin's nurse truthfully relates all the details of Robin's death. Empathy would have made Robin's nurse weak. For Robin's nurse to share the human feelings of Robin's parents would have made her duty unbearably painful. She is strengthened in her duty by apathy. She finds in the absence of feeling a sort of strength. If empathy among persons is a virtue, then this context does not call for the truth. But if submission to the duty to tell the truth is a virtue, then empathy is a vice. There is no benevolent purpose served by Robin's parents hearing the truth. The consequences of the nurse's truth telling are entirely evil. But, for a deontologist, context, consequences, empathy, and purposes are all irrelevant.

The truth a nurse tells may strengthen and encourage a patient. Or it may discourage and terrify him. Neither is the purpose of the deontologist. Truth is not a value which one tells for the sake of one's patient. It is a burden that a nurse bears for no purpose beyond itself.

Kant, in his essay "On a Supposed Right to Tell Lies from Benevolent Motives," demonstrated that if it were permissible to tell a lie to save the innocent victim of a murderer, anything would be permissible. If deontology permitted the benevolent lie, it would have no logical foundation. According to Kant, "it is wrong to tell a lie even to save another man's life. Moral rules . . . are universally valid and admit of no exception" (Edwards, 1972, p. 102). If a deontologist cannot lie to save an innocent life, she surely cannot lie to save parents the anguish of hearing of their daughter's final horror.

From a nondeontological perspective it must seem that, if ethics was ever devised for the benefit of humanity, somewhere it lost its way. For a deontologist, however, this is what ethics is all about—this and only this.

Deontology and Privacy. If deontology guides the actions of a nurse, then her patient can never know whether his privacy will be respected. It depends on where her loyalties lie. If they lie with her patient, then perhaps he can depend on his privacy being protected and his confidences being kept. But a patient can never know this. A nurse may just as easily give her loyalty to a patient's family, to the physician or hospital, or to anyone or anything else.

A deontologist has no internal or logical reason to respect her patient's privacy. She, herself, is not a private person. She is owned by her duties, not by herself.

If a dying patient asks his nurse not to reveal that he has spoken to his lawyer about changing his will, she may not. But then again she may. It depends upon where she feels her duty lies. This puts the patient in a peculiar position. He can have no more confidence in his nurse than he could if she had no moral standards whatever.

Deontology and Beneficence. For a deontologist duty *with* attention to consequences is a logical and practical impossibility. On the other hand, beneficence *without* attention to consequences is a logical and practical impossibility. There is no particular reason why an act done from the promptings of duty cannot result in someone's benefit. But in relation to duty, that benefit is an accidental by-product of the deontologist's actions.

Benevolence—the urge to beneficence—in a deontologist is the sign of a moral failing. It is an indication that she is emotionally uncommitted to her ethical position.

✂ **DILEMMA 5-8**   Mr. Rogers is suffering from a rare disease. Verna, his nurse, knows of a hospital that has been successful in treating this disease. She feels an aching desire to inform Mr. Rogers of the existence of this hospital. However, Mr. Roger's physician does not want Mr. Rogers to have this information. Verna has always believed that a nurse has a duty not to interfere with the patient/physician relationship. It is easy to see that Verna's desire reveals a lack of commitment to the ethical standard that motivates her. Her humanity places an action (her desire) in conflict with the passion (her duty) that deontology forces on her. From the perspective of deontology this is the sign of a moral failing on her part.

Beneficence and duty are, obviously, two directly opposed methods of ethical decision making. An ethical agent motivated by beneficence is interested in the meaning of his actions in relation to the situation in which he acts. He is oriented to see the situation in an ethical context. He acts to "help or at least to do no harm." A person inspired by duty is, of necessity, apathetic toward the context and the people in it.

Apathy and beneficence cannot coexist.

Deontology and Fidelity. The violation of any standard for the sake of duty is, at the same time, a violation of fidelity. Because every standard is presupposed by the nurse/patient agreement, every standard is an item of the agreement.

At the same time there are various reasons why duty cannot be the source of the agreement that a nurse makes with a patient.

First, there is no standard of justification in a deontological context except duty itself. Yet, if duty were a sufficient justification, there would be no need for the agreement. The agreement is formed for specific purposes. Deontology has no commerce with purposes. Therefore, the nurse/patient relationship can be conducted according to one or the other — but not both. Fidelity to a rule and fidelity to an agreement are not at all the same sort of thing. A deontologist often finds that they conflict.

Second, fidelity to an agreement is chosen. Fidelity to duty is unchosen. The terms of the agreement are subject to contextual reasoning and analysis. The demands of duty are not. By its very nature duty takes precedence. This makes an intelligible and stable agreement impossible. Deontology does not allow for analysis, and analysis is the condition *sine qua non* of objective judgment. Without objective judgment — without cognitive intercourse between an agent and the real world — two people cannot form the specific details of an agreement.

✖ DILEMMA 5-9   Marge, Mrs. Collins' evening shift nurse, has an order to give Mrs. Collins a sleeping pill every evening. At 10:00 P.M. Marge finds Mrs. Collins sleeping. She does not awaken her. Mrs. Collins needs rest. Marge believes that her agreement with Mrs. Collins requires her to provide Mrs. Collins with the best possible care. This does not include waking Mrs. Collins up to give her a pill that will put her back to sleep.

Betty, Mrs. Clay's evening shift nurse, has an order to give Mrs. Clay a sleeping pill every night. At 10:00 P.M. Betty finds Mrs. Clay sleeping. She awakens Mrs. Clay and gives her a sleeping pill. Betty believes that giving Mrs. Clay a sleeping pill is a duty. She also believes that she has a duty to do her duty.

For a deontologist an agreement must be an out-of-context absolute. A change in the context would not allow a deontologist to make adaptations in keeping the agreement. Regardless of the consequences, the deontolgist's agreement is unrelated to the actual context.

Utilitarianism

Utilitarianism is the most widely accepted ethical theory in our culture. That is to say, no ethical theory receives more lip-service in our culture than utilitarianism.

A wall of confusion surrounds this theory, and there is a certain vagueness built into that wall. It seems almost essential to an influential ethical theory that it be covered in vagueness. Indeed, the lack of clarity may explain the popularity of utilitarianism. Its vagueness also makes utilitarianism an unworkable theory (Le Bon, 1895; Mackay, 1841).

First there is the problem of who constitutes "the greatest number." There is a practical limit to how many people an ordinary agent can provide for. There is also the difficulty of choosing one group over another when precise numbers are not known. It has been suggested, no doubt with tongue in cheek, that a universal war of all against all, fought with clubs and stones, is the only fair method for establishing who is and who is not to be included in "the greatest number."

Then there is the problem of what constitutes "the greatest good." It may be that the question "What is the greatest good for the greatest number?" is very much like the question "What is the greatest food for the greatest number?"

It is obvious that there is no answer to this question. Although the term "greatest" in "greatest number" can be defined, at least in principle, the term "greatest" in "greatest food" cannot.

Five hundred is a greater number than four hundred and ninety nine, and the "greatness" of any number can easily be determined in relation to the "greatness" of any other number that is known. But is the "greatest" food the most nutritious food? The most delicious food? The food most immune to spoilage? The least fattening food? The most easily produced food?

It is obvious that the term "greatest" in the phrase "greatest food" is (even contextually) indefinable. The term as used in the phrase "greatest good" is even more obscure.

The question of the nature of the greatest good is very much like the question "What is the greatest place on earth to live for the greatest number?" No answer to either question can be found. The discovery of either good would ruin it.

Suppose that this "greatest place to live" were identified. Then, of course, the utilitarian would want to move the "greatest number" to that place. This geographical area would be their "greatest good." Imagine what a nightmare this would create. With one person for every 2 or 3 millimeters of space "the greatest place to live for the greatest number" would become the worst place on earth to live. There is no reason to suppose that "the greatest good for the greatest number" is not of precisely the same nature.

A nurse ought to pause and ponder before she gives up the opportunity of an objective ethical agreement with her patient. What she loses will not be balanced out by the joys of pursuing "the greatest good for the greatest number."

On a very abstract level everyone would desire "the greatest good for the greatest number," if there were such a thing. It is pathological not to wish for an end to suffering, disease, poverty, ignorance, injustice, war, and other human evils. But the way these goals have been pursued has seldom led to "the greatest good for the greatest number."

If every person in the world could be hooked up to a lie-detector and asked "Would you like to know that everyone in the world is as happy as possible?", the overwhelming majority would sincerely answer "yes." If they were then asked "Would you like to know that everyone *you know* is as happy as possible?", the number who could sincerely answer "yes" would severely decline. No one alive does not know some people whom he or she thoroughly dislikes.

This is the location of the vagueness. "Everyone in the world" is a very broad abstraction. The phrase is merely suggestive. It does not point to anything or anyone of whom we have direct experience. If the phrase were "someone in the world," it would not be vague. We have a direct experience of someone in the world. We have no direct experience of "everyone." We live with *someone* in the world. We know him or her. We do not live with everyone in the world. We do not and cannot know *everyone*. Concerning ourselves with "everyone" only deflects our attention from the people we actually do know and with whom we interact.

There is always a temptation for utilitarianism to be used as a way to escape ethical responsibility. A person can concern himself with the total population of the globe and tell himself that he is morally upright, while at the same time he remains unconcerned with the real people with whom he forms implicit or explicit agreements. He never comes to grips with the real and immediate dilemmas with which he ought to deal. He never produces the happiness he might bring to others and gain for himself.

Most ethics texts directed toward nurses advise nurses to adopt the utilitarian standard. None suggest the extreme ethical reorientation which this would involve. Actions guided by a concern for individual integrity and justice are very different from actions guided by a concern for "the greatest good for the greatest number." In turning from one to the other it is necessary to restructure one's conception of effective ethical action.

It is a very common situation for a person not to know that he is failing to act effectively. If a person does not know that his action is failing, it seems to him that his action is succeeding. But these two things, the unawareness of failure and the fact of success, are not the same thing. So, in order to clear up the confusion surrounding it, let us examine what utilitarianism is not:

1. It is not a feeling of general good will. A feeling of general good will does not necessarily make one a utilitarian. Nor is every utilitarian necessarily possessed of a general good will.
2. It is not concerned with the needs and desires of individuals. Nursing, since nurses deal with individual patients, seems particularly unsuited to a utilitarian standard. People who enter nursing "to serve humanity" suffer a confusion which will have a very negative impact on their career satisfaction. All the time they spend with individual patients is time taken away from the pursuit of their chosen moral standard. This is a direct pathway to ethical discontent and burnout.
3. It is not a way of effectively extending the benefit of a nurse's action over a greater number of beneficiaries. When a nurse's actions toward a patient's family violates the patient's self-ownership, this is not a wider spread ethical action. It is a devaluing of the patient and a violation of the nurse's ethical agreement.
4. It is not a way of guaranteeing the benefit of every individual involved. The individual cannot be the center of the utilitarian's concern.
5. It is not a way of clarifying basic ethical concepts. It involves only a pragmatic demand for "the greatest good for the greatest number."
6. It is not an effective way of escaping the problems of deontology. Eventually it collapses into deontology.
7. It is not a way of averting ethical dilemmas and problems. At best it can only relocate ethical dilemmas and problems.
8. Like deontology, it is not a way of protecting a patient against harm. And, like deontology, it is not a careful way to protect one's license to practice.

Let us examine how utilitarianism interfaces, or fails to interface, with the contemporary bioethical standards.

Utilitarianism and Autonomy. Autonomy, as a standard, is the recognition of a person's right to his own unique individuality. Autonomy as a fact in the world is the individual uniqueness of every person.

There is nothing in utilitarianism that concerns itself with the uniqueness of persons — not to the extent that utilitarianism is true to its essential viewpoint.

There was a time when patients were treated with much less regard for their individuality than they now enjoy. For example:

- Every patient age 65 and over was subjected to having the side rails on his bed pulled up at night.
- Visiting hours were standardized for everyone. No consideration was given to different people in different situations.
- Patients were not told the risks of various procedures. The idea was that patients would be unnecessarily stressed by hearing this information and would not want to know the risks.

It is extremely unlikely that utilitarianism was the inspiration for these practices, and yet each one had a utilitarian rationale: *What is good for the majority of people is good for each individual person.* This is an unjustifiable (and currently unfashionable) idea that happens to be central to utilitarianism.

A utilitarian's first moral action must be to reject autonomy as a standard. Respect for autonomy is the contrary of dedication to "the greatest good for the greatest number." In pursuing the good of the greatest number one must reject the uniqueness of every person. A utilitarian cannot concern herself with persons or with uniqueness.

Utilitarianism and Freedom. To put her ethical theory into practice a utilitarian would have to ignore the autonomous wishes of those with whom she deals. In the case of a health care professional she would have to adopt paternalism rather than informed consent as her guiding principle. A utilitarian, in order to be a utilitarian, must reject the right to free action in favor of the "best interest" standard.[2]

Utilitarianism is the implicit basis of many disputes. Typical among these are disputes concerning a patient's living will. When a patient becomes unable to speak for himself, except through his living will, it is expected, at least by the patient, that his wishes will be followed. Contemporary practice is often otherwise. If a patient's family is not in favor of the terms of his living will, many physicians will follow the family's wishes, and the nurse is compelled to become a party to this violation of a patient's freedom.

The standard of freedom has no meaning unless it concerns a person's freedom to act on his own individual desires. Freedom is freedom to pursue one's own purposes. In an interpersonal context the standard of freedom presupposes that everyone has the same right except where this right is limited by an agreement. This right is entirely foreign to the letter and the spirit of a consistent utilitarianism. Utilitarianism recognizes only an agent's pursuit of the purposes of others as justifiable ethical action.

In a utilitarian context only collective purposes are relevant. The pursuit of individual purposes would make a utilitarian context unintelligible and impossible. A utilitarian must hold the pursuit of individual purposes as a vice. If it were not a vice, there would be every reason for a utilitarian to pursue his own individual purposes and to let others pursue theirs (Machan, 1975).

This poses a dilemma for a utilitarian. If it is not good or right for a person to acquire that which is good, then a utilitarian should not pursue it, even for another. If it is good and right for a person to acquire that which is good, then there is no reason why a utilitarian should not pursue it for himself.

This dilemma and any possible solution to it lead us to an inescapable paradox of utilitarianism. Utilitarianism only works if some people are not utilitarians.

Imagine a desert island with only three inhabitants. All three are sincere and dedicated utilitarians. Each sets out to direct his actions toward the greatest good for the other two. But it is impossible, under these circumstances, to produce any good. Suppose Helen were to desire to benefit Kay and Annette with some good. Kay would regard only that which would benefit Helen and Annette as a good. Annette would recognize as good only that which would benefit Helen and Kay.

Obviously there is a vicious (or a vacuous) circle at work here. No good could be produced on the island because none of its inhabitants would have any conception of (an individual and personal) good. This also means that no one would hold any ethical values. For anything to be good it must be good for, at least, one autonomous, nonutilitarian individual. No one on the island would benefit from receiving something for herself. No one desires anything but an empty abstraction.

No one, on the other hand, enters a health care setting to pursue an empty abstraction.

Utilitarianism and Veracity. A utilitarian must reject the standard of truth, and truth itself, in holding to the greatest good standard. Suppose an accusation were brought against a utilitarian by two perjurers. If their accusation stands, each perjurer will gain more than half of what the utilitarian will lose. Assume that the utilitarian considers himself as worthy as either perjurer. His standard of ethical judgment demands that he not defend himself against their accusations. Their gain and his loss, and only this, produces the greatest good for the greatest number.

The necessity of pursuing the greatest good demands that the utilitarian ignore the truth. Truth is the enemy of his moral code.

Historically utilitarians have had a problem fitting truth into their system. An attempt to solve this problem was made when utilitarians adopted William James'(1842-1910) "pragmatic" theory of truth. The pragmatic theory of truth holds that:

1. A proposition or belief is true only when acting on it has a desired result.
2. A proposition or belief is false if acting on it brings about an undesired result.

According to James, "the true is only the expedient in the way of our thinking, just as the right is only the expedient in our way of behaving" (James, 1910, p. 84).

The value of truth telling, for a utilitarian, depends on who will or will not benefit. A patient must be told the truth only insofar as this is beneficial, not to the patient himself but, to the greater number. A utilitarian, insofar as he *is* a utilitarian, is interested only in this final goal.

In the past families often did not want a patient to be told the truth about his diagnosis. The family did not want to deal with the patient's awareness. In light of this they convinced themselves that not knowing was best for the patient. This desire was, until very recently, honored.

A nurse who lies to a child in order to gain his cooperation has recourse to the pragmatic theory of truth. This theory presupposes an ethical principle that has justified more injustice than all others combined: "The end justifies the means." It has been observed that a nurse can easily use this theory to justify anything — including, of course, the unjustifiable (Bunting and Webb, 1988).

Utilitarianism and Privacy. The question of whether a utilitarian would violate a patient's privacy would depend entirely on the effect this action would have on the group. The concept of "privacy" does not exist in a pure utilitarian context. In a purely utilitarian society the concept would wither and fall away.

There is no way an agreement could be made between nurse and patient without a preexisting recognition of the patient's right to privacy. Agreements are not made with those who are insignificant. There is no way a person is significant if his self-ownership is insignificant.

✖ DILEMMA 5-10   Harry is in the hospital. He is dying. Harry's family is unaware of the fact that he is dying. He does not want his family to know. Harry's son has been discharged from the army and is returning home. The family intends to surprise Harry with his son's return when he arrives home. What should be done?

A utilitarian would say that Harry's family should be advised of his prognosis, even against his wishes. They need to know this in order to decide what they desire to do. They are the greater number.

Yet the standard of privacy would inspire Harry's nurse to keep her agreement with her patient. His right to privacy would compel her to reveal the fact of his son's return and let Harry decide what he desires to do.

But for a utilitarian any claim of "the greatest good for the greatest number" is a sufficient reason to divulge anything or to conceal anything. Obviously this is incompatible with the nurse/patient agreement as that agreement is usually understood.

Utilitarianism and Beneficence. In keeping with the utilitarian theory an ethical agent ought to put aside beneficence toward the individual in order to practice beneficence to the group. However, beneficence is not important in utilitarianism. Numbers are important. This concept radically devalues the standard of beneficence. It makes the possibility of a nurse/patient agreement, and beneficence arising from the agreement, inconceivable.

Any form of medical experimentation might produce results that would have beneficial results for someone. It is generally agreed that medical experimentation conducted on innocent victims without their consent is ethically unthinkable. Yet, this form of beneficence should be acceptable to, and even approved by, a consistent utilitarian.

Utilitarianism and Fidelity. For a utilitarian the question is not "Who will benefit?" but, rather, "How many will benefit?" He must remain unconcerned with the question of who will benefit. Therefore, he cannot in good faith give any promises or make any agreements.

From the perspective of fidelity utilitarianism is viciously paradoxical. Tomorrow a utilitarian might have to turn on and injure, at least by violating fidelity, the group he is benefitting today. The next day he might benefit a larger group, and these benefits might require the betrayal of the second group—*ad infinitum*.

SUMMARY

Obviously there are severe and far-ranging conflicts between the contemporary bioethical standards of nursing and the traditional ethical theories. It is also quite evident that the traditional ethical theories must be laid aside if nursing ethics is to have any logical connection to nursing. At the same time actions guided by an inconsistent deontology or utilitarianism cannot be *justifiable* ethical actions.

However, a nurse ought not reject the ideals of deontology and utilitarianism out of hand. A nurse can be courageous and steadfast in her ethical actions without embracing deontology. She can strive to extend beneficence as widely as possible without becoming a utilitarian.

She probably cannot reject the contemporary bioethical standards and practice what is recognized, in our culture, as the role of a nurse.

NOTES

1   A behavior can be said to be any movement or change which a thing undergoes. Thus we can speak of the behavior of a person or an animal. We can also speak of the behavior of nails in the vicinity of a magnet or the behavior of a raindrop running down a window pane. Strictly speaking, however, a *behavior* is a movement or change in a conscious being.

An *action* is a volitional behavior. It is a behavior taken for a purpose and directed toward a desired goal. According to this definition a purposeless behavior—a behavior taken without the desire to reach a goal—is not an action.

A behavior that does not originate in the desire of an agent is a passion. A passion is a behavior that a patient is compelled to take by factors outside himself. A patient is a person whose behavior is, essentially, passive—pushed along, as it were, by outside forces.

A nurse fluffing her patient's pillow illustrates this action/passion distinction. The nurse's behavior arises from inside herself; it is not compelled from without. Her behavior is chosen and purposive—it is an action. The patient's behavior (being lifted off the pillow, etc.) is determined from without. It is determined by his nurse. The patient is passive—his behavior is a passion.

In ethics the action/passion distinction arises very often. It is central to ethical theorizing. In order to be an effective decision maker it is not necessary that a nurse understand all the ins and outs of this distinction. But she must understand that there is a distinction. Otherwise she would be unable to understand the very real ethical differences between herself as agent and her patient as patient.

2 The best interest standard is the idea that the physician (or some authority figure) knows what is best for an individual regardless of the affected individual's purposes or desires. Because the authority knows best and because the best ought to be done, the affected individual has no voice in the decision.

REFERENCES

American heritage dictionary. (1985). (2nd college ed.). Boston, MA: Houghton Mifflin.

Angeles, P.A. (1981). *Dictionary of philosophy.* New York: Harper and Row.

Aroskar, M.A. (1987). (Commentary). Case studies: Nurse's appeal to conscience, *Hastings Center Report, 17*(2), 26.

Bernal, E.W. (1987). (Commentary). Case studies: Nurse's appeal to conscience. *Hastings Center Report, 17*(2), 25-26.

Bunting, S.M., & Webb, A.A. (1988). An ethical model for decision-making. *Health Care Issues, 13,*(12), 30-34.

Edwards, P. (Ed.). (1972). *The encyclopedia of philosophy* (Vol. 2). New York: Macmillan.

Hoover, P.S. (1987). (Commentary.) Case study: Nurse's appeal to conscience. *Hastings Center Report, 17*(2), 25-26.

James, W. (1910). *The meaning of truth: A sequel to "pragmatism."* New York: Harper & Row.

Le Bon, G. (1960). *The crowd.* New York: Viking Press. (Original work published in 1923).

Machan, T.R. (1975). *Human rights and human liberties.* Chicago: Nelson Hill.

Mackay, C. (1971). *Memoirs of extraordinary popular delusions.* New York: Noonday Press. (Original work published in 1841).

McKeon, R. (Ed.). (1941). *The basic works of Aristotle.* New York: Random House.

Minogue, B.P. and Taraszyewski, R. (1988, October/November). The whole truth and nothing but the truth. *Hastings Center Report, 18*(5), 34-36.

CHAPTER

6

The Ethical Context

Imagine this scene:

Your name is Alice.
You are the Alice in Lewis Carroll's Wonderland.
You work in a kitchen in Wonderland.
The ethic of the kitchen is harsh, badly proportioned, and unfair.
If you drop an egg, and fail to report having dropped it, an unhappy child will go to bed hungry.
So, if you drop an egg and want to prevent a child's unhappiness, you ought to report that you have dropped it.
Last time one of the kitchen workers dropped an egg and reported it, the Queen of Hearts had her beheaded.
You are in a perilous situation—one where you ought to think very carefully before reporting the loss of the egg.

Very seldom is the context of an ethical situation as clear cut as this. But, in a very basic way, the context is relevant to every ethical decision and action.

If you decide to report the fact that you dropped the egg, this will be an ethical decision. It may make a child very happy. It may also be the last ethical decision you will ever make.

Imagine the character of a child who would be happy about your decision if he or she knew the particulars (the context) of it.

If you decide not to report the fact that you dropped the egg, this will also be an ethical decision. Unlike many ethical decisions it would be a contextual, well-proportioned, and rational decision.

THE NATURE OF A CONTEXT

A context consists of two distinct but dynamically interrelated elements.

The *context of the situation*: The aspects of a situation that are helpful to understanding the situation and to acting effectively in it.

The variables that a nurse finds within her patient's situation forms the context of the situation. Every time a nurse takes on the care of a patient this action places her in a context—although not necessarily an ethical context. Such factors as the patient's history and physical, the diagnosis of the physician, the patient's family situation, the laboratory results, the emotional state of the patient, the age and sex of the patient are all aspects of the context of the (nursing) situation.

The *context of knowledge*: An agent's[1] awareness of the relevant aspects of a situation that are necessary to understanding the situation and to acting effectively in it. The forming of a context of knowledge is the purpose of the nursing assessment. A nurse needs to become aware of the relevant aspects of the patient's situation. She needs this knowledge so that she can give care based on *this* patient's actual situation. She uses her knowledge to group and prioritize the relevant aspects (the context) of the situation. In order to formulate an individualized plan of care a nurse uses her context of knowledge to evaluate the context of the situation.

Solving a problem requires that the elements of the problem be understandable. If they are not understandable then some way must be found to make them understandable. Facts need to be identified, collected, sorted, and put into a meaningful pattern (Polanyi, 1958).

The Context of the Situation

The agent's context of knowledge, including his awareness of relevant standards and principles, enables him to recognize the context of the situation. The context of the situation provides the criteria that guide him in the application of ethical standards and principles. Attention to the aspects of the situation that are relevant to his purposes makes it possible for an agent to relate his ethical actions to his ethical purposes.

If an ethical agent could take actions without reference to the context of the situation, the situation would be irrelevant to her actions. Her actions would also be irrelevant in relation to the situation.

For this reason a discussion of ethical issues in isolation from a context can never lead to a meaningful ethical decision. The issues are, of necessity, disjointed, unrelated to real life situations or to each other.

When issues in isolation form a context, the context is sufficient only to lead a nurse to a predetermined conclusion. For this reason discussions of ethical issues often serve, not to strengthen and expand a nurse's knowledge, but to harden her prejudices. She is thrown back on the nebulous ethical notions that she has acquired, without analysis, through random cultural influences. It is possible to discuss such issues as organ transplantations, abortion, euthanasia, the use of fetal tissue, genetic engineering, treatment of anecephalic infants, human experimentation, and so on and come away fundamentally uninfluenced by the discussion and with nothing to apply to a real-life dilemma.

The context of the situation is those aspects that are relevant to a person's understanding of the situation. The aspects of the situation relate to the purposes of the people acting in it. To act according to the context of the situation means, first and foremost, to act with an awareness of the situation. It is for an agent to guide his actions according to that which is implied by the situation in relation to his purposes. Without an awareness of the context of the situation a person has no reason to act. This is not simply in the sense that whether or not a person acts is a matter of indifference. Unless there is a perceived context of the situation, no ethical action is possible. "[T]he perceptual grasp of a situation is context dependent; that is, the subtle changes take on significance only in light of the patient's past history and current situation"(Benner, 1984, p. 5).

For a nurse to maintain awareness of the context of the situation while she is acting, means to maintain an awareness of the demands and promises of the situation. It means to maintain an awareness of her plans in regard to her purposes. It also means to maintain an awareness of changes in those contextual factors that must shape her actions if she is to act effectively.

Tina has promised to take a group of chronically ill pediatric patients to the zoo. Her purpose is to share their enjoyment. The children—their desires and their handicaps—form the essential context of the situation. While Tina is preparing for the trip, she discovers that Brucie, the sickest of the children, is scheduled for surgery the next day and will not be able to go on the trip.
Tina is not motivated by a sense of duty. Nor is she devoted to the greatest good for the greatest number. This change in the situation causes her to cancel the trip. She would not enjoy the trip knowing that Brucie could not come with them. She hopes the children would not want to go without Brucie and will be content to wait until later for the trip.

Tina maintained an awareness of the context. This enabled her to be aware of a change in the context and the influence this change had on her purpose. Then, however, Tina discovered another fact in the situation—a fact that changed the context of the situation for her again. She discovered that Brucie was afraid of animals and really did not want to go to the zoo. So Tina explained the situation (less than the entire truth) to the children. Brucie was spared an embarrassing moment, and everyone had a wonderful time at the zoo.

The Context of Knowledge

The context of the situation provides a person with an awareness that there is something to be done. It often provides him with an awareness of what is to be done. "Keeping the context" is the act of maintaining an awareness of the factors relevant to a person's ethical actions and changes in these factors. Keeping the context is the first order of ethical action. The context must shape a person's actions if he is to act effectively.

The fact that there is a situation accessible to the purposes of an agent is not enough for the existence of a context. There must be an agent who recognizes the nature of the situation. In addition, the agent must have a desire to act within the situation. He must see it as either (a) requiring action to prevent some undesirable consequence, or (b) possessing aspects necessary to the accomplishment of a desired goal.

This awareness on the part of an agent presupposes that he is able to put the relevant aspects of the situation together into an intelligible form. This is what a nurse does each time she makes a nursing diagnosis.

Every decision which an agent makes, if he acts "in (or according to) the context" must be made according to:

• His knowledge
• That which is relevant in the situation

His knowledge enables him to recognize that which is relevant in the situation. That which is relevant in the situation enables him to apply his knowledge. Both together enable him to act to accomplish his purposes.

Every decision the agent makes must be made with regard to changes in the situation if he keeps (acts with an awareness of the basic nature of and relevant changes in) the context.

An agent's context of knowledge is his awareness of those aspects of the situation that invite action. His awareness of the possibilities for success in the realization of that which is intended by his action is also part of his context of knowledge.

An agent's keeping the context of knowledge involves maintaining both an awareness of changes in his knowledge and an awareness of the emergence of new factors that threaten the realization of his purposes, which offer new ways of realizing them, or which offer new values worthy of pursuit.

In reference to ethical decision making a context of knowledge is both a body of prior knowledge and a state of present awareness. A person's knowledge and his awareness must be relevant to the attainment of fundamental, vital, and long-term goals. The context of knowledge is the knowledge of a decision maker—an agent acting for his own interests. It can also be the context of one person who is acting as the agent of another—as a nurse acts as the agent of her patient. Finally, it can be the context of a person who acts to assist or guide the decision making process of another—as nurses often act to assist or guide the decision making processes of their patients.

THE INTERWEAVING OF CONTEXTS

Efficient ethical decision making requires an interweaving of the context of the situation into the context of knowledge in a way that leads to an appropriate conclusion.

On any given day in order for a person to decide whether he ought to wear a coat to go outside, he must have a preexisting[2] body of knowledge. He ought to know, in general, what weather conditions call for a coat. He must determine what the actual weather conditions are outside at this time. It is desirable for him to determine what changes in the weather are in store.

Whether or not he will wear a coat is his dilemma. Knowing what weather conditions, in general, mandate the wearing of a coat is the preexisting part of his context of knowledge. It is that part which he brings to the situation. The weather conditions as they are outside right now is the context of this specific situation.

His awareness of these conditions is that part of his context of knowledge which he acquires directly from the situation.

In the form of a syllogism the decision would be made like this:

If it is below 40° F, I ought to wear a coat.

It is now below 40° F.

Therefore I ought to wear a coat.

This decision is based on an interweaving of the context of the situation into the context of the agent's knowledge. It is a logically justifiable decision.

A nurse, in her role as nurse, must be aware of changes in her patient's condition. In the same way a nurse, in her role as ethical agent, must be aware of changes in the ethical context.

Knowledge of ethical principles is an inner resource that an agent brings to a situation. A systematic awareness of this resource is necessary if it is to function beneficially. An agent's awareness must make it possible for him to analyze that which is known in a logical, step-by-step process. The analysis enables a decision maker to view the situation as an intelligible whole. An agent seeing the situation as an intelligible whole that is relevant to his purposes is seeing it as a context. Purposes determine contexts. This enables an agent to interweave the elements of the situation and thereby act in an optimally appropriate way. Attention to the context enables a decision maker to act with maximum efficiency in bringing about a desired outcome. It can enable a nurse to act with maximum efficiency in laying the groundwork to help her patient to arrive at the best decision for him to make at any point in time.

A decision made out of context can never, except through pure chance, be a correct decision. Without attention to the context, there is no way to know whether or not the decision is ethically justifiable. Regardless of how well an ethical agent understands the logical interconnections of abstract ethical concepts, outside of the context there is no way to know whether a decision is appropriate to the context.

THE STRUCTURE OF A CONTEXT

For a nurse a context of knowledge is formed by:

1. Her awareness of her purposes.
2. Her awareness of the aspects of a situation which are relevant to her purposes.
3. The relevant preexisting knowledge she brings to the situation.

A context, in and of itself, does not provide a ready made decision. It will not compel a nurse to take effective and justifiable actions. Only the active application of her knowledge to the situation can do this.

An ethical situation also demands this interplay between the context of knowledge and the context of the situation. It is a nurse's awareness of the relevant realities of a situation and her knowledge of effective and justifiable ethical principles that makes effective and justifiable ethical actions possible. Success follows upon effective action. Effective action follows upon active awareness.

Only the ethical context involves ethical principles. Aside from this, every context is basically similar.

Take the context of a student studying for an examination: Knowing the material a test is going to cover will not compel a student to take the time to study. It will not even *help* a student take the time to study. Only the student's own purposeful action can do this. Knowing what a test is going to cover, however, will enable a student to study what is relevant. If his purpose is to study, then knowledge of what the examination will cover will help him.

Ethical action is like the action of taking time to study. Being aware of the context of the ethical situation is like being aware of the material a test is going to cover.

The study habits of most people are much more efficient than their powers of ethical analysis. Their study habits are (usually) guided by reason and purpose. Their processes of ethical analysis are guided by the traditional ethical theories, which means that their analysis is guided by duties, "instincts," words, and rules carried over from childhood.

THE PARADOX OF CONTEXT

Most ethical agents take the validity of the traditional ethical theories for granted. For this reason their understanding of an ethical context is paradoxical.

A context of one sort or another is the most common item of everyone's experience:

- Whenever any person desires or values something, he is in a context. His desire and that which he desires give birth to the context.
- Whenever a person has a purpose, his state of mind and the object of his purpose form a context.
- Whenever a person acts, his action and the object of his action places him in a context.

Everyone is always in a context. Everyone is not always aware of the nature of the context he is in. Attention to the rules and goals of the traditional ethical theories leads a person's mind away from the context. This makes the subject of context appear paradoxical. Most ethical agents sense that the context is somehow relevant to ethical decisions and actions. But the presence of ethical theories in their attention keeps them from seeing what relevance it has. By means of the contemporary bioethical standards biomedical professionals can get through the traditional ethical theories into a bioethical context.

However, if the bioethical standards are joined to the traditional theories, they become out-of-context ethical abstractions. Autonomy ceases to be a fact to be discovered and analyzed in regard to every patient. It becomes a rule that is precisely similar in regard to all patients. The ethical theory hides the contradiction. Veracity becomes a duty to be exercised without regard to benefit or harm. Fidelity becomes, not a bond between a nurse and her patient, but a bond between a nurse and a rule.

Nurses are often in a potential ethical context. They are familiar with the experience of being in a context. At the same time they often do not recognize the context *as a context*.

If a nurse does not recognize the nature and importance of the context, she will make her decisions according to these out-of-context abstractions. These abstractions have no relevance to the immediate and proper purposes of a nurse. They have no necessary value to a patient and no concrete relationship to nursing.

It is a paradox that the ethical context is the most familiar item in the experience of ethical agents and the one they understand least. There are three reasons for this paradox:

1. The ethical theories by which people guide their ethical actions lead to confusion and self-contradiction. Whenever an ethical agent is blocked by confusion or a self-contradictory desire, he will act on duties or instincts or rules. The ethical theories reinforce an agent's confusion. Confusion reinforces his reliance on the ethical theories. His reliance on the ethical theories blocks his perception of the ethical context.
2. The ethical theories do not involve the desires, values, and purposes of the acting agent. No ethical context outside of the desires, values, and purposes of the acting agent is possible. A context is formed by the interrelation between an agent's present state of desire and the final state of affairs he acts to bring about.
3. The ethical theories are not concerned with specific agreements made between agents. They are entirely concerned with ethical abstractions — fairness, honesty, etc. They are concerned with duties or with an indeterminate number of unknown beneficiaries whose desires are unknowable.

Each of the major theories of ethics provides the outline of a non-contextual ethic. For deontology the rules that are to be applied to different situations override concern for the ethical context. For utilitarianism the "greatest good" and the "greatest number" replace the ethical context. The contemporary bioethical standards and the major theories of ethics are incompatible.

There is a reason why the contemporary bioethical standards and the major ethical theories cannot be brought into harmony. The theories require out of context decisions, choices, and actions. "The greatest good for the greatest number" has no connnection to the here and now. The dutiful decisions and actions that may turn out quite well in some situations will have a disastrous effect in others. On the other hand the bioethical standards cannot be practiced out of context. The bioethical standards directly relate the decisions, choices, and actions of an ethical agent (a nurse) to her individual patient.

The bioethical standards are an obvious effort to relate bioethics to the biomedical context. They are the principles of a contextual ethic. Various factors, not the least of which is a series of costly lawsuits, have forced biomedical professionals into the bioethical context. Ethical decisions and actions taken out of a sense of duty or for the benefit of the greater number prove impractical. They are taken without regard for the patients affected by them. They fail to consider the *relevance* of what is happening and to whom it is happening. This is a luxury that biomedical professionals can no longer afford.

ETHICS IN CONTEXT

Whenever a nurse makes an ethical decision or takes an ethical action, the context is important. The context, once again, is the useful knowledge she brings to a situation (context of knowledge) and the relevant facts she finds there in the situation (context of the situation). For her to be guided by the context is for her to be guided by that which is relevant to her purpose. To ignore the context is to ignore something that is relevant to her purpose.

A patient facing surgery for a fractured hip will experience a certain amount of fear. A patient whose mother died during an operation for a fractured hip will probably experience more fear than most. A nurse who ignores this fear cannot engage in ethical communication with her patient. She fails to recognize his autonomy. In ignoring the truth of the situation she violates the standard of veracity. She acts toward him without benevolence. She fails to fulfill the nurse/patient agreement.

THE SCOPE OF THE CONTEXT

> In ethics everything is contextual; and the context of every action is unique and unduplicable, with the result that even a small difference between two situations may yield a difference in our moral verdict. (Hospers, 1972, p. 63)

Driving 55 miles/hour in a 55 mile/hour zone is ordinarily quite justifiable. It is not justifiable if the road is covered with ice. What is and what is not justifiable entirely depends upon the context.

A practical system of ethical decision making is one which inspires justifiable actions. No noncontextual system is practical. If a system is to inspire justifiable actions, it must be oriented to the context in which the action is to take place. Ethical actions are justified by reference to ethical purposes. Ethical purposes are justified by reference to ethical goals. An agent's purpose is brought to a situation by the agent. The interweaving of a situation and a purpose forms a context. The facts that are relevant to a purpose—to an agent's decisions and actions—will be found in the situation. This is the interweaving that brings the context into existence.

Every ethical action has meaningful effects lasting beyond the immediate moment. Otherwise it would not be an ethical action. Ethical actions are actions taken in the pursuit of vital and fundamental long-term goals.

Every interpersonal ethical context arises in the midst of human interactions. The nature of the best outcome is contained in the context and revealed through attention to the context. A situation lacking the possibility of any good or any harm being brought about by human agency cannot be an ethical context. There is no such thing as a neutral ethical context.

Mrs. Chan is critically ill. She talks frequently to Rhonda, her nurse, about her daughter. Mrs. Chan and her daughter became estranged many years ago. They had a violent argument over Mrs. Chan's son-in-law.
Mrs. Chan does not seem motivated to get well. She says that she has nothing to live for. Her husband is dead, and her only child does not speak to her. Rhonda finds out where Mrs. Chan's daughter lives and calls to tell her about her mother's illness.

Rhonda's overarching ethical goal is the well-being of her patient. Rhonda believes that a reconciliation between Mrs. Chan and her daughter would have a beneficial effect on Mrs. Chan's well-being. Calling Mrs. Chan's daughter gives Rhonda a chance to effect this reconcilliation. Rhonda's action (calling Mrs. Chan's daughter) can be justified by reference to her purpose (to effect a reconciliation). Rhonda's purpose (to effect a reconciliation) is justifiable by reference to her ethical goal (Mrs. Chan's well-being).

Rhonda observes the context of the situation. Then she reasons as follows:
"My ethical goal is the well-being of my patient.
"A reconciliation would serve the well-being of my patient.
"The only way I can bring about a reconciliation is by calling Mrs. Chan's daughter.
"I will call Mrs. Chan's daughter.
In the ethical context this is perfectly justifiable reasoning and action.

CONTEXTUAL ACTION

A person cannot live without acting and cannot act without some awareness of the situation within which he acts. A context begins, at one extreme, in the mind of an agent. It begins with a state of self-conscious awareness.

Jack is aware of his desire to recover his health and leave the hospital setting.

Sue is aware of herself as a nurse. She is conscious of her commitment to act as Jack's agent while he is a patient. Her final goal is the same as Jack's.

A context proceeds through the aspects of a situation that offer the possibility of loss or gain.

Jack has numerous compound fractures from a skiing accident. If Jack does not recover, he will not be able to pursue his occupation. He will not be able to do many of the things that he now takes for granted.

In order to help Jack recover, Sue must see to it that no decubiti are formed, traction is kept in alignment, adequate circulation is maintained, and infections do not occur.

The forming of a context requires that an agent become aware of his situation.

Jack is informed of the particulars of his condition. He becomes aware that he will need an extended period of bed rest followed by rehabilitation.

In order to adequately care for Jack, Sue must become aware of the extent of Jack's injuries and the part she will need to play in his recovery.

A context includes the alternative actions that the aspects of the situation make possible.

Jack can either undergo the steps necessary to his recovery or he can refuse to do what is necessary for his full recovery. Sue can live up to the nurse/patient agreement, or she can fail to do this.

A context ends up at the other extreme, which is the potential outcomes of these actions.

If Jack becomes a partner in his care he will achieve an optimum recovery. If he does not, he may be left with permanent disabilities.

If Sue lives up to her agreement, she will help make Jack's recovery less burdensome and more free from anxiety. If she does not it will make Jack's stay in the hospital more unpleasant. It will make Jack less able to gain the benefits of the health care setting.

SUMMARY

Achieving awareness of the context means integrating that which a person experiences into all the relevant knowledge that he possesses. Achieving awareness of the context is, in effect, a process of "converting"the context of the situation into a context of knowledge. Losing awareness of the context means ignoring relevant items of knowledge or relevant aspects of the situation.

To ignore either context in arriving at a decision is to make the correctness of the decision a matter of pure chance. Losing awareness of the context is the worst possible way to begin a decision making process. Not having awareness of the context makes it impossible to justify a decision.

When a nurse retains awareness of the bioethical context, she and her patient are most apt to gain the maximum benefit of ethical action. For anyone, in any ethical context, to benefit from ethical action it is necessary for him to retain a clear awareness of the context.

NOTES

1   In an ethical context an agent is a person who initiates action. In any ethical relationship between any two people, generally, each functions as an ethical agent. In a relationship between two nurses, or between a nurse and a physician, each functions as an agent. The relationship between a nurse and her patient is rather uncommon. A nurse, by definition, is one who performs the role of agent. To a greater or lesser extent a nurse becomes the agent of her patient. A nurse

does for her patient what he would do for himself if he were able. A nurse is essentially and uniquely an ethical agent.

2   An agent's preexisting knowledge is that general knowledge which she brings to the situation as opposed to the information that she gains from her experience of the specific factors of the situation. Thus a nurse's recognition of a patient's right to autonomy is part of her preexisting knowledge. How that recognition relates to this specific patient will depend upon the character of the patient. A nurse will discover the requirements of her patient's individual freedom by discovering the nature of his values and desires. This she learns from the situation. The knowledge that he has a right to individual freedom is part of her preexisting knowledge. Preexisting means, quite simply, applicable to an ethical context but possessed by an ethical agent prior to experience of a specific context.

REFERENCES

Benner, P. (1984). *From novice to expert.* Menlo Park, CA: Addison-Wesley.

Hospers, J. (1972). *Human conduct: Problems of ethics.* New York: Harcourt Brace Jovanovich.

Polanyi, M. (1958). *The study of man.* Chicago: The University of Chicago Press.

7

Context and Ethical Action

A context is very much like a sweater. All the strands making up the sweater are interwoven. Likewise all the facts and beliefs making up the context are interwoven. The interweaving of the sweater is what keeps the strands together and makes it a sweater. The interweaving of the strands of a context is, likewise, that which keeps it together and makes it a context.

A context is the interweaving of three things:

- The situation a person faces insofar as the situation is related to his desires, purposes, and actions. A situation is a group of related facts. A group of facts can be part of a context—the context of the situation. This group of facts that form the context are those facts that can assist or hinder the desires, purposes, and actions of the person dealing with them.
- The person's awareness of the facts is the context of his knowledge. This awareness is an awareness of the situation and of how the situation will assist or hinder his purposes and actions.
- The ethical beliefs that an agent brings to the situation. (These beliefs may very well be unrelated to the context of the situation or the context of the person's awareness.)

JUSTIFICATION OUT OF CONTEXT

To justify an ethical decision or action, in context, is to explain that decision or action as it relates to an ethical purpose, and show that it is appropriate to the situation in which the decision is made or the action is taken.

Gertrude, Rita's patient, complains to Rita that her son has not written to her for several weeks. She tells Rita that she has decided to break off all contact with him. Rita can understand Gertrude's feelings. The same thing happened to Rita a few years ago. Based on her own experience Rita agrees with Gertrude's decision.

Contextually Rita's advice is inappropriate. Rita's evaluation of Gertrude's situation is based on her own situation, not Gertrude's. If Gertrude followed this out-of-context advice, it would undermine the value of her relationship with her son for the sake of a short term feeling of "getting even."

Rita's advice is based on one single thread of Gertrude's context (the fact that her son has not written to her). Gertrude's context is much more than this one single thread. There is no contextual justification for Rita's advice. There is, therefore, no ethical justification fo Rita's advice. Rita has no right to get this far out of context.

Gertrude's decision should be based on a much wider context. She might express hurt to her son over his failure (if it was a failure) to write. To break off contact with him would be all out of proportion to his not having written.

Gertrude's strong feelings imply that she wants to establish contact with her son. Breaking off contact with him, in this context, would not make sense.

Let us look into another context:

Jean's light is flashing while Janet, her nurse, is having a very pleasant conversation with Greg, a new patient on the unit. By the time Janet answers the light, Jean is dead.

Question: What is Janet's best defense?

- In the past she was able to save the lives of several patients by answering their light.
- In the future she will be much more attentive to her patient's call light.
- At the hospital across town where she worked previously she never failed to answer a patient's light.

Answer: None of the above.

None of these replies relates to the context. The center of this ethical context is Jean. Take Jean out of the context, and there is no context. What Janet did in the past, what she will do in the future, or what she did in another place does not relate to Jean at all.

Consider this situation:

April is the charge nurse on a unit where medications are being tested. The subjects of this study have all been given a hypoglycemic agent. The resulting side effect in 90 percent of the subjects is flatulence and cramps. In addition to this, one of the subjects, Joe, has a slightly elevated temperature. This elevated temperature is caused by the onset of appendicitis. April takes no action in regard to Joe. She does not discover Joe's elevated temperature until his appendix ruptures. Joe arrives in the operating room much later than would be desirable. What should April have done?

From this, very limited, context there is no way to answer this question. But, now, look what happens when the context is expanded.

If April could have been expected to discover that Joe has an elevated temperature and that his temperature is a symptom of appendicitis, then she is blameworthy for not discovering this and for not acting.

If, on the other hand, April could not be expected to discover this, then she *cannot* be blamed for not knowing and not acting.

Suppose that April did discover the fact of Joe's elevated temperature.

If she might be expected to recognize this as symptomatic of appendicitis and she did recognize it, then she is neither blameworthy nor praiseworthy.

If April recognized the meaning of Joe's symptom and she could not, reasonably, be expected to recognize it, then she is praiseworthy.

The fact by itself tells nothing. The fact in context tells everything there is to be told. Whether April is blameworthy or praiseworthy depends not only on the actions she took but also on the context of the situation and the context of her knowledge.

To repeat John Hosper's observation:

> In ethics everything is contextual; and the context of every action is unique and unduplicable, with the result that even a small difference between two situations may yield a difference in our moral verdict. (Hospers, 1972, p. 63)

STANDARDS IN CONTEXT

The standard of freedom involves a patient's right to determine for himself the meaning and importance of a context, form his own purposes, determine his own actions, bring about changes in his own circumstances, and pursue his own goals.

Freedom, as a bioethical standard, implies that a health care professional has an obligation not to interfere with a patient's choices and decisions.

It is easy for a nurse to understand the meaning of the concept of "freedom." She can understand and accept the fact that each individual has a right to think, decide, and act for himself. She may still come upon dilemmas involving freedom. There may be any number of situations in which she does not know how the standard of freedom is to be applied. How does the standard apply to a patient who suffers from intermittent confusion? How does the standard apply to a child? How does it apply in cases of abortion and euthanasia?

Dilemmas arise that cannot be solved rationally by reference to abstract standards taken out of context. The bioethical standards cannot be understood apart from the broad and specific contexts to which they apply.

Every bioethical standard calls for action on the part of a health care professional. The concept of "action," like every concept related to ethics, is far from being simple. For instance, an action cannot be understood simply by an abstract analysis of the word that signifies the action (Polanyi and Prosch, 1975).

The word "run" is a simple word and easy to understand. It abstractly signifies a particular type of action. We take note that a number of actions are similar. We see Jane run, Jack run, Jim run, a horse run—and we capture and retain every action of this type in the concept "run." Once we have learned the concept "run," we can use it to think and to communicate. But, taken by itself, in abstraction, it tells us almost nothing. The concept "run" signifies too many actions to be useful simply by itself. People run, animals run, motors run, rivers run, noses run, and stockings run. "Run" is a *very* general abstraction.

Every concept signifying actions is very general. To be useful a concept or a standard must be related to a context. To be meaningful and useful a concept must be applied to a specific situation.

Taken by itself in abstraction, every action—theft, lying, benevolence, justice—has a specific nature. But the conditions within which the action takes place are supremely important. They determine the moral meaning of that action to a beneficiary and to the agent who performs it. We understand the specific meaning of any word or of any action from the actual context in which it occurs.

Except for a formalism[1] carried to its utmost extreme, hiding a fat man's table is much less evil than stealing a hungry widow's plate. Giving false testimony against an innocent defendant is much worse than lying to a child about Santa Claus. In and of themselves, and considered abstractly, each of the first two actions is theft; each of the second two is lying. Yet one of each pair is, at worst, a trifle, while the other action is morally abominable. The difference is entirely in the context.

The goal for which a person acts may, in one context, secure and enhance his life. In another context it may secure or enhance the life of another. In a different kind of context it may threaten life or lessen the quality of life. Narcotics for pain control after an operation greatly enhance a patient's life.

Narcotics used for recreation threaten and lessen the quality of an addict's life.

Whenever a person wants to act on a desire, he needs to analyze his desire. Whenever he makes an ethical choice, he needs to analyze that choice. He must consider the possible effects of the actions that will follow upon that choice. This need for ethical analysis involves a further need. All ethical analysis requires attention to the context.

ETHICAL ACTION IN A NURSING CONTEXT

The more data a nurse can gather and systematize, the better her chance of taking actions that will lead to her desired goal. Likewise the more complete the context she can build, the greater are her chances of resolving a dilemma correctly.

Bioethical standards can be utilized by a nurse in one of two ways: to replace a context or to delineate a context.

Replacing a Context

A bioethical standard can be used to replace a context. A nurse can perform certain formalistic actions that, she believes, will satisfy the requirements of the standard.

In the name of "autonomy" a nurse may comment on and force long hours of discussion of her patient's uniqueness.

In the name of "freedom" a nurse may allow a young patient who loves acid rock to fill the halls of the hospital unit with MTV.

In the name of "veracity" a nurse may tell a patient the truth and cause him great harm.

In the name of "privacy" a nurse may keep a confidence that should be broken.

In the name of "beneficence" a nurse may let a patient fail to perform his range-of-motion exercises.

In all these cases the nurse fails to make her actions appropriate to the context. She replaces the context with a bioethical standard. This action makes her actions, at best, irrelevant to the context—and to bioethics.

Delineating a Context

Ethical standards can form a sort of lens through which the outlines of a context can be seen. They can identify what is meaningful and important to human purposes in any ethical circumstance.

The standard of autonomy can help a nurse to analyze the desire of an athlete to risk an experimental operation in the hope of being able to return to his sport.

The standard of freedom can help a nurse accept a patient's decision not to undergo treatment.

The standard of veracity can give a nurse the confidence that she is right in giving a patient the information he needs in order to make a vital decision.

The standard of privacy can help a nurse to understand a patient's unwillingness to share certain items of information about himself.

The standard of beneficence can help a nurse to understand the need to balance potential good against potential harm.

The bioethical standards are those ethical abstractions that have been found to be most relevant to the health care professions.

An effective ethical agent applies her knowledge of relevant ethical standards to those facts of the situation of which she is aware. In the same way a nurse applies her knowledge of patterns, nursing diagnosis, goals, and nursing actions in the nursing process. The steps of the nursing process enable a nurse to form her nursing context. In the same way the bioethical standards enable a nurse to form her ethical context. In order to form either context she must gather and systematize data from the actual situation.

THE DIVIDED CONTEXT

The most common way a nurse can lose the broad context is through forming two distinct and separate contexts.

One of the contexts which she forms will be a nursing context. She will attempt to act as efficiently as possible in this context. She will strive to be able to justify every nursing intervention.

The other context which she will form will be her ethical context. In this context she will direct all her actions toward an ethical abstraction chosen without any particular reference to the nursing context. There will be no connection between her context as an ethical agent and her context as a nurse.

She may be aware of her patient's need for privacy and confidentiality. On some level she may believe that privacy and confidentiality are his right. Despite this she believes that her first loyalty must be to, for instance, the standard of "honesty." She will be honest in her efforts toward her patient and honest toward the world in general. She is determined that she will be able to justify her ethical actions. She will do this by showing that she behaved "honestly."

✕ DILEMMA 7-1   Adam is in the hospital to be treated for a degenerative nerve disease. His employer, Carl, comes in to visit him. Laura, Adam's nurse, is an old friend of Carl's. Carl asks Laura whether Adam's condition is going to interfere with the quality of his work. Laura, who is totally devoted to honesty, replies that the quality of Adam's work will probably suffer as a result of his condition.

Quite obviously, through Laura's methodology, the ethical context—and her patient—will suffer. Any ethic that keeps a nurse's nursing context and the context of her ethical action in strict isolation from each other cannot be an effective nursing ethic. If one looks at it carefully, it is apparent that it cannot be a *nursing ethic* at all.

HOW STANDARDS COME INTO THE CONTEXT

Most people do not form ethical concepts. They acquire an equivalent of ethical concepts. They memorize words. They never learn the meanings of these words from the situations to which they apply in the real world. They then apply these words to ethical situations that are far too complex to be grasped in a word. As a result they are entirely ineffective in applying these words to the real world.

In order to form an ethical concept a person must begin by observing basic facts in the world. He must then come to understand these basic facts and their relationship to human purposes. A person observes that no one with whom he comes in contact is identical to anyone else. Rather, everyone is unique and different. He finds that he must interact with everyone according to the person's uniqueness. He can find no reason to justify a demand that everyone should be the same. Therefore, when he perceives the importance of a person's uniqueness in relation to that person's vital and fundamental goals, he realizes that "autonomy" is an ethical concept.

He notes that it is impossible to form agreements and interact with other people apart from a recognition of their autonomy. Therefore he adopts autonomy as an ethical standard.

An ethical concept cannot be formed and it cannot be understood apart from its relation to the purposes of ethical agents. It can no more be understood than an artifact from a distant civilization can be understood by a person who has no knowledge of the purpose of the artifact.

Thus, for instance, "honesty" cannot form part of a nursing ethic. It is a duty-based concept. It is not essentially related to human purposes in general or the purposes of patients. All the things that "honesty" cannot do "beneficence" can. Beneficence is a kind of honesty. It is honesty exercised with purpose and intelligence.

A nurse notes the differences in the health care setting between those situations where nurses interact beneficently with patients and those where they do not. She sees that the purposes of the health care setting—the health and well-being of a patient—are best served by beneficent interactions. She notes that beneficence increases the pride of a nurse in herself and her profession. Based on this experience she adopts beneficence as an ethical standard.

So it is with every ethical standard she forms on an independent and first-hand basis. She forms ethical standards from her experience of situations where those standards were needed. A standard which a nurse *understands* is one which she knows how to apply and why she should apply it. She learns this from the ethical context.

Ethical actions are actions taken in the pursuit of vital and fundamental goals. They are actions intended to make an important difference in a person's life. Ethical action requires:

- An interplay between a person and a situation.

This situation must either offer the person the possibility of achieving some value or it must threaten the loss of some value.

✖ DILEMMA 7-2 Vladimir, a concert pianist, has sustained an injury that may affect his ability to play the piano. There are two operations that could be performed. One operation has a 90 percent chance of restoring gross movements of the hand and eliminating pain. Another, experimental operation is showing about a 10 percent success rate in restoring fine motor coordination. However, if this operation were to fail, Vladimir would lose much of the gross movement of his hand. Vladimir must make a decision. The decision regards the possibility of achieving a value or the loss of a value. The value of being able to play the piano must be considered in the context of other activities that Vladimir values. The decision which Vladimir must make is an ethical decision. The action he will take, based on this decision, is an ethical action.

- A knowledge of how the situation can guide the person's action in the pursuit of his purpose.

Vladimir must take into consideration these two essential facts: The success rate for one operation is 90 percent; for the other, it is about 10 percent.

- A set of ethical principles held explicitly or implicitly.

When making his decision, Vladimir must consider the value he places on his ability to play the piano. He must also consider the disadvantages of losing gross motor coordination.

By means of these principles Vladimir can judge the relative desirability of both operations.

In order to interact effectively with Vladimir his nurse will have to understand and get into Vladimir's ethical context.

THE NURSE'S ETHICAL ATTITUDE

The demands of a situation, the preexisting knowledge through which a person understands a situation, and the interaction between a person and a situation form the context. The art of applying the ethical standards well to these demands consists in knowing what ethical standards apply to a certain situation and how they apply, and being capable of acting and capable of justifying actions.

Objectively justifiable actions require a knowledge of what ethical standards involve. The justification of ethical actions requires something more than this. It requires an awareness of the relationship of ethical standards to the vital and fundamental goals of the people engaged in the action.

For a nurse the possession of these skills is never acquired automatically. It involves:

- A sincere willingness to accept the autonomy of her patient.
- A willingness to accept her patient's right to freedom of choice, decision, and action.
- A concern that her communication shall serve, not any extrinsic and sacrosanct ideal of truth, but the well-being of her patient.
- A psychological acceptance of her patient's self-ownership.
- A consistent beneficence, motivated by good will, toward the beneficiary of her actions.
- An unwavering, but contextual, commitment to the agreements she has made with her patients.

Perfecting skillful ethical action requires a nurse to open herself to the experience of the situation. A nurse is the agent of her patient. Before a nurse could discuss Vladimir's situation with him she would have to know the meaning of the situation to him. In order to know this she must come to understand his evaluation of the things he may achieve and the things he may lose. She can come to understand this by reference to her knowledge of the bioethical standards.

There is only one way that she can understand the meaning and importance of things in the lives of her patients. She understands this through her knowledge of the meaning and importance of things in her own life. The meanings and the relative importance of things are what brings a context into being—and into focus.

Solving a problem requires that the various aspects of the problem be understandable. If they are not understandable then some way must be found to make them understandable. The aspects of an ethical problem become understandable through the application of standards to the ethical context. An ethically competent nurse must understand the nature and purpose of the bioethical standards. The bioethical standards serve human purposes.

THE ABANDONED CONTEXT

Imagine that you live on an island. This island is ruled by a disoriented and ill-directed king. The king of the island is passionately interested in increasing the happiness and contentment of his subjects. This poses a serious threat to them.

At this time there are exactly 100 inhabitants on the island. A panel of experts has informed the king that 10 of his subjects are the happiest and most contented 10 percent on the island. Another 10 are the 90th percentile. And so on down to the unhappiest and most discontent 10 percent of his population.

The king reasons that without this unhappiest 10 percent of the population the society he rules would be, statistically, happier. And so the king has the 10 least happy citizens of his island kingdom drowned.

Now, assuming you were not one of the unhappy 10, let us continue. When this statistically unhappy 10 percent is disposed of, the island society, on a mathematical basis, is about 5.5 percent happier and more content. At the same time, you will notice, your mood is entirely unchanged. It is the same with everyone on the island. Not one individual is happier or more content by an eyelash.

A disinterested observer might discover a number of flaws in the king's decision-making process:

1. A context can enable a person to begin to solve an ethical dilemma. It cannot, by itself, serve to solve the dilemma. The king assumed that the dilemma, in effect, solved itself. He applied no ethical standards to the context. He simply observed the context and applied a mathematical equation.

2. The king was not aware of the difference between the nature of a group of 100 individual women and men and the nature of a single individual woman or man.

   This is the central reason why he failed to solve the dilemma he perceived. He failed to maintain the context of his knowledge. Before a person becomes a king—or an ethical agent—he should know the difference between a percentage and a person. The king did not maintain an awareness of the difference between concrete realities (the individual women and men who lived on the island) and mental abstractions (the percentages studied by his panel of "experts").

3. He failed to maintain the context of the situation. If there are two people on an island and one dies, the sum of his happiness will not accrue to the other. His death may very well diminish the happiness of the other. What holds true of two people, in this context, holds true of a hundred.

   The king's action was entirely irrational. In order to maintain the context a person must differentiate between the rational and the irrational. The king did not.

4. The king did not maintain an awareness of simple causal factors. There are values that make people happy and content and losses that make them unhappy and discontent. Other people on the island had died without their deaths influencing the happiness or unhappiness of the entire citizenry. There is nothing in the nature of individual people or happiness or death such that the death of the unhappy increases the happiness of the living.

5. The king kept himself unaware of the nature of a fundamental interpersonal ethical concept. He maintained an unawareness of the rights of his subjects. The right to autonomy, individual freedom, and privacy cannot be the right of a percentage. All rights are the rights of individuals.

   The king remained unaware of the fact that rights — the right not to be killed — accrue to people because of their human nature. The belief that a person loses his right to life when he becomes unhappy is absurd. There is nothing in the nature of individual people, of rights, or of happiness to justify this belief.

   The king would not have made a good biomedical professional. For him a group of 100 people, *as a group,* is a reality no different from an individual man or woman.

Ethics, and especially bioethics, has to do with individuals. Nursing dilemmas are, essentially, dilemmas concerning individual nurses and patients. The nursing context is an interpersonal but individual context. It is not a solitary context. But neither is it a group or a statistical context.

ETHICAL INDIVIDUALISM AND THE LAW

Every patient who enters the health care system, concerned for his survival and well-being, enters as an ethical individualist. Many lawsuits have originated over the failure of the health care system to recognize this. Virtually every law that relates to these issues sanctions the patient's ethical individualism.[2] The law recognizes (among other things):

- A patient's legal right to give an informed consent. No one has a legal right to treat a patient without his consent. No one has a legal right to obtain a patient's consent without the patient knowing what he is giving his consent to.
- A patient's legal right to refuse treatment.
- A patient's legal right, post mortem, to be protected against the "harvesting" of organs.
- The legal right of children to medical attention regardless of the wishes of their parents.
- A patient's legal right to confidentiality.

- An individual's legal right to refuse to donate organs, for example, bone marrow, to a relative.
- A patient's legal right not to participate in research against his wishes.
- A patient's legal right to be protected against malpractice or wrongful death.

THE PATIENT AS THE CENTER OF THE CONTEXT

A context is the interwoven aspects of a situation including a person's awareness of those aspects that are necessary in order for him to understand the situation and to act effectively in it. For a nurse, the range and the nature of a context is set by the needs of a patient and her role as nurse in relation to her patient. It is set by a nurse's agreement with her patient and the relevant applications of that agreement.

Once it is formed by a nurse, the context guides her in the application and justification of the standards she applies. Awareness of the context enables a nurse to judge the adequacy and appropriateness of a standard to the situation, to her patient's rights, and to their mutual purposes.

For instance, nearly every nursing context calls for a nurse to tell her patient the truth. However it is sometimes better (more beneficent) for her to exercise a controlled response and lie to her patient.

Ellen has suffered three myocardial infarctions. She is in the hospital for an emergency coronary bypass. Her nurse, Judy, is preparing her preoperative medication. Word is received that Ellen's husband has been killed in an automobile accident on the way to the hospital. Ellen asks Judy why her husband is not at the hospital. There are several reasons, in this context, why Judy ought not tell Ellen the truth, at this time.

There is nothing in the nurse/patient agreement that permits a nurse to harm her patient for the sake of an out of context ethical abstraction. No ethical abstraction can be the logical center of a bioethical context. The context comes into being with the patient. In the nature of things *only* the patient can be the focus of the bioethical context. The nurse/patient agreement, on the part of a nurse, is an agreement to enter into the context of her patient. If an ethical standard interferes with the nurse/patient agreement, then it is taken out of context. If it is taken out of context, it is inappropriate to a biomedical situation.

Let us take "honesty" again:

Frank's condition is very grave. All the factors are in place for a stressful shock to put him in a state of, probably fatal, cardiac arrest. Frank might ask Amelia, his nurse, about his condition. Here "honesty" would certainly be against the spirit—and the letter—of the nurse/patient agreement.

Amelia knows that in order to give a truthful reply she would have to abandon the context. A truthful reply would be "All the factors are in place for a stressful shock to put you into a state of, probably fatal, cardiac arrest." This reply might very well come to Frank as a stressful shock. The proper application of every standard, and especially veracity, is thoroughly context dependent. Honesty, like a joke, can be carried too far.

The bioethical standards cannot be effectively applied without a thorough awareness of the context. Without this awareness the bioethical standards cannot even be understood.

CONFLICTS WITHIN THE STANDARDS

The bioethical standards will guide the actions of a nurse in an ethical context. They will even help shape the context. However, difficulties can arise in the application of the bioethical standards. Until these difficulties are resolved, it is impossible to act effectively *in the context*. Within each standard there is a possibility for dilemmas to arise:

Autonomy

Problems with autonomy are problems with self-image, character, and personality structure. Nurses sometimes have to care for children who want both a tube of lipstick and a teddy bear. At times they care for children who want to be cuddled while they want to be thought of as football players. Nurses often find it difficult to know what part of the child's self-image they are interacting with.

There is often a clash between a patient's physical, emotional, or intellectual capabilites and his self-image or desired life style. This poses a series of ongoing dilemmas for a nurse. A nurse must deal with the uniqueness of her patient. She must deal with different aspects of and changes in her patient's personality.

Freedom

There can be a clash between a patient's freedom to ambulate and his freedom to take indirect action to protect himself from injury. This action he takes through his nurse, who is his agent.

This is the case with an aged, infirm, disoriented, or debilitated patient who has come into a health care setting in order to recover from an illness or injury. The patient can no longer endure confinement. He wants to get out of bed and move about. At the very same time he wants his nurse to see that he does not sustain an injury. She must decide on her course of action. Will she ally herself with his freedom to act on his desires, or will she draw him toward accepting a more realistic view of his freedom?

The limitations of a nurse's agency — where her obligation to decide ends and her patient's right to decide begins — is an ongoing dilemma.

Veracity

A patient will sometimes ask a nurse not to tell a third person the specifics of his condition. If this third person asks the nurse about the patient's condition, she must lie or she must break her promise. Breaking a promise is also a form of lying. She cannot escape lying.

Dilemmas arise around the standard of veracity that cannot be resolved simply by reference to that standard.

Privacy

A patient has been given a terminal prognosis. He asks to be left alone. An error in his diagnosis is discovered. To inform him of this immediately would be a violation of his privacy. Here the standard of privacy seems to conflict with common sense.

> **✖ DILEMMA 7-3**   A patient exercises his self-ownership by bringing himself into a health care setting. He comes into the hospital for a liver condition. While he is in the health care setting, he becomes quite friendly with his nurse. One day he swears his nurse to secrecy. Then he informs her of a certain fact regarding his condition.
>
> During the course of his treatment the patient becomes incapable of making a decision. This poses a dilemma for his nurse around the standard of privacy. She has promised to maintain the confidentiality of their communication. The information the patient gave her is now needed by the physician to treat him effectively. But she has no reason to believe that her patient would release her from her promise now.

On the other hand the patient's purpose in coming into the health care setting was to have his condition treated.

This is a dilemma centering on the standard of privacy. It cannot be resolved simply by reference to that standard. The context provided by the standard of privacy, in isolation, is too narrow for this to be possible.

Beneficence

The philosopher Plato points out the strange difference between the attitudes of people toward the baker and the physician. Everyone loves visiting the baker; no one enjoys visiting the physician. The baker gives us cakes and pies, delicious-tasting delicacies which make us sick. The physician gives us noxious and bitter-tasting medicine and painful treatments of various sorts, which make us well.

Both the baker and the physician, each in his own way, treat us with a form of beneficence. What is and is not beneficent is often hard to recognize. It is radically context dependent.

Plato's parable raises some very interesting problems for biomedical professionals:

- In regard to beneficence what is the function of a nurse?
- In regard to beneficence are the functions of a nurse the same as those of a physician?
- Is the beneficence of a physician entirely expressed in his attempts to heal his patient?
- Is the beneficence of a nurse entirely expressed in her attempts to comfort the patient and ease his immediate suffering?

There are dilemmas that arise within the standard of beneficence that cannot be resolved simply by reference to that standard.

Fidelity

A conflict within a standard or any conflict between two standards is a conflict involving fidelity. These conflicts cannot be resolved by reference to fidelity nor to the standard(s). If they could, there would be no conflict.

✂ **DILEMMA 7-4**   A biomedical professional promises a patient that if he becomes comatose and experiences a cardiac arrest, no extraordinary means will be used to resuscitate him. One day the patient slips into a coma. The next day a cure for his condition is discovered. The following day the patient arrests. Of course, he should be resuscitated, but if he is this will violate the standard of fidelity.

It seems that the standard of fidelity is capable of clashing with optimal medical practice

SUMMARY

Every decision is made either in a solitary context or an interpersonal context. (A solitary context is a context in which no one except the person himself will be significantly affected by his decision and subsequent actions. An interpersonal context is a context in which one or more others will be affected by an agent's decisions and actions.) If a person loses his awareness of a solitary context, he loses his ability to take appropriate actions. This undermines his efficient pursuit of his own most important goals. If a person loses awareness of an interpersonal context, he loses his ability to communicate effectively with the other people involved in the context. This means that he cannot rationally interact with the other people.

Ethical decisions and actions must be justified according to their appropriateness to the situation. In a solitary context their appropriateness depends upon the person's purposes and desires. In an interpersonal context it depends on the terms of the agreement that forms the context.

A decision or action is ethically justified if it is appropriate to the ethical aspects of the situation in which it occurs. A person can justify his decisions and actions if he can show that they are appropriate. An ethical agent must recognize the aspects of the context by which he is guided in his decisions and actions. Otherwise his decisions and actions will not be justified or justifiable. This is true whether the ethical agent is a nurse or the patient himself.

Anyone who takes ethical actions ought to recognize:

1. The nature of the situation—that it is a situation calling for ethical action and why it is, that it is a situation involving vital and fundamental goals.
2. The desires and purposes operating within the situation which structure the specific ethical aspects of it.
3. The present condition of the people involved in the situation.
4. The desires of the people involved in the situation—the conditions to which they are aspiring.
5. The factors which can facilitate their efforts in realizing their purposes, and the factors which might hinder them.

The art of ethical decision making consists in knowing what ethical standards apply to the various types of ethical situation. It involves knowing how and why they apply.

In a pluralistic society there is no substitute for experience and thought in acquiring the skill to make justifiable ethical decisions. There is no criteria by which to judge ethical decisions except the nature of human beings and the challenges which reality thrusts at them.

NOTES

1 Formalism is "rigorous or excessive adherence to recognized forms..." (*American Heritage Dictionary*, 1985, p. 526). An ethical formalist is one who concentrates entirely on the abstract category into which an action can be placed, without regard for the context or the effects of the action.

The spirit of formalism in deontology is captured in the Latin maxim: "One should tell the truth though the heavens fall."

If, in a certain country, there were many rich people and very few poor ones, a Robin Hood who robbed from the poor to give to the rich would be practicing a utilitarian formalism.

2 This is not to suggest that ethical individualism is desirable and proper because it is sanctioned by the law. Individual rights are not produced by law. Rather laws are purposeless and unintelligible if they are not derived from individual rights. Contemporary medical law is desirable and proper because it is sanctioned by ethical individualism.

REFERENCES

American heritage dictionary. (1985). Boston: Houghton Mifflin.

Hospers, J. (1972). *Human conduct: Problems of ethics.* New York: Harcourt Brace Jovanovich.

Polanyi, M., & Prosch, H. (1975). *Meaning.* Chicago: The University of Chicago Press.

Conflicts Among the Bioethical Standards

Most conflicts between the contemporary bioethical standards are not open to easy solutions. They are, in fact, acutely difficult. But a nurse cannot hope to be capable of consistently objective ethical thinking and effective ethical action if she is unable to resolve them.

An ethically effective nurse is one who performs well within the context of the nurse/patient agreement. The actions and attitudes of an ethically effective nurse are structured by the bioethical standards. This has always been true. It was true even before the contemporary bioethical standards became contemporary.

There is no possibility of a nurse making consistently effective ethical decisions without some principles, such as the bioethical standards, to guide her. There are a number of reasons for this. That which seems to be good is not always the same as that which is good. Some *means* is necessary to enable a nurse to note the difference between that which seems and that which is.

This means is the context. The bioethical standards, unfortunately, are not sufficient, by themselves, to place a nurse firmly in the context.

Velma has learned that patients like seeing a sunny, smiling nurse. Therefore it seems that Roger, who has been in a car crash would enjoy seeing a sunny, smiling nurse. But Roger's wife was killed in the car crash. Now, here, there is a difference between what seems and what is.

Velma has learned that patients like being partners in their treatment. Therefore it seems that Tom would like being a partner in his treatment. But Tom would prefer that biomedical professionals make the decisions concerning his treatment for him. Here again there is a difference between what seems and what is.

Velma can see no reason to clutter Peter's mind with the reasons for doing range-of-motion exercises. It happens that by knowing the reasons Peter will be more likely to be motivated to do them. Once again there is a difference between what seems and what is.

Velma assumes that David enjoys her dropping in to chat when she has time. But David is working on a problem and does not enjoy chatting. So Velma fails to differentiate between that which seems to be the case and that which is the case.

Velma assumes that Maude wants to be left alone. In fact Maude wishes Velma would stop in so they could discuss her surgery. Once again Velma fails to differentiate between that which seems and that which is.

In making her ethical decisions and choosing her actions no nurse can hope to be infallible. No nurse has complete and certain knowledge of what is good in every situation.

Without the guidance of ethical standards the nurse/patient agreement would be undermined. Decision and choice would be turned over to the arbitrary whims of the nurse and/or her patient. But a nurse needs to know the reasons for the bioethical standards. She needs this knowledge in order to know when and how the standards are to be applied.

EFFICIENT NURSING AND THE BIOETHICAL STANDARDS

A nurse must be conscious of the fact that her ethical interactions involve another person. She is bound to this other person by agreement. This other person is a unique and autonomous individual.

Every nurse is called upon to care for a wide spectrum of individuals and a wide spectrum of types. She is called upon to care for female infants and elderly males, male infants and elderly females. The differences between these types are far-ranging and profound. The differences between the individuals who make up these types are, in different ways, even wider ranging and more profound.

A nurse cannot interact with a type. A "type" is a mental abstraction, and a person cannot interact with an abstraction. If a nurse does not interact with the autonomous individual, and according to his uniqueness, she fails at ethical interaction. She fails, quite simply, because she does not *interact* at all. A nurse cannot interact with the idea of a patient that she has in her mind. To interact with her patient she must interact with the real person. This involves interacting with the unique and autonomous person he is.

An effective nurse accepts the fact that her patient is capable of making decisions and taking actions; she *expects* him to make decisions and take actions. Insofar as a patient is capable of acting, of course, he is his own agent. He is a patient only to the extent that he is incapable of acting.

Nurses act as agents of their patients because of the nurse/patient agreement. If patients did not make their own decisions and take actions for themselves, no agreement would be possible. A patient must decide and then act to make an agreement. To make an agreement a nurse must accept the fact of her patient's freedom. She must interact with him on the basis of his freedom. Without this acceptance there is no other basis upon which they can interact.

A nurse and patient can and should discuss the patient's choices and decisions, and the actions he plans to take. These discussions are one of the reasons why there are nurses. An amateur can always profit from discussion with a more knowledgeable professional. An experienced and conscientious nurse is a professional. In certain situations she is much more knowledgeable and much better able to make an objective judgment than a patient. She is able to help a patient arrive at a more objective judgment than he might reach alone, without her aid. Every patient is placed into a circumstance where he is an amateur.

But, in the final analysis, every patient has an absolute right to make his own decisions and choices. He has a right, by nature, to act in what he perceives to be his own best interest. This is the central factor in the contextual interaction of nurse and patient.

An effective nurse recognizes her patient's autonomy and his freedom, which means that she relates to him with objectivity. Her awareness is determined by the actual nature of the *external* reality which is her patient.

If a nurse respects the autonomy and freedom of her patient she will feel obliged to relate to him with veracity. A patient cannot exercise his right to free choice and action unless he knows the truth. If he desires to exercise his freedom, his nurse violates this right unless she tells him the truth he needs to know.

An effective nurse also deals with her patient from the perspective of beneficence. No patient goes into a health care setting expecting to derive no good and looking forward to the possibility of harm. Even the patient who knows he is dying expects to gain something. He expects to gain a peaceful death by being in the health care setting. Beneficence is expected by the patient and is a person's reason for becoming a nurse. It forms part of the nurse/patient agreement. Whatever forms part of the nurse/patient agreement forms part of the nurse's ethical context.

In order to deal competently and contextually with the ethical aspects of nursing a nurse respects the self-ownership—the privacy—of her patient. It is impossible to respect a patient's autonomy and freedom without recognizing the fact that he is in possession of himself—by right.

Everyone has a right to enjoy some degree of isolation from others. Without the freedom from distraction provided by this isolation a patient could not maintain his well-being and function effectively. This is what motivates a patient to come into the health care setting—the desire to regain his health and his power to take (unimpeded) actions.

Then, again, no contextual interaction is possible without privacy because no *context* is possible without privacy. The situation in a beehive is unchanging. Bees do not enjoy self-ownership. What the bees are doing now is what they have done, and will do, over and over, endlessly. There are no contexts in a beehive.

CONFLICTS AMONG THE STANDARDS

Actions that are ethically appropriate in relation to one patient at a certain time and in a certain way may not be appropriate in relation to another patient. Or the same actions may not be appropriate to the same patient at a different time or if the actions are taken in a different way.

Nurses can use the bioethical standards as ethical instruments. There are two problems that arise for a nurse in her use of the standards:

1. She can be uncertain as to the application of a bioethical standard. This uncertainty produces a dilemma.
2. She can feel a greater confidence in the application of a standard than is justified. This feeling can block the resolution of a dilemma. It can leave a nurse with the realization that the decision she made was not the best decision, when it is too late.

These problems arise because it is possible for conflicts to arise among the standards. We will now turn to those conflicts.

Autonomy and Freedom

The standards of freedom and autonomy are often confused. They are not the same.

A person's *freedom* is his ability to take independent actions. His *right to freedom* is his right to make independent choices and decisions and to act on these choices and decisions. The *standard of freedom* involves his right to take uncoerced actions, actions motivated by his own independent purposes and judgment. A biomedical professional's refusal to accept a patient's decisions and choices is a violation of the bioethical standard of freedom. Her efforts to coerce actions from her patient is another form of the same violation.

A person's autonomy is his independent uniqueness. His right to autonomy is his right to be what he is. Every form of intolerance is directed against someone's autonomy.

The difference between autonomy and freedom is shown by a consideration of the way each standard is violated.

Violation of Autonomy. In order to violate the standard of autonomy a person must (1) take some action against another which he or she ought not take; or (2) fail to take some action for the benefit of another which he or she ought to take.

The first action is an act of aggression. The second does not involve aggression; it involves the failure to take an action.

In either case this aggression or failure to act is motivated by an intolerance of the autonomy — the differences — of the other person.

Anna is the head nurse on a busy medical-surgical floor in a large hospital in the city. Dolores is an assistant director in a small community hospital. Anna and Dolores graduated from the same high school in the same year. In school they were in bitter competition with each other. Dolores was voted Homecoming Queen. This event was very painful for Anna, who had expected that she would be Homecoming Queen.

Anna, on the other hand, was appointed head cheerleader of the football team. Dolores had expected to be head cheerleader and was very resentful of Anna's success.

One day George was brought onto Anna's floor. It was George's misfortune that Anna discovered that he is the brother of Dolores. Anna arranged to have George placed in the least desirable room on the floor.

This was her way of getting even for the supposed injustice she suffered at Dolores' hands. The action Anna took was an unjustifiable violation of George's autonomy.

As fate would have it Anna's brother, Harry, became a patient in the hospital where Dolores worked. Dolores discovered that Harry is Anna's brother. Dolores pulled strings to have Edna appointed as Harry's primary nurse. Edna is under observation for possible substance abuse.

In this way Dolores took her revenge for being denied the position of head cheerleader. Dolores' action, motivated by a desire other than the desire for Harry's health and well-being, was an inexcusable violation of Harry's autonomy.

Violation of Freedom. A violation of a person's freedom, on the other hand, always involves an *interference* with that other person's decisions, choices, or actions.

Don wants to find out about his upcoming operation. He asks Audrey, his nurse, what he can expect on the day of his scheduled surgery. Audrey, however, is expecting a phone call from an old friend and wants to stay close to the phone. She gives Don his sedative so that he will go to sleep and she will not be bothered by him.

Audrey's refusal to discuss the operation with Don is a violation of his right to freedom. A nurse is the agent of her patient. The freedom of a patient involves the "freedom" to expect cooperation from his nurse. It is the freedom to take actions through his nurse. Her failure to cooperate is a form of interfering with his action.

If autonomy and freedom were the same, then actions that violated one would violate the other. But this is not the case. These standards are different. The difference between these two standards makes it possible for conflicts to arise between them.

✖ **DILEMMA 8-1**   Rick is a professional football player. He has sustained a severe concussion during spring practice. He has a headache and is experiencing vertigo. He is on strict bed rest. But Rick is attempting to get out of bed and walk around.

If Glenda, Rick's nurse, interferes with his efforts, she will be interfering with his freedom to take action. If she does not prevent him from getting out of bed, he may injure himself by falling. Or he may do himself permanent damage by causing an increase in his intracranial pressure. Either may diminish his physical capabilities and force a radical change in his life style. Either injury may be harmful to Rick's physical capabilities and self-image. If Glenda permits this injury to Rick, and could have prevented it, she has failed to respect his autonomy.

Here then is a conflict between two standards that apparently cannot be resolved by reference to either standard or to both together. Whatever resolution is possible must come from outside of the standards. It must come from outside of the nurse/patient agreement — insofar as that agreement is understood solely in terms of the bioethical standards.

Consider another situation:

✖ **DILEMMA 8-2**   A health care professional is determined that a patient shall exercise his right to make decisions regarding his treatment. The patient wants the health care professional to make the decisions.

It can be argued that:

• The patient is exercising his freedom by delegating responsibility to the professional.
• The nature of this patient's autonomy is such that this is the best way he can exercise his freedom.

- A patient's relationship to a health care professional always, to some extent, involves this delegation of responsibility.

It can, just as plausibly, be argued that:

- The patient is not exercising his right to freedom in refusing to exercise it.
- The patient is not expressing his autonomy but abandoning it.
- In matters concerning the course of his life it is ethically desirable that a patient delegate as little responsibility as possible.

In the life of a nurse a large number of conflicts between freedom and autonomy arise. They sometimes arise out of a failure to differentiate between the two. These conflicts cannot be resolved within the confines of "freedom" and "autonomy."

Autonomy and Veracity

A nurse has an ethical obligation to recognize the fear of a patient who is more fearful than most. This is one way a professional recognizes the autonomy of her patient. Each patient has a right to be who he is, and this patient is more fearful than most.

> **DILEMMA 8-3**   Rachel has a patient, Ken, who is dying. She and Ken are old friends. Rachel knows that Ken is probably unaware of the seriousness of his condition, and she knows that Ken is terrified of dying. She also knows that Ken has many business and personal affairs that he would want to get in order if he knew of his condition.
>
> Rachel is, as the saying goes, caught on the horns of a dilemma. If she reveals his condition and incites terror in him, she will be ignoring Ken's present personality structure. This would be a violation of his autonomy. If she does not tell him and enable him to get his affairs in order, she will be violating the standard of veracity.
>
> Since they are old friends, Ken might expect Rachel to tell him that he is dying. At the same time his behavior might have given her no opportunity to do this.
>
> But, Rachel's behavior might lead him to believe that he is not dying, which is not true. If she knew that her behavior might mislead him and she could have prevented this, then, in respecting his autonomy, she violated the standard of veracity.

Note that, whatever Rachel does, she must find some way to apply what she does know to what she does not know.

Rachel is in a double bind. Neither autonomy nor veracity will enable her to work her way out of this dilemma.

Autonomy and Privacy

An individual person's right to privacy is an outgrowth of his autonomy, an outgrowth of his "right"[1] to be what he is. One thing that every person is, regardless of other differences or similarities, is an independent individual. Every person is private—by nature. One cannot deny (violate) the privacy of another without, at the same time, denying (violating) his autonomy. Nor, of course, can one violate the autonomy of another without violating his privacy. If a nurse rigorously accepts a patient's autonomy she cannot violate his privacy.

Autonomy is individual and independent uniqueness. A person's right to autonomy is that moral property whereby he has the right to be dealt with according to his uniqueness. A person's right to privacy is his right to self-ownership, which includes his right to be free of undesired and undesirable interactions or relationships.

Any conflict that arises between autonomy and privacy is not a real but a merely apparent conflict. The conflict arises only because one or both terms ("autonomy" and/or "privacy") is ill defined.

Mohan and his wife are asleep when their house catches on fire. Mohan manages to get out of the house. He is taken to the hospital in an ambulance. For a long time Mohan can get no information on what has happened to his wife. Finally he is told that she is dead. He begins to cry. He asks Kathleen, his nurse, to see that he is left alone.

Mohan's physician is contacted by the coroner about arrangements for the disposition of the body of Mohan's wife. Mohan and his wife were Hindu and no one knows what should be done.

The physician instructs Kathleen to ask Mohan what he wants done. Kathleen tells the physician that Mohan is crying and wants to be left alone for the time being. The physician angrily orders Kathleen to go and get the information he asked for. Now Kathleen faces an apparent conflict between an aspect of Mohan's autonomy (the fact that he is a Hindu) and his privacy (the fact that he wants to be left alone).

If Kathleen breaks in on Mohan's mourning, this will be a violation of his autonomy. The only way it could be otherwise would be if Mohan does not enjoy self-ownership but is owned by his physician, or, perhaps, by his religion. That he is owned by his religion suggests that the autonomy that ought to be respected is not Mohan's uniqueness but only one facet of his uniqueness—his religion. It suggests that Mohan has a right to be dealt with, not according to *his* uniqueness, but, according to the uniqueness of his religion.

The idea that Mohan's uniqueness might be the property of his physician is even more absurd. There is no way to make the idea that Mohan is owned by someone or something other than Mohan himself ethically intelligible.

On the other hand Kathleen would also violate Mohan's right to privacy. She would do this because his physician decided that the practices of Mohan's religion are more important to Mohan right now than his experience of the loss of his wife. In asking to be left alone Mohan made a decision concerning his privacy. If he has a right to privacy, then, of necessity, he had a right to make that decision concerning his privacy.

It might be argued that it is not Mohan but his physician who decides what interactions Mohan finds desirable or undesirable. There is no reason whatever to believe that Mohan would order his priorities in this way or turn his self-ownership over to his physician in this context.

The conflict between Mohan's autonomy and his privacy is merely apparent. Both have been violated. There has been no conflict between them.

No conflict between autonomy and privacy is possible.

At least two other relevant series of events are possible here:

1. Kathleen does not disturb Mohan. The coroner takes the body of Mohan's wife and handles it through the usual procedures. In this case, apparently, Mohan maintains his privacy but his right to autonomy may be violated.

   Surely there must be a conflict here.

   But, if we look at this series of events as it is, this is what we find. It is not Kathleen, nor even the physician, who violated Mohan's rights. If, in fact, anyone violated Mohan's rights, it was the coroner. Furthermore, note that no conflict between privacy and autonomy arises because the coroner does not become involved with Mohan's privacy. Depending on other factors — the context of his knowledge, and the intentions that motivate his actions — the coroner may or may not be guilty of violating Mohan's autonomy. But, even if Mohan's autonomy is violated, it is not Kathleen who violates it.

2. It is possible that Mohan may require nursing and/or medical interventions. In this event Kathleen must use careful contextual judgment. She must balance the importance of honoring Mohan's rights against the importance of the nursing or medical interventions.

   If all Mohan needs is morning care, it would be absurd of Kathleen to break in on his privacy. If he needs a vital medication, it would be absurd not to.

   One does not have rights desire by desire, but in the context of one's life and over the whole span of one's life.

   Whatever Kathleen does, she cannot escape a need for keen ethical judgment. No ethical agent can ever escape a need for ethical judgment.

The bioethical standards, themselves, are *not* ethical judgments. They are *standards* of ethical judgment.

This points up a central flaw in both deontology and utilitarianism. Deontology provides no standards or guideposts for determining *the nature* of one's duty. Utilitarianism provides no standards or guideposts for determining *the nature* of the greatest good. They do not because they cannot — not if they are to remain deontology on the one hand and utilitarianism on the other. If deontology were to propose a standard of duty, or utilitarianism were to propose a standard of utility, then this standard would displace duty or utility as the agent's ethical motivation.

The fact that duty and utility are undefined is a tragedy inherent in the traditional ethic. It is a flaw that makes either utterly inappropriate as a bioethic. A biomedical professional, in ethical interactions, must interact. Biomedical professionals must know what they are doing and why they are doing it. They must know the exact nature of the benefit their actions produce.

Autonomy and Beneficence

Perhaps no ethical dilemmas that a nurse faces are more common than those that arise through conflicts between the requirements of beneficence and the recognition of autonomy. For the biomedical professions as a whole the most difficult and the most severe dilemmas arise through conflicts between these two standards.

DILEMMA 8-4   The classic case of a conflict between autonomy and beneficence is the case of a comatose Jehovah's Witness who needs a blood transfusion. His autonomy demands that, since he cannot explicitly communicate his wishes, it be assumed that he would not want the transfusion. The standard of beneficence, on the other hand, demands that the professional act to bring about good. To allow a patient to die when he could have been saved is a very great failure to bring about good. Still and all to give a patient a transfusion and save him, under these circumstances, would violate the standard of autonomy.

DILEMMA 8-5   A patient is taken to the physical therapy room against his will by the "gentle coercion" of his nurse. He is frightened and depressed. His nurse has violated his autonomy. His long-term well-being requires that he take physical therapy. If he does not, in the future he will come to regret it. He will be left with a permanent disability. So, it seems, this "gentle coercion" is demanded by a rational beneficence.

Let us move ahead, to what may now seem quite difficult, in order to illustrate this. Later on an approach to these dilemmas will not seem so forbidding, although their analysis will never be easy:

DILEMMA 8-6   A certain patient is comatose. There is no predictable chance that he will recover from his condition. Some time in the past he expressed a wish that he be allowed to die if he were in these circumstances. How are autonomy and beneficence to be applied here? It can be argued that:

- He must be allowed to die. The unique individual that he once was no longer exists. The recognition of his right to autonomy includes a recognition of the fact that there is no autonomous being to be kept alive.

- He must be allowed to die on the basis of beneficence. Biological survival in the sense of the preservation of electrochemical processes are in no way whatever the equivalent of a human life. If there were any foreseeable possibility of his attaining even the lowest level of a human existence, the demands of beneficence would be entirely different. There is no hope for a worthwhile and human existence and respect for his once human dignity requires that he be allowed to die.

On the other hand:

- He must be kept alive. One possesses life only once and life is precious above everything else. Without life nothing whatever is of any value. The patient's staying alive is a tribute he pays to himself and to his life. Beneficence demands that he be assisted in staying alive.
- He must be kept alive since no one has a right to terminate the life of an autonomous individual. What the patient was in the past is no longer relevant. His autonomy now is the unique nature of his present existence. Recognition of his present autonomy demands that his life be preserved.

The recognition of a patient's autonomy and the motivation of a nurse's beneficence do not necessarily lead to one exclusive and justifiable decision. This is because the bioethical standards, as we have seen, should not, by themselves, inspire a feeling of perfect confidence in *any* decision.

Autonomy and Fidelity

The primary responsibility for fulfilling the agreement between nurse and patient naturally lies with the nurse. It cannot be otherwise. The patient is a patient—one who is, to a greater or lesser extent, passive—unable to initiate action. Agency, the unhindered ability to initiate action, resides in the nurse.

This poses a remarkable dilemma.

✖ **DILEMMA 8-7**   Henry, Irene's patient, has a low tolerance to pain. Henry is very high-strung and fearful. He makes such demands on Irene's time and energy that she cannot adequately attend to her other patients. Does Irene's recognition of Henry's autonomous nature demand of her that she ignore her responsibility to her other patients? Or does fidelity to her agreement with her other patients override her obligation to recognize Henry's autonomy?

The ethical situation which Irene faces here is a dilemma that cannot be resolved by reference either to autonomy or to fidelity. The conflict here is not merely apparent, it is real.

Freedom and Veracity

A conflict between the standards of freedom and veracity can arise whenever two or more people are interacting.

✖ **DILEMMA 8-8**   Bobby is 4 years old. He has a problem with bedwetting. Bobby has asked Marilyn, his nurse, not to tell his parents, and she has agreed. Bobby's parents are, perhaps, overly concerned with his bedwetting. When his parents come to visit, they ask Marilyn, whether Bobby has been wetting the bed. If Marilyn tells them the truth, this will be perfectly in line with the usual understanding of the demands of the standard of veracity. It may also interfere with the spontaneous and positive interaction between Bobby and his parents. It will interfere with the actions Bobby wants to take. Instead of being open and accepting, Bobby's parents may be harsh and forbidding.

In order to facilitate Bobby's freedom of action, Marilyn would have to practice deception. She would have to lie to Bobby's parents.

One bioethical standard requires Marilyn to facilitate her patient's freedom of action. Another places a moral obligation upon her to tell the truth. The two together pose a dilemma for Marilyn.

The dilemma cannot be solved by use of either standard alone.

Freedom and Privacy

If any person enjoyed total and complete privacy, no question as to his right to take free action could arise. If he had total and complete privacy, he would have no occasion to interact with another person. If he had no occasion to interact with another person there would be no one to interfere with his freedom of action.

But patients are in a situation where they cannot expect to enjoy complete privacy. A patient's nurse can have no greater respect for his privacy than his medical condition and her nursing functions permit.

Whenever one person "invades" the privacy of another, it is possible that this person will interfere with the freedom of the other person. Linda stops a former patient passing in the street to ask how he is. This is a way of interfering with her former patient's freedom of action, but it is an entirely blameless way. It is not a violation of his privacy.

This form of interfering with a person's freedom is of no ethical importance. Interruptions of a patient's freedom of action through an invasion of his privacy can occur in two ways:

1. Linda interrupts a patient's action even though the goal of this action is one upon which the patient places a high degree of importance.
2. Linda does not interfere with any important action her patient wishes to take. However, she subjects him to a constant series of minor interruptions. She violates his privacy and his freedom simply by the repetition of minor obstructions to his freedom.

Occasions can arise when not interfering with an agent's action will mean a loss of his privacy. There are also occasions when not invading a patient's

privacy will result in his losing his freedom of action. This occurs, for instance, every time a nurse wakes a patient (invades his privacy) in order to
give him his medication (and thus enhance his future freedom to act).

A dilemma involving the standards of freedom and privacy could occur in
this way:

⚖   **DILEMMA 8-9**   A caller phones the nurse's station and speaks to Lotte,
Ray's nurse. The caller tells Lotte that he is Ray's lawyer. He tells her that he was
to come in today for Ray to sign his new will, but he is unable to get there today.
He asks Lotte if he might come in the next day to see Ray. Lotte knows that there
is a strong possibility that Ray might not live that long.

If she tells the caller of Ray's condition, she violates the standard of privacy. She
has no way of being certain that the caller is Ray's lawyer. There is a definite
possibility that the caller is a speculator who could use a prior knowledge of Ray's
impending death to profit by undermining the value of Ray's corporation. If she
does *not* tell the caller of Ray's impending death, there is a possibility that this will
interfere with Ray's freedom to take actions that are vitally important to him.

It will require a particularly keen attention to the context to resolve this
dilemma.

Freedom and Beneficence

A conflict between freedom and beneficence is a conflict in which a patient's
desire to act is placed in opposition to his well-being.

⚖   **DILEMMA 8-10**   Yvonne is treating Steve, a recovering stroke patient.
Steve is having difficulty feeding himself. If Yvonne takes time to feed him, this
might certainly be interpreted as an act of beneficence. It also might be interpreted
as an act of interfering with his freedom. In order to exercise his freedom in the
future Steve must learn to feed himself.

On the other hand if Yvonne tells Steve that she cannot help him, that he is going
to have to feed himself, this might be interpreted as a failure of beneficence. It might
also be interpreted as an act by which Yvonne supports Steve's freedom of action.

The ethical context produces the ethical dilemma, and it is by reference to
the context that an ethical dilemma is resolved. Yvonne's context (and every
context) has three aspects:

- The situation which Yvonne faces, and which calls for her to take some
  ethical action.
- Yvonne's awareness of the nature of the situation.
- Yvonne's preexisting beliefs concerning the elements of ethical action.

Yvonne's situation calls for an ethical response. None of the bioethical
standards provide the elements necessary to securely guide Yvonne's response.

✖ **DILEMMA 8-11**   Margaret is 87 years old. She is very feeble, and is kept restrained in a wheelchair. She complains to Sandra, her nurse, that she wants to be "untied" so that she can walk around. Sandra knows that there is a very good chance that if Margaret were to walk around she might fall. If she fell, she could severely, painfully, and permanently injure herself. This would cause her to lose the safe freedom of action she already enjoys. "Untying" Margaret would violate both beneficence and freedom.

Assume, however, that the only freedom Margaret could enjoy, since she cannot sit for any length of time, would be to walk around. A small change in the context changes a fairly clear-cut situation into an ethical dilemma. A minor change in the context will often have major ethical repercussions.

Freedom and Fidelity

✖ **DILEMMA 8-12**   Charlie, a heart attack patient, is having a heated argument with a business associate. He regards the favorable resolution of this argument as being of extreme importance to his career. Ingrid, Charlie's nurse, wants to call a halt to this argument, but Charlie wants to continue it. Ingrid believes, rightly, that this argument places Charlie's health and, possibly, even his life in jeopardy.

It's Charlie's life to do with as he will. If Charlie has a right to live, then he has a right to take chances. Life requires one to take chances.

At the same time Ingrid has had Charlie's medical care placed in her hands. Her knowledge of the requirements of effective medical care is much greater than Charlie's. She has a responsibility to protect Charlie's life and health.

If Charlie exercises his right to take free action, Ingrid cannot exercise fidelity to her agreement. In order to exercise fidelity to the nurse/patient agreement, she must interfere with Charlie's freedom of action.

Nurses, generally, tend to argue in favor of Ingrid's right to interfere with Charlie. At the same time they tend to argue against Sandra's right to interfere with Margaret.

But there are no fundamental differences between the two cases. In principle these cases are identical. Each case places a patient's right to take certain actions in opposition to a nurse's responsibility to protect his well-being.

This poses a question: Does a nurse have the right to protect a patient against himself? This question cannot be answered simply by reference to the bioethical standards.

The difference in the decisions that the nurse arrives at is not caused by any difference in the cases themselves. It is caused by a difference in the approach the nurse takes to the two cases.

Veracity and Privacy

If a nurse is to defend her own right to privacy—her own right to self-ownership—she must take certain positive actions. She must actively maintain her right not to disclose any fact if this disclosure would threaten her right of self-ownership. If a nurse is to defend a patient's right to privacy, she must have the same attitude toward her patient. She must maintain her right not to disclose any fact when she is aware that this disclosure would threaten her patient's right of self-ownership.

Two nurses, Sybil and Janet, work together and maintain a friendly relationship with one another. This relationship includes their going out to dinner occasionally.
Sybil and Janet are both aware that at some future time they may be in competition for the position of head nurse. This awareness has never before influenced their relationship.
One evening Sybil tells Janet that a mutual friend has said that Janet is a recovering alcoholic. She asks Janet if this is true.
In fact Janet is a recovering alcoholic. Janet can affirm that she is a recovering alcoholic. Or she can deny it. Or she can refuse to discuss the topic. If Janet does not deny this fact, or if she refuses to discuss the topic, then Sybil will have every reason to believe that the information she has received is accurate.
It is quite possible that Sybil could use this information to prevent Janet's being considered for the position of head nurse. Then again, Sybil might never use the information in this way. It is very possible that Sybil is simply "making small talk" and is not at all thinking of violating Janet's right to privacy.

Janet faces a dilemma. If she tells the truth, and friends have a "right" to expect truth from each other, she surrenders her right to privacy. If she decides to maintain her privacy, she will have to lie to Sybil.

Let us look at a different situation:

✖ **DILEMMA 8-13**   Karen has entered the hospital and had an abortion. Her husband, Steve, a salesman, has been out of town. He locates Karen's nurse and asks her why Karen is in the hospital.
This presents a dilemma. Karen's nurse knows nothing about the circumstances surrounding the relationship between Karen and Steve. If she tells Steve that Karen has had an abortion, she may be violating Karen's right to privacy. If she does not tell him, she is violating the standard of veracity — and probably for no reason. If she refuses to tell him anything, her refusal might cause Steve great anxiety. It might also sow the seeds of distrust in his mind.

It would be very desirable if a nurse had a way to deal with such dilemmas before they arose. The bioethical standards, unfortunately, do not provide such a way.

Veracity and Beneficence

Conflicts between veracity and beneficence produce a great number of ethical dilemmas for nurses.

�֎ **DILEMMA 8-14**   Hugh is dying. Lucy, his nurse, believes that his death is imminent. She remembers that Denise, his wife, had expressed a desire to be with her husband when he dies. Hugh and Denise had agreed to be with each other at the end so that the person who died first would not die alone. Lucy calls Denise to tell her of her husband's condition. It is a rather long time before Denise arrives at the hospital. Denise is blind and she must find someone willing to drive her to the hospital. By the time she arrives Hugh has died.

Before Lucy takes her into her husband's room, Denise expresses how glad she is to have arrived before his death. She spends several minutes in the room with her husband. She does not know that he was already dead when she arrived. If Lucy tells Denise that her husband died before she arrived, she honors the conventional standard of veracity but fails the test of beneficence. If Lucy tells her that she was with her husband while he was still alive, Lucy violates the standard of veracity but meets the test of beneficence.

This poses a dilemma.

Veracity and Fidelity

By the nature of things conflicts between the standards of veracity and fidelity will arise very seldom. Fidelity to the nurse/patient agreement will normally entail veracity. But in some unusual cases a conflict can arise:

✖ **DILEMMA 8-15**   Ike is Joan's patient. Ike's prognosis is poor. For reasons known only to himself Ike does not want his wife Helen to be told of his prognosis. There are a number of legal and practical arrangements that must be made, and Helen needs to know the facts of Ike's condition.

If Joan reveals Ike's prognosis to Helen, she violates the agreement she has with Ike. And then she has lied to Ike.

But Joan also has an ethical, and possibly a legal obligation to Helen. If she does not tell Helen the truth, it will mean an unnecessary future hardship for Helen. Joan is not certain that Ike understands this.

Joan faces a dilemma that cannot be resolved either by reference to veracity nor by reference to fidelity.

Privacy and Beneficence

Taken to the extreme either privacy or beneficence would make the exercise of the other impossible.

If any person had the isolation of perfect privacy, it would not be possible for any other person to act benevolently toward him. For one person to act benevolently toward another he must know something of the other person's situation and values. But a person's perfect privacy would preclude anyone from knowing anything about him. So a person's perfect privacy would make another person's benevolent action toward him impossible.

At the same time if one person's actions toward another were consistently and dependably benevolent, the first person would have only the most rudimentary need of privacy from the other.

Let us look at another dilemma—a common dilemma:

✖ **DILEMMA 8-16**   Doris brings Shawn, her 5-year-old son, into a clinic to be treated for injuries sustained through a fall. Alice, the nurse who treats Shawn, recognizes that his injuries are much more consistent with battering than with a fall.

Beneficence seems to demand that Alice report her belief that Shawn is a battered child. She cannot do this, however, without creating an invasion of Doris' privacy. Whatever she does, she ought to do it only with full awareness.

Neither privacy nor beneficence, nor both together, can make this awareness possible.

Privacy and Fidelity

A nurse has a moral obligation to remain faithful to her agreement with her patient. However her obligation to exercise fidelity does not end with her obligation to her patient. As an ethical agent and as a nurse she also has an obligation to exercise fidelity toward her colleagues and toward her employing institution.

Conflicts between the standards of privacy and fidelity are rare, but here is one possibility:

✖ **DILEMMA 8-17**   Art enters the hospital as a charity patient. Wilma, the nurse assigned to him, recognizes him as a wealthy recluse from a neighboring town.

Wilma has an obligation to remain faithful to her unspoken agreement with her patients. Part of that obligation involves maintaining her patient's privacy. Another part of Wilma's obligation is to the hospital where she works. It is very seldom, perhaps never, justifiable for Wilma to keep the truth from the hospital.

Wilma faces a dilemma.

Beneficence and Fidelity

There are no conflicts between beneficence and fidelity.

A hypothetical conflict would take something like this form:

John is going to have his leg amputated. Suddenly he changes his mind. He asks not to be anesthetized. Marilyn, his nurse, is determined that he shall receive the benefits for which he entered the hospital. The operation is performed.

Such an event, of course, could never occur. For this reason no actual conflicts between beneficence and fidelity can arise.

For Marilyn to maintain fidelity to her agreement by coercing John into going through with the operation would involve an absolutely unjustifiable breach of his freedom. The agreement cannot be met in this manner.

The case is implausible and uninteresting.

SUMMARY

The bioethical standards can place a nurse in the bioethical context. They can make it easier for her to resolve ethical dilemmas. But conflicts among the bioethical standards can arise. They cannot be resolved in the context they have created. A wider context must be formed by elements more basic than the bioethical standards. Very soon we shall turn to these elements.

But first we shall give a final consideration to the very real importance of the contemporary bioethical standards.

NOTE

1   Strictly speaking every right is the right to take an action. To be what one is, for example, a male, a redhead, a schizophrenic, or a hypertensive, is not an action. One does not act to be male, redheaded, schizophrenic, or hypertensive; this is simply what one is. The phrase "the right to one's autonomy" is not just a figure of speech. It denotes the ethical propriety of accepting the autonomy of any person with whom one interacts.

Not to accept the autonomy of another person is ethically improper since no one is ethically responsible for that which he did not act to bring about. No one ought to be praised or blamed because he is a male or redheaded or schizophrenic or hypertensive.

CHAPTER

9

Agreements Without Standards

There are situations when the proper application of a bioethical standard is ambiguous and difficult:

- Should a nurse talk to her frightened pediatric patient about being a football player, or should she cuddle him?
- Should a nurse respect her patient's freedom to ambulate, or should she act on his behalf in order to prevent him from injuring himself?
- Should a nurse lie to her patient if his knowing the truth might cause him harm?
- What are the limits of a nurse's responsibility to protect her patient's privacy?
- Does beneficence call for the nurse to moderate her patient's therapy so that the therapy will not be painful? Or is it more beneficent to subject him to stringent therapeutic regimens if this will result in a faster or a more complete recovery?
- What is the nature of the nurse/patient agreement? What does the nurse/patient agreement cover? To whom does the nurse/patient agreement apply? Is the nurse/patient agreement necessary?

Bioethical standards are, of necessity, very broad abstractions. They have been derived from legal and biomedical experience. They have been found, through this experience, to make the ethical interaction between biomedical professionals and patients optimally harmonious. Their scope, however, covers needs much more basic than harmony. The fact that these needs are so basic and so relevant to the biomedical context is the reason why they produce harmony.

Nonetheless a nurse cannot confidently rely on the bioethical standards alone. For the bioethical standards to be reliable guides, a thorough understanding of their meaning in relation to her patient is needed.

A nurse, like anyone else, can make herself believe whatever it is convenient for her to believe. It is easy to rationalize the application of the standards. Then she can apply them in any way that suits her convenience.

Even with the best intentions, it is difficult to know when and how the standards ought to be applied. It is also difficult to know *why* they ought to be applied in a particular way in a particular case.

The efficient application of the bioethical standards requires careful attention to the context. But the bioethical standards, taken simply by themselves, do not provide the outlines of a clear and complete context. Taken by themselves the standards do not even reveal the *ethical* context. The bioethical standards, taken by themselves, do not answer questions such as the following:

- *Why* should one person respect the autonomy of another? Why should a person prize his *own* autonomy? ("A person just should!" is not an answer.)
- *Why* should one person respect the freedom of another? Why should a person value his *own* freedom?
- *Why* should a person deal truthfully with others? Why should a person deal truthfully with *himself*?
- *Why* should one person respect the privacy of another? Why do people value their *own* privacy?
- *Why* should people deal with each other beneficently? (It seems obvious that people should, but this question does not answer itself.)
- *Why* should people exercise fidelity in their dealings with each other? *Why* should a nurse honor the nurse/patient agreement?

These questions cannot be answered by reference to the standards. Their answers depend on deeper and more fundamental ethical principles.

THE STANDARDS AS A BIOETHICAL MODEL

[A] model is an instrument for learning about some feature of the world but it is not this feature itself. [A model has] heuristic intentions. (Herstein, 1983, p. 7)

That is to say, a model is an instrument that is intended to serve as a guide to the analysis and the solution of problems (ethical dilemmas). It is an instrument for dealing with the world. A model is *not* the world itself.

The bioethical standards are an ethical decision-making model, an instrument for dealing with an ethical context. All too often, however, they are treated, not as an instrument for understanding the context, but as the context itself.

If a nurse asks herself, "What is needed by my patient?" or "What would be an ethically appropriate action in this context?", she can use the standards in order to arrive at her answer.

If a nurse asks herself, "What does the standard of privacy demand?", or if she tells herself, "Whatever I do I must maintain the standard of veracity!", she is abandoning the bioethical context in favor of a bioethical standard. But a standard has no use outside of a context.

The first nurse is like a person who wants a 6-foot board. This person takes his saw and his tape measure and looks for some boards. When he finds them, he measures 6 feet on one board and saws off the excess. Then he has his 6-foot board.

The second nurse is like a person who also wants a board 6 foot long. This person takes his saw and his tape measure and looks for some boards. When he finds them he throws them away and begins to examine his tape measure. He is never successful in coming home with a 6-foot board.

THE USES OF A BIOETHICAL MODEL

The bioethical standards form an incomplete ethical decision-making model. They can be looked at and used as absolute rules — unrelated in themselves to the nurse, to the patient, or to the context.

This makes the ethical function of a nurse one of interaction with the standards rather than interaction with her patients. The needs of her patient are one thing. The importance of the standards is an entirely different thing, unrelated to the needs of her patient. The model that the standards form is not an instrument used by a nurse for dealing with the patient's needs. The bioethical standards are one level of the nurse's concern. The needs of her patient are an entirely different level.

Dora has been assigned to Bernice, a battered wife. In the middle of the night Thorsten, Bernice's husband, comes to visit her. He is flushed from intoxication and, in the hand where many men carry flowers, Thorsten has a hammer. He demands to know where his wife is.
Dora was raised to be truthful and honest. When she discovered that veracity was a bioethical standard, she adopted it very easily. Dora has the highest respect for the standard of veracity. Her highest ethical ambition has always been to tell the truth.
Bernice, on the other hand, needs to be protected, or at least hidden, from Thorsten.

In this situation Dora may violate the standard of veracity as she under-stands it. Or she may follow the deontologists in regarding the standard as an absolute rule superseding every other consideration. If she does this, she will overlook a very important question: If the bioethical standards are not to be held subservient to a patient's needs, what possible reason could there be for the bioethical standards to be *bioethical* standards? The bioethical standards would be measures with nothing to measure.

The bioethical standards are instruments to analyze what is out in the world. However, they are not, *themselves*, what is out in the world. Nor are they that final object that needs to be analyzed.

The bioethical standards are to be used for the benefit of a nurse and her patient. They can be used by a nurse as instruments for analyzing the needs and rights and desires of her patient. They can help to guide a nurse in her ethical choices, decisions, and actions.

Ingrid, a nurse who works with Dora, makes an ethical analysis of each of her patients. She proceeds in this way:

She seeks to learn the autonomy of her patient. She does this by learning about her patient. She does not do this by examining her concept of autonomy. She knows that her ethical interaction will be with an autonomous patient. It will not be with the idea of autonomy that she carries around in her mind.

She seeks to learn the areas of her patient's desire for freedom. She does this also by learning about her patient. She does not reflect on the concept of freedom in her mind. She will be engaging in ethical interaction with a person. She will not be engaging in ethical interaction with a concept.

She engages in a close analysis of the context. She does this in order to determine if and where she might harm her patient by stumbling over the standard of veracity. She seeks to discover where her patient will benefit by receiving some truthful information. She does not bother to closely examine the nature of truth. Her patient is the center of her ethical attention.

She attempts to determine areas of the patient's life where he will desire privacy while he is in the health care setting. Again she begins with her patient. She does not begin with an abstract idea of privacy.

She stays on the alert for areas where she can do her patient some good. She stays alert for areas where she might do him harm.

Dora's center of attention, on the contrary, is the standards and not her patient. She regards the standards as deontological rules. In ethical matters she gives her attention to the standards rather than to her patient.

Dora's process of ethical discovery is not governed by the nature of her patient's situation. She feels a responsibility to the standards themselves. The standards, and only the standards, possess ethical relevance for her. Used in this way the bioethical standards make it impossible for her to stay in tune with the context.

Ingrid's use of the standards assumes that the efficiency of a nurse's ethical actions is measured by the benefit the nurse's actions yield. Since she assumes this, the center of her ethical context cannot be abstract ethical rules. The center of her context must be the nature and the needs of her patient. Ingrid does not attempt to benefit a standard.

The bioethical standards are means to ends *beyond* themselves. They are not ends *in* themselves. This is why dilemmas among the standards can arise. If two friends want to visit Los Angeles, no conflict can arise as to where they want to visit. If one wants to get there by plane and the other wants to go by train, then it is very likely that a conflict will arise. Los Angeles serves as an end in itself. Travel by air or by rail are different means to that end. This is where the conflict arises.

There is no way, in the standards themselves, to show that the standards have any value. It is of no value to a stone to have its autonomy recognized. Veracity is of no value to a tree. The standards have no value in and of themselves. They have value only in relationship to individual women and men who are motivated by desires.

Bob is an elderly, feeble, senile man who has entered the hospital for diagnostic studies. On her shift Dora cares for Bob, and Ingrid cares for him on hers.

Bob wants to get up and ambulate. Ingrid quiets him but does not allow him to ambulate. Dora does allow Bob to ambulate. Bob falls and fractures his hip.

Dora claims that the reason she allowed Bob to ambulate was out of respect for his right to freedom. Unless this happened in a very peculiar biomedical context, Dora's claim does not justify her action. She placed the well-being of freedom above the well-being of her patient.

Ingrid claims that the reason she did not allow Bob to ambulate was through a fear that he would fall and injure himself. Unless what she did took place in a very peculiar biomedical context, Ingrid's claim does justify her action. Ingrid placed the well-being of her patient above the well-being of freedom.

It is often difficult to know where and how a standard ought to be applied. It is very often difficult to know which standard ought to be applied to an ethical situation. Rational ethical action on the part of a nurse without reference to the bioethical standards is impossible. On the other hand, the bioethical standards alone do not and cannot outline the ethical context.

It is possible for the standards to conflict. Therefore they are, in themselves, an inefficient model. They do not provide the way for a nurse to keep the nurse/patient agreement. A nurse cannot be consistently certain of being able to take ethical action if she begins with the bioethical standards. For she cannot be certain of beginning within the context.

The bioethical standards are very broad abstractions, and some way must be found to bring them into a context.

AGREEMENT AND CONTEXT

The center of the nurse's ethical context cannot be posterity or the environment or cultural "values" or anything but the individual patient. The boundaries of a nurse's ethical context arise entirely within the agreement she has with her patient.

Without the nurse/patient agreement no ethical context would ever arise. The nurse's and the patient's situation and interactions would be unintelligible. Only in the context of the agreement do they become intelligible. Only through an agreement does a nursing situation become a context.

Nursing, as an activity, has a nature entirely its own. It is different from all other types of activity. Nursing is an activity oriented toward specific purposes. It is characterized by specific interpersonal interactions. The nature of these interactions is determined by the nature of nursing as a science.

Within the interpersonal relationship of nurse and patient there is an interweaving of expectations and commitments. These expectations and commitments form the terms of the relationship for both nurse and patient.

This complex of expectations and commitments between nurse and patient forms an agreement between them. Each agrees to satisfy, to one extent or another, the expectations of the other. Both agree to live up to the commitments each has made to the other. Their agreement is a recognition by each of the expectations and commitments existing between them.

Interactions between people must be based on expectations and responsibilities that are known by each. Otherwise there will be no pattern to their interactions. Without intelligible patterns of interaction between nurse and patient, nursing would not be a specific activity. The word "nursing" would refer to nothing.

Whenever an agreement exists between two people, each has expectations and responsibilities as a result of that agreement. This is true of the nurse/patient agreement, as it is true of every agreement. His expectations motivate a person to take on the responsibilities of an agreement.

THE STANDARDS AND THE AGREEMENT

There are two ways in which the standards and the agreement are interrelated that are of paramount importance.

Preconditions of the Agreement

The bioethical standards are preconditions of the nurse/patient agreement.

A nurse or a patient cannot enter into an objective agreement without a recognition of the bioethical standards. The standards of ethical interaction that are recognized as the contemporary bioethical standards are preconditions of *any* agreement between rational beings.

It is possible for a nurse or a patient not to *explicitly* recognize her or his reliance on the bioethical standards. It is not possible that a nurse or patient can enter into an objective agreement without, at least, an *implicit* recognition of the standards. If one person enters into an agreement with another, he assumes that that other is autonomous, free, truthful and dependent on truth, private, beneficent, and faithful. If the second person were not all these things, he could not enter into an objective agreement.

Terms of the Agreement

The bioethical standards are terms of the nurse/patient agreement.

- The terms of the nurse/patient agreement are set by the autonomy of the parties to the agreement. In any objective agreement people agree to the exchange of values. The values a person desires depends upon his unique character structure. In this way the autonomy of each party becomes an intrinsic part of the agreement.
- In order for a person to make an objective agreement he must be free to make an agreement. In order for him to carry out the agreement, he must be free to do so. Every party to an agreement must depend on the freedom of the other parties. Every party to an agreement implicitly promises the other parties that he has the freedom to carry out the agreement. Each party promises that he will exercise his freedom. In these ways freedom becomes one of the terms of every objective agreement.
- In order to enter into and carry through on an agreement, each party to the agreement must have a true knowledge of the terms of the agreement. Thus when the parties to the agreement set the terms, they implicitly promise veracity to the other parties to the agreement. Without the assurance of veracity no agreement would be possible. Veracity is one of the terms of every possible agreement.
- In order to make an agreement one must own himself and his efforts. No one can commit himself to an agreement unless he owns himself. No one could be responsible for carrying through on an agreement unless he owned himself. Every party to an agreement is expected to be responsible for carrying out his end of the agreement. The other parties to the agreement depend on this. Privacy is one of the terms of every agreement.
- Everyone enters into an agreement depending on the beneficence of the other parties. Everyone enters into an agreement depending on some benefit to accrue from the agreement. Each party to the agreement recognizes this. This is why each party makes the agreement. In this way beneficence becomes one of the terms of every agreement.

- Every agreement consists in the specific terms of that agreement and an implicit promise by each party to the agreement that he will be faithful to it. Without this implicit promise there simply is no agreement. Fidelity is one of the terms of every agreement.

AGREEMENT IN THE ABSENCE OF THE STANDARDS

There is a way to see the relationship between the standards and the nurse/patient agreement with perfect clarity. First it is necessary to examine what an agreement would be without each standard. This is difficult to do. In order to make the examination the reader will have to use the fullest resources of his or her imagination.

It is difficult to imagine a person making an agreement without recourse to any of the standards. There is no human being who does not bring a right to the standards to an ethical interaction. Patients do not acquire a right to the bioethical standards when they enter the health care setting. They bring this right with them.

Let us examine what the condition of an agreement would be in the absence of each standard.

We can begin by using our imagination in order to build a thought experiment:

Let us pretend that there is a club with a very peculiar membership. All the members of the club are on a skiing vacation. They are staying at a cabin in the mountains. There has been a blizzard followed by an avalanche. The members of the club are trapped in the cabin. There is not enough food, water, and fuel for them to survive. Immediate action must be taken to escape the cabin.
Rose, the most resourceful member of the club, begins to make plans to escape. She finds herself faced with some very remarkable hindrances.

To continue our thought experiment:

Agreement in the Absence of Autonomy

Rose sees one course of action open to her. She decides to enlist the cooperation of Art, one of her fellow club members. Art has a very remarkable character flaw. He cannot function on his own. He can only adopt the desires and motivations, and mimic the actions, of someone else. He entirely lacks autonomy.
Rose attempts to discuss their situation with Art. All he can do is echo her words. She proposes a course of action to him and proceeds to demonstrate what she means. She wants to dig a hole through which they can escape. Art adopts her motivation. He decides he also wants to escape—because Rose wants to escape. An irreconcilable difference (or

lack of difference) arises between Rose and Art. Only one person at a time can dig through the snow. Rose wants Art to begin to dig. Art's motivations are the mirror image of Rose's. Art wants Rose to begin to dig. Rose decides that she will begin to dig. Then Art, predictably, becomes determined that he will begin to dig.

It is very lucky that nature has, in fact, made everyone unique and different. Otherwise, as we can see, no agreement — no exchange of values — between people would be possible. Quite obviously no cooperation between Rose and Art is possible.

The crucial point to be established is that the autonomy — the individual uniqueness — of each party to an agreement is a necessary precondition of *any* agreement between them. Art lacks autonomy. Because of this Rose cannot make an agreement with him. Without an agreement no genuine cooperation between them is possible.

Agreements between people are possible because *every* person possesses autonomy. If no one possessed autonomy, no *interaction* between people would be possible. Everyone would spend his life waiting for someone else to take the first step.

On the other hand the existence of an agreement between two people logically establishes the autonomy of each.

Everyone with whom a nurse establishes a nurse/patient agreement possesses autonomy. Otherwise there could not be an agreement. The nurse accepts the fact of autonomy in making the agreement. Every patient possesses the right to have his autonomy respected or he possesses no rights at all.

The existence of an agreement between nurse and patient logically establishes the autonomy of each. For, if each did not possess autonomy, no agreement could exist between them.

For either to violate the autonomy of the other is to act as if no agreement does exist between them. For this is, implicitly, to deny a necessary precondition of the existence of an agreement. If no agreement exists, then no stable and intelligible relationship can exist between nurse and patient. If no stable and intelligible relationship can exist between nurse and patient then there can be no such thing as nursing.

Agreement in the Absence of Freedom

Let us suppose that one of the skiing party, Mike, is peculiar in a different way:

Mike can make no free choices or decisions and he cannot take free actions. For Rose to attempt to make an agreement with Mike in order to escape the snowbound cabin will be a waste of time. If he cannot make free decisions and choices, he cannot freely decide and choose to make an agreement with Rose. The making of an agreement is, by definition, a free act. If Mike cannot take free actions, he cannot freely act to make an agreement with Rose.

If Mike and Rose are able to reach an agreement, then the situation is very different. Of necessity, each must possess the power to make agreements. This power to make agreements is nothing but the power to take free actions.

Whenever two people reach an agreement, each implicitly assumes that the other possesses the power and the right to decide, choose, and act for himself. This is a necessary precondition of their agreement.

If a nurse remembers the necessary preconditions of an agreement, this gives her an ethical resource. For, in the very nature of nursing, every nurse has an agreement with her every patient. Freedom is a necessary precondition of the nurse/patient agreement, as it is of every agreement.

A nurse should never forget that a patient has the right to free decision, choice, and action. To forget that a patient has this right is to forget that there is a nurse/patient agreement. If there were no nurse/patient agreement, there would be no nurse/patient relationship. If there were no nurse/patient relationship, the nurse would have no right to take any action whatever in regard to the patient.

Agreement in the Absence of Veracity

One person cannot make an agreement with another person unless he has a right to expect to hear the truth from that other person. There can be an agreement only where there is a meeting of the minds. Each party to the agreement must have an informed (true) knowledge of the terms of the agreement. Without this knowledge a person, obviously, could not be party to an *agreement*. Each party to the agreement must be certain of the terms of the agreement. He can be certain of the terms of the agreement only if he has an assurance that he has access to the truth concerning the terms of the agreement.

Suppose Rose were to state, "I have an agreement with Herb. However, when we made the agreement, Herb was not truthful with me." It is obvious that Rose would be wrong. She could not have an agreement with Herb if she could not know (the truth concerning) the details of the agreement. She could not know the details of the agreement if Herb was not being truthful with her.

There cannot be an agreement between people if one person does not know what the agreement is all about. A person cannot function in an agreement without knowing the truth. An agreement in which a person cannot function is no agreement at all.

Just consider how foolish Rose would be if she turned to Herb and attempted to make an agreement with him. In order that there would be no misunderstanding between them she would have to agree not to expect their communications to be truthful. Under these circumstances there cannot be a "meeting of the minds."

Rose would want to establish an agreement with Herb. To do this she would allow the absence of veracity between them. She would allow a condition that would make an agreement between them impossible.

If a nurse wished to have an agreement with a patient and was unconcerned with the standard of truth, she would be guilty of the same contradiction. The wish for an agreement to exist cannot be fulfilled without the conditions that make the existence of an agreement possible. The existence of the nurse/patient agreement implies that nurse and patient have a right to, and function on the basis of, veracity.

Agreement in the Absence of Privacy

Individuals must enjoy some degree of isolation from one another. Without the freedom from distraction provided by this isolation an individual could not maintain his integrity or function effectively. A patient comes into a health care setting in order to maintain or to regain his integrity and his capacity to function.

Everyone has a need for privacy—for a certain degree of isolation. This isolation is essential for a person's self-awareness. It is also essential for the exercise of a person's freedom. This isolation is the value that the standard of privacy offers the individual.

If a person has no right to privacy, then there is no such thing as self-ownership. If one has no right to self-ownership, he has no right to make an agreement. One cannot make an agreement for the disposition of that which he does not own. He cannot agree to exert effort if he does not own and control his effort. He cannot agree to devote time if he does not own his time. No one who is not a private person has a secure hold on his time and effort. Everyone who has a secure hold on his time and effort is a *private* person.

It would be folly for Rose to attempt to make an agreement with Fred. Fred is a peculiar person in that he is entirely public. Fred does not own himself. If Rose wants an agreement, she must go to whomever owns Fred at that moment in order to make the agreement. Fred cannot make an agreement on his own. With Fred there is no "on his own."

An agreement with Fred would be as unstable as a figure in a cloud. Fred might make an agreement with Rose. He might devote several moments to fulfilling his agreement with Rose. Then he might very well run off to meet some other demand that has been made on him.

Agreement in the Absence of Beneficence

Every individual person has a need to achieve good and avoid harm. Beneficence is a bioethical standard (and, more generally, a standard of ethical action) because humans are beings who can impede and injure as well as benefit one another. The standard of beneficence arises when ethical agents have attained a sufficient degree of rationality to recognize the advantages of doing good or at least doing no harm.

People can impede and injure one another. This is proved by the fact that they do impede and injure one another. They can also agree on and exercise beneficence toward one another. This is proved by the fact that they do exercise beneficence toward one another. The biomedical sciences are a concrete expression of this beneficence.

Agreements serve a purpose in human lives. This purpose is the benefits that people gain through cooperation. Through cooperation ethical agents are able to achieve good and to avoid harm. It contradicts the nature of an agreement, then, that people would form an agreement and, within the confines of that agreement, refuse to do good or at least do no harm to one another.

It is easy to see that Rose would not even attempt to make an agreement with Bert. Bert's peculiarity is the fact that he cannot recognize the difference between beneficence and maleficence.[1] Rose is aware that there is no value in an agreement with Bert. She cannot confidently expect good from Bert, nor can she be certain that he will do her no harm.

In the same way if patients cannot expect beneficence from nurses, there will be no value in the existence of nurses. If nurses were maleficent, then only a fool would have a nurse.

Agreement in the Absence of Fidelity

It is a very easy matter to see that no agreement between two people can be maintained if the standard of fidelity is not maintained. Fidelity is an outgrowth of the other standards. To gain the benefits of interaction individuals must be able to rely on each other. This reliance is made possible by the tacit and explicit understandings upon which their interaction is based. Fidelity is fidelity to these understandings.

A denial of the relevance of any of the bioethical standards to the agreement cannot be logically justified. In one way or another the denial would make a claim that, if it were true, would undermine all possibility of an agreement. To greatly simplify the matter, it is rather like someone declaring, "I don't speak a word of English," when the very fact that this claim is made *in English* falsifies it.

Fortunately, we can assume that Rose is too bright to attempt to make an agreement with Pete. Pete is someone who has no power to remain faithful to an agreement. To be able to make an agreement while being unable to remain faithful to it is an impossible situation. A person is either able to make an agreement and to remain faithful to it, or he is unable to remain faithful to an agreement and, therefore, unable to make an agreement.

Fidelity is fidelity to an agreement. We cannot imagine Rose saying "There is an agreement between Pete and me but we feel no obligation to be faithful to this agreement." Their situation would be no different than the situation between two people who had no agreement at all.

It is no less absurd to say, "There is an agreement between Bert and me, but we feel no obligation to extend beneficence to one another." If there is no obligation to extend beneficence, then the agreement places no obligation on either party. The obligation would be an obligation to extend some form of beneficence. An agreement that places no obligation on either party is, very obviously, no agreement at all.

It is equally absurd to state, "Fred and I have an agreement but neither of us is a private person."

It is absurd to declare, "Herb and I recognize the existence of an agreement between us, but we see no reason to be dependably truthful with each other." This is worse than saying, "Herb and I have an agreement, but we do not know what the terms of the agreement are."

It is absurd to declare, "Mike and I have made an agreement, but I do not believe that Mike has the right to exercise free action."

It is absurd to state, "Art is totally lacking in autonomy and there is an agreement between Art and myself."

It is absurd to declare, "As a nurse I have an implicit agreement, with every patient, to fulfill my role as nurse. But I do not admit the necessity of recognizing my patient's right to the bioethical standards."

If a nurse is one who makes an implicit, but specific agreement with a patient, then a nurse must, in her attitude and behavior, be guided by the bioethical standards. A nurse who would reject any of the bioethical standards is, quite simply, not a nurse. Her claim, explicitly or implicitly, is that she is a nurse and, at the same time, she is not a nurse. But nothing in the world can be a nurse and, at the same time, not be a nurse.

SUMMARY

We have established that

- Nursing as an intelligible activity relies on the nurse/patient agreement.
- The nurse/patient agreement presupposes the bioethical standards.
- The bioethical standards reflect those aspects of human nature that make the nurse/patient agreement desirable and *possible*.
- The existence of the nurse/patient agreement implies the appropriateness of the bioethical standards as standards.

Every person is unique. So is every bullfrog and every waterfall unique. And every group of persons is unique.

The uniqueness described in the bioethical standard of autonomy is not the uniqueness of bullfrogs, waterfalls, or groups. It is the uniqueness of individual people.

The freedom described in the bioethical standard of freedom is a freedom to choose, decide, and act. This is a freedom only possessed by individual people.

Veracity is a biological device whose purpose is the well-being of individuals.

Privacy, clearly, is the privacy of individuals. One defining characteristic of a group is the absence of privacy.

Beneficence is a value that benefits. Any value that benefits is a value that benefits individual persons.

Fidelity is a virtue that can be practiced only by individuals, one by one.

Wherever nursing has a logical foundation, it is an activity essentially involving individual nurses and their individual patients. Every other nursing activity (education, administration, research, etc.) is an outgrowth of this.

The bioethical standards, as we have seen, are implied by the nurse/patient agreement. But, as we have also seen, they are not sufficient, by themselves, to govern the relationship between nurse and patient. We will now turn to the bridge between the bioethical standards and the people to whom they apply.

NOTE

1   If beneficence is "to do good or at least do no harm" (Hippocrates), then maleficence will be to do harm or at least to refuse to do good (where one might reasonably be expected to do good).

REFERENCE

Herstein, G.L. (1983). Form-value triva-
   lent logic. *Synapse*, 39, 7-9.

PART TWO

BIOETHICS AND THE NATURE OF INDIVIDUAL AUTONOMY

CHAPTER

10

Aspects of Human Nature as Elements of Ethical Knowledge

Socrates was one of the most famous of philosophers. Libraries of books have been written about this great ethicist. Yet Socrates himself wrote nothing. Virtually everything the modern world knows about Socrates is learned from Plato, his student. Indeed, it is not absolutely certain that Socrates was a real person. However, a Greek playwright of the time, Aristophanes, wrote *The Clouds*, a play in which Socrates is a character. This gives added weight to the probability that he was an actual person and not just a creation of Plato's literary imagination.

Aristophanes depicts Socrates and the other Greek philosophers of his time as floating around in the skies, spinning vast patterns of airy thoughts out of clouds.

This picture of ethicists is not too far from the mark. Almost every ethicist, as physician Leon Kass declares, is guilty of dealing with vague and nonessential abstractions:

> In the practice of ethics today . . . the action is mostly talk . . . . Philosophical ethics . . . spends little time on . . . motives and passions . . . matters . . . not simply reducible to [speculation]. It, by and large, ignores real moral agents and concrete moral situations. (Kass, 1990, p. 6)

There is an overwhelming temptation to treat ethics as an impractical and speculative science. It is all too easy to make even the bioethical standards empty and useless abstractions woven out of clouds. People do this by simply splitting the standards off from the purposes of moral individuals acting in concrete moral situations.

There is a way to bring the standards down out of the clouds and to keep them from floating away again. This can be done by analyzing all the bioethical standards in terms of individual autonomy. We will, so to speak, define the standards in terms of the elements that constitute the autonomy of individuals. First, we will discuss the reasons why ethical abstractions are so subject to abstract and irrelevant speculation.

WHY THIS CLOUDY SPECULATION?

There are several reasons why the bioethical standards are made objects of speculation unrelated to the ethical purposes of biomedical professionals and patients:

1. Patients are viewed as collections of characteristics. There is no wholistic view of the individual.
2. A professional often fails to recognize the difference between a professional ethic and childhood training. The professional assumes that all that is needed is the application of his or her childhood training to the profession. This failure makes it impossible for the professional to form a context as complex as the bioethical context can become.
3. There is the failure to which Dr. Kass points—the failure to distinguish between different levels of ethical knowledge. These various levels are:
   a. The level of very broad abstractions—the nature of autonomy, the reality of human freedom, etc.
   b. A narrower level of abstractions—a patient's right to autonomy, a patient's right to exercise his freedom, etc.
   c. The concrete level of ethical applications—Harry's unique nature, George's way of exercising his freedom, etc.
4. The professional fails to differentiate between the solitary and the interpersonal ethical context. This generally occurs when the solitary context is ignored.
5. The professional tends to develop ethical knowledge without reference to the understanding to be gained through introspection; this single failure will diminsh every ethical success.

This last failure is the most tragic of all ethical failures. This is an agent's failure to reflect upon self, inner awareness, and evaluations. In order to gain understanding through introspection a nurse must both reflect upon herself and the meanings that things have for her, and reflect on her inner aware-ness—her evaluation of different people and events.

KNOWLEDGE OF NATURES VERSUS KNOWLEDGE OF CHARACTERISTICS

Childhood training is, generally speaking, training in obedience to rules. It is an intertwining of very broad ethical abstractions (rules) and the rights or supposed rights of others. It has no relationship to any agreement between ethical agents.

Nurses sometimes fail to properly apply the standards because, as the saying goes, they "do not see the forest for trees." They see a few of their patient's characteristics but do not see the whole unique person.

The bioethical standards are values that a patient seeks in the biomedical setting. They are also specific expressions of a patient's rights.

A nurse can learn what her patient's rights are by memorizing what she is told by others. Then, through the understanding of his rights which she gains in this way, she can infer what he is. This odd but often used approach is equivalent to a student studying technical skills without learning the clinical skills. She learns what nursing is only from books and lectures. Then she goes directly from the classroom into the health care setting. Ask yourself what the results of her nursing interventions would be.

There is no reason why the same sort of results cannot occur in ethical contexts. In fact the same poor results do occur in ethical contexts; it is simply not as easy to perceive their tragic nature. It is easier to rationalize them away: I was doing my duty. I was thinking of the greater number. I was being honest.

Nurses, like other professionals, often make flawed ethical judgments. They do this by applying broad ethical generalizations to ethical situations when these generalizations are inappropriate. There are unique features to the situation which the nurse overlooks. These unique features make any generalization inappropriate.

Rita has been told that her patient Sam has a right to his autonomy, to freedom to make his own decisions, to receive truthful communications from her, to privacy, and to beneficence from her. Rita comes to know Sam, on an ethical level, through this knowledge. She knows that Sam possesses these rights. She knows only the characteristics of Sam. Even this she knows only on an abstract level. That is *all* Rita's education has taught her about Sam. She learns nothing about Sam from Sam.

Betsy knows, by introspection, the inner nature of her patient Saul. Saul is a living being motivated by desire. Saul is a being who determines his actions through reason. His actions are purposeful. He values his agency—his capac-ity to take actions.

INTROSPECTION

An Exercise

Introspection is the observation of one's self and one's mental states and processes. It is an examination of one's thoughts, feelings, and evaluations. It is a reflecting back on one's self.

Here is an ideal opportunity to practice a little introspection on a most basic level. Ask yourself these questions:

Am I, the reader, a living being?

(If you have asked yourself this question, you may be quite certain that the answer to it is yes.)

Am I motivated by desire?

Am I a being who must determine my actions through reason?

(This question does not assume that a person is *forced* to act through reason. It simply assumes that a person can act *effectively* only when he or she directs his or her actions by reason.)

Am I a being whose actions are purposeful? Do I act to accomplish things?

Do I desire to retain my capacity to take actions?

Betsy asked herself these questions. She knows these desires, actions, and states of being to be true of herself. She knows them, also, to be true of Saul. She knows what they mean to Saul by being aware of them as true of herself.

How a Nurse Gains Bioethical Understanding

Through introspection a person will discover two types of facts:

1. One will discover aspects of oneself that are peculiar to oneself. These are facts such as: I enjoy the city better than the countryside. I am afraid of butterflies. I would like to learn three foreign languages.

    The person has experience of other people and discovers that these facts are not true of everyone.

2. One person will discover aspects of oneself that are common to all people. These are facts such as: I am motivated by desire. I cannot act effectively without exercising a prior process of reasoning. I experience my actions as purposeful. I act toward goals.

The object of a nurse's ethical understanding—the nature of her patient as an ethical agent—is a very complex state of affairs.

Betsy discovers her own characteristics through introspection. Through her awareness of Saul, she discovers that these are also his characteristics. Far more important she discovers the inner nature of these characteristics. She discovers them, so to speak, from the inside.

Rita's knowledge of Sam is a knowledge of Sam's rights and characteristics. It is a relatively superficial knowledge—like knowing of trees that they are very large plants.

Betsy's knowledge of Saul is based on a much deeper and more thoughtful understanding. It is based on her knowledge of the autonomy, the uniqueness, of Saul.

Betsy's understanding of Saul allows her to infer a great number of facts about him. Rita understands Sam as a being possessing a right to certain ethical standards, yet this knowledge allows her to infer nothing about Sam as an individual person. It is very little knowledge and no understanding at all.

Let us examine this on a different, much simpler, and nonethical level:

Someone, looking out of a window, tells you, "There is something in the street out there." You ask, "What is it?" The reply you receive is, "I cannot tell you that, but I will tell you that it rolls."

To know that a certain thing rolls is to know almost nothing about it.

Balls roll. Wheels roll. Coins, marbles, and stones roll. Children roll. Logs roll. Pencils, bottles, dogs, and pieces of candy roll. To know that something rolls is not enough to have an adequate knowledge of what it is. To know that something is a ball or a child is to have much more knowledge of it. To know that it is a golf ball or an 8-year-old girl is to have even more knowledge of it.

So it is also with ethical knowledge. Knowledge of a person is a higher form of ethical knowledge than knowing the characteristics of people in general. To know the characteristics of people, in general, however, is a higher form of ethical knowledge than to know a word signifying an ethical abstraction.

SOURCES OF ETHICAL KNOWLEDGE AND THE CONTEXTS THEY PRODUCE

Nurses sometimes fail to properly apply the standards because they fail to get into the bioethical context.

Sometimes, in order to understand one context (the bioethical context), it is useful to examine a different, simpler context. It will be necessary once again to call upon the resources of your imagination. We are now going to examine a simple, nonethical context in order to illuminate the more complex bioethical situation.

A wine-tasting gathering is a particular type of party. It is a party where a number of people get together and taste samples of perhaps six to twelve different wines.

Imagine that you are at a wine-tasting party. Your host tells you, "One of the eight wines in our tasting tonight will be stronger and more assertive than the others. Let's call this "excessive." One of the wines, this evening, will be excessive in comparison to the other wines."

As you taste the different wines, you discover that one wine is, indeed, much stronger and more assertive than the others. It is, indeed, "excessive."

Eight wines, one "excessive" in relation to the others, are all that is needed to form a situation. It is not all that is needed to form a context. Something more is needed for this.

If you enjoy strength and assertiveness in a wine you will, probably, enjoy this wine. If you do not; if you find it harsh and unpleasant — let us call this, also, "excessive" — then you will not enjoy the wine.

Your enjoyment, or lack of enjoyment, allows for an examination of the context:

You have found one wine "excessive" in relation to the other wines. It is much stronger and more assertive than the other wines.

It requires a separate judgment to discover whether you find it "excessive" in relation to yourself. This judgment is an evaluation.

It is obvious that you cannot discover whether the wine is "excessive" in relation to yourself simply by examining the situation. You have to look into yourself — into your own experience and evaluation. When you do, then a context comes into being.

So it is with an ethical context.

In a solitary ethical context you must examine the situation plus your experience of it, your prior knowledge, and your evaluation of it in relation to yourself. In an interpersonal ethical context a nurse ought to examine the situation plus the values and purposes of the other moral agents in the context.

This is the way a nurse must function in the biomedical context. That this is so can be discovered through introspection. Ask yourself these questions:

- Would I feel confidence in the ethical actions of a person who was guided *entirely* by memorized abstractions — freedom, veracity, privacy, and so on?
- Would I feel ethically understood by someone who understood me only as a being possessing a right to freedom, veracity, privacy, etc., and whose understanding had nothing to do with my present purposes?
- Would I feel confidence in a nurse if her ethical actions toward me were determined only by her childhood training?
- Would I feel ethically at home with someone whose ethical interactions with me were guided by "lessons" she had learned from others?

If your answer to these questions is no, you might remember that your patient would answer in the same way.

THE LEVELS OF ETHICAL KNOWLEDGE

Nurses sometimes fail to properly apply the bioethical standards because they fail to distinguish between different levels of ethical knowledge.

Vague and out-of-context ethical generalizations are at best chancy and at worst counterproductive.

To "know" that:
Humans are autonomous beings, or
Humans are beings possessing freedom, or
Humans are, unlike bees and ants, private beings, or
Humans are beings with a need to possess truth

is to know next door to nothing about what is necessary to guide ethical decision making and action.

Remembering that conflicts can arise among the standards, ask yourself this: A nurse knows that "Humans are beings possessing freedom." Based on this knowledge alone, is this nurse capable of making a dependable ethical judgment?

No.

To know, in addition to the above, that:

Jane has a right to have her autonomy respected, or
Jane has a right to make free choices and take free actions, or
Jane has a right to privacy, or
Jane has a right to interactions based on truth

is to have much more knowledge about the ethical decision-making process.

Ask yourself this: A nurse knows that Jane has a right to freedom of action. Based on this knowledge alone, is this nurse capable of making an efficient ethical judgment in regard to Jane?

By no means. Not knowing what Jane's desires are, the nurse could not know what Jane's freedom consists in.

If a nurse knows, in addition to the above, that:

Jane is unique in certain specific ways, or
Jane is motivated to make certain specific choices and take certain specific actions, or
Jane desires privacy in certain specific areas, or
Jane needs certain specific truths in order to make her choices and actions

then the nurse has enough knowledge to make effective ethical decisions.

In order to master these stages of knowledge a nurse needs to go through an ethical evolution.

Suzy drops in on Larry, her colostomy patient. Larry asks Suzy about potential problems he might encounter with his colostomy. Suzy is feeling "up" today and does not want to discuss dreary subjects. But she reminds herself that humans are beings who need to possess truth. So sadly, almost begrudgingly, Suzy counsels with Larry about his colostomy. In this context there is only a wisp of the ethical. Using the truism that "Humans are beings who need to possess truth," Suzy is able to make a decision. She does not think of what information would be appropriate for Larry to have, based on his unique situation and desires. She is not able to know why the decision is right — not in this context. She has gained nothing to bring to another similar context.

A few years later Suzy drops in on another colostomy patient, Terry. Terry asks Suzy about potential problems he might encounter with his colostomy. Again Suzy is feeling "up" that day and would rather not discuss dreary subjects. But by this time Suzy has grown into her role as a nurse. Part of this role is imparting to a patient certain information that he needs and that she has. Suzy knows that Terry has a right to interactions based on truth. She is aware of the existence of an agreement between herself, as a nurse, and Terry, as her patient. This agreement places on Suzy the responsibility of putting Terry's right to truth above her mood. It places a responsibility on Suzy to communicate information to Terry.

Suzy knows that what is ethically right and wrong, on her part, depends upon her fidelity to the terms of their agreement. This much is self-evident.

With Terry, Suzy is much more competent. She has a better understanding of ethical decision making than she did when Larry was her patient. She is far less likely to take unjustifiable ethical actions based on a faulty decision-making process.

A year or two later Suzy drops in on Paul. Paul is also a colostomy patient. Paul asks Suzy about potential problems he might encounter with his colostomy. Again Suzy is feeling "up" but now there is no conflict between her mood and her obligation to her patient. She has come to think of her patient's disability as her adversary and her patient as her friend.

Suzy gives Paul the information he will need to deal with the problems he might have with his colostomy. She bases this information on Paul's situation and life style. She gives Paul the specific information that *he* needs to make choices and to take actions.

Originally Suzy's ethical understanding was centered on ethical abstractions. This is where she began. Then she grew to the point where her ethical understanding became centered on the rights of patients. This was Suzy's ethical adolescence. Now Suzy's ethical understanding is based on knowledge she acquires of her individual patient. She now has a much better understanding of her patient's rights. She also has a much greater understanding of what these ethical abstractions mean — how they relate to the outside world. She has grown into ethical maturity.

Suzy knows that the fundamental characteristic of patients is that they are reasoning beings. Because of this she knows that she must communicate with them and interact with them truthfully and objectively.

She knows that each of her patients is motivated by unique desires. That is to say: Every patient comes at the world from a unique vantage point. A person's uniqueness determines the way he experiences and expresses his desires (his affective life).

Suzy knows that every patient is, by nature, an agent, a being who acts independently for his or her own purposes. She knows, therefore, that every patient needs respect for self-ownership. Every patient has a right to privacy.

She knows that her patients enter the hospital because they are motivated by the desire to escape harm and pain and regain their health and well-being.

She knows that, in ordinary circumstances, her patients act to overcome adversities. She knows that her function as a nurse is to act for a patient in order to overcome adversities of a kind that he cannot overcome alone.

Suzy knows that every patient is a living being of a specific kind. She understands this kind of being through her self-knowledge. Her patient is the same kind of being as she is. Therefore she knows that it is appropriate for her to interact with him beneficently. It is ethically appropriate that she interact with him in a way which will bring him good or at least bring him no harm.

She knows that her patients, in common with all people, pursue values and possess rights. She knows that they enter the health care system in pursuit of the values of health and well-being. She knows that they have rights before they come into the health care system. She knows that they do not lose these rights while they are there.

She agrees to interact with her patient according to the unique person he is. This is what people who enter the health care system expect — and have a right to expect — and do not always find.

In her role as nurse Suzy exercises fidelity to the agreement that she has with her patients. This is because she understands her patients. She understands them as beings like herself. She feels empathy with them. She has a personal desire to exercise fidelity to the agreement.

INTROSPECTION AS AN ETHICAL ASSET

Suzy knows all of this through observation combined with introspection. Introspection gives her a knowledge of ethical agents and agency by giving her access to her own human nature. Introspection is not something that has to be learned. Everyone introspects. Without the power of introspection it would be impossible for a person to take appropriate actions in relation to his or her world.

Very often a nurse may have the experience of doing precisely the right thing. She will do this one right thing for precisely the right reason. She will have an insight into the nature and desires of her patient. She will perceive the whole context, and she will know exactly what the context requires. Her effective ethical action will be made possible by introspection. She will know what her patient wants because she will know what, in these circumstances, any person would want. She, in turn, will know this because she will see what she would want — not as Suzy, but simply as a human being.

An obvious example:

Suzy comes into Oscar's room. Oscar is the athletic father of two. Oscar was in an automobile accident and he is on a respirator. Suzy sees that the respirator is malfunctioning. If Oscar is to live, she must act immediately. She begins to manually operate the respirator. Then she calls for emergency assistance. Suzy spends no time deliberating. She knows that, in this situation, she would want to live. She knows that the probability that Oscar wants to live is overwhelming. In a situation this clear cut, the bioethical standards are irrelevant — except as a subconscious backdrop to her context of knowledge.

SOLITARY CONTEXTS AND THE INTERPERSONAL CONTEXT

Nurses sometimes fail to properly apply the standards because they fail to differentiate between the solitary and the interpersonal context.

The nature of an ethical context is brought into being and determined by the nature of an ethical agent. An ethical agent often acts within an interpersonal context. Every interpersonal context, however, begins in a solitary context. It is in a solitary context that an individual evaluates and acts to gain that which he or she sees as good and avoid that which he or she sees as evil. The individual enters into an interpersonal context whenever he or she sees cooperation as being the best way to gain values or to avoid evils.

Every ethical agent gains *knowledge* of good and evil, however, in a solitary context.

A certain nurse, Nora, acquired her bioethical understanding in the interpersonal context of nursing. It came to her in the form of disconnected generalizations. She learned, in a manner of speaking, what was good through group approval. She learned of evil through group disapproval. Her bioethical understanding never became an integral part of her life. She had no first-hand way of relating it to her inner life or to the inner life of her patient.

In a solitary context she could have gained ethical knowledge through observation and through introspection. In this context she would learn by referring her experience of the desires and aversions of others to the reasons for her own desires and aversions. Her bioethical understanding would have begun with a first-hand knowledge of her patients.

Another nurse, Agatha, acquired her ethical knowledge in a solitary context. She acquired her ethical knowledge by thinking about her life and the lives of other people. Agatha was able to acquire the essentials of bioethics even before she became a nurse. She first learned about her own ethical nature. From this she learned what is generally true of ethical agents. Then she applied this to the nature of her patient. Her patient became, for Agatha, like "another self."

Agatha acquired her foundational knowledge of ethics very much like a person might acquire a thorough knowledge of, to give a simple example, apples.

The best knowledge of apples a person could acquire would come through direct experience. A person learns what an apple is by looking at it, feeling it, smelling it, and tasting it. Finally, perhaps, the person learns what an apple tastes like in a pie.

Acquiring ethical knowledge in an interpersonal context is like learning about the apple by hearing descriptions of it, but without ever seeing or feeling or smelling or tasting a real, three-dimensional apple.

In the solitary context a person acts as agent and as observer:

- She begins by perceiving an ethical context. This context promises to bring her some good or it threatens her with some harm.

Elaine is a nurse on a neurologic unit. She wants to get to the hospital before Walter, her favorite patient, has his operation. When she leaves her home, she discovers that her car has a flat tire. This threatens the possibility of her getting to the hospital before Walter goes to surgery. The flat tire interferes with Elaine's exercising her freedom of action.

- She moves to act within the context which promises benefit or to avoid the context which threatens harm.

Elaine calls the auto club to come and change the tire.

- She observes the results the context has on her purposes.

The result of the flat tire is that Walter is taken into surgery before Elaine arrives at the hospital.

- Through an examination of the effects that the context has on her purposes, she judges what their quality would be in an ethical context.

Elaine's problems in getting to the hospital form a nonethical context. The tire did not choose to be flat. Nonetheless the effects of the flat tire are undesirable. The flat tire interferes with Elaine's taking an action that is important to her.

In an ethical context, when someone chooses to interfere with an important action, the effects are an ethical evil. The effects of this interference are no more undesirable than the effects of the flat tire. But they are avoidable. Therefore they are relevant to ethics.

Elaine realizes that unjustifiable interference with the actions of another *ought* to be avoided.

- She stores away her understanding of this in the form of a useful generalization, an item of ethical knowledge.

Elaine, of course, cannot violate her own right to freedom. Nor can Elaine's flat tire violate her rights. If, however, another ethical agent chose to interfere with Elaine's ethical action this would violate her rights.

- Elaine then applies this understanding to the interpersonal context.

Elaine realizes that, if she interferes with the free action of another person, this is a violation of that person's rights. She decides that, in her interactions with others, she will not interfere with their freedom of action.

The evolution of a nurse's ethical understanding to the point where she can have an actual *knowledge* of the bioethical standards will always proceed, more or less, in this way. If, in her earliest years, a nurse has given attention to her experience and her evaluation of things, it will be easy for her to understand the value of the bioethical standards. If she has not, it will be more difficult.

If the nurse has not thought of the meaning of things in relation to herself, she will have a difficult time understanding the meaning of things in relation to others. She will learn the bioethical standards by being told of them. She will learn them without taking them into her inner experience and making them part of herself. Because of her limited understanding she will always regard the bioethical standards as rules.

If the nurse has prepared the way for her understanding of the bioethical standards, they will become a part of her self-understanding. This self-understanding can be gained only in a solitary context—while she is *with* herself.

For this reason nurses, and people in general, need and value privacy. They need privacy to experience, to think and to learn about themselves and their values.

A person completely lacking self-knowledge could not have any motivation to ethical interactions, and thus would have no reason to act. This person would have no motivation to form agreements with others. There would be no values to be pursued and nothing to be communicated to others.

This person would not find this particularly stressful because he or she would have no motivation to communicate.

All ethical understanding begins in self-understanding. All ethical interaction begins in an agent's privacy. From the vantage point of an individual person, ethical interaction is shared privacy.

A person's most basic ethical actions occur in a solitary context. In the solitary context, if an individual acts successfully, according to his or her nature, the person attains that which is good and avoids that which is evil. People sometimes find they can attain good or avoid evil by acting together. For this reason they make agreements. Through these agreements a solitary context becomes an interpersonal context.

It is a value to a nurse to understand the nature of the patient with whom she is interacting. In order to do this it is necessary for her to come to understand the nature of her patient as a human being like herself.

It is inconceivable that any nurse would ever gain a knowledge of the nature of her patient as a human being, and as an ethical agent, unless she had first gained this knowledge of herself.

If the nurse learns of human nature through introspection, through the acquisition of self-knowledge, she will be learning of it by, so to speak, seeing it, feeling it, tasting it, touching it, and hearing it. If she gains all her knowledge of human nature from others, she will not be learning of human nature as a natural reality. She will learn only the disconnected characteristics of ethical agents.

To know that something rolls is to know almost nothing about it. To know that someone cries is to know almost nothing about that person — unless you know what crying is. If you do know what crying is, you have not learned it merely by watching someone cry.

INTROSPECTION AND ETHICAL KNOWLEDGE

Nurses sometimes fail to properly apply the bioethical standards because they have learned nothing about ethical action through introspection.

An adequate knowledge of the nature of human beings must be gained through an examination of one's self and one's own nature. A person has no access to the inner and personal world of another. The inner world of another can be understood only by beginning with what one finds to be true of oneself.

To learn about others a person begins with his or her own characteristics. Then, through observing others, the learner identifies what characteristics people have in common. After this the only task is to determine how these characteristics are expressed in each individual person. This determination will reveal the meaning of these characteristics to the person in whom they are expressed.

At the same time, in order for a person to gain this awareness and, with it, a knowledge of his or her self, it is necessary to have the knowledge of human personality gained by observing other people.

This seems to present a dilemma:

> A person needs an understanding of other people in order to understand his or her own self.
> *But*
> A person needs an understanding of himself or herself in order to understand other people.

If both of these assumptions are true then, it seems, no one can ever understand self or understand other people.

In order to resolve this dilemma we will consider it as a much simpler, nonethical problem, one described and resolved by the ethicist, Benedict Spinoza (cited in Gutman, 1949).

Spinoza proposes two facts, apparently contradictory to each other.

- In order to make a hammer it is necessary for a person to be able to work iron.
- In order for a person to be able to work iron he needs a hammer.

Therefore it seems that no one can work iron and there can be no such thing as a hammer.

For a person must *have* a hammer in order to make a hammer.

But, a person must be able to *make* a hammer in order to have a hammer.

Therefore, it seems, it is impossible either to make or to have a hammer.

And yet, people do have hammers. People are able to work iron and to make hammers.

Hammersmiths began with whatever assets they had ready at hand, perhaps stones. They perfect these assets, more and more, until they have a primitive type of hammer. With this they are able to work iron . . . primitively.

The better they become at working iron the better hammer they can produce. The better hammer they can produce the better they can work iron.

So it is also with ethical understanding.

A person looks into his or her self and gains a better understanding of others.

Then the person observes others and gains a better understanding of his or her self.

This process continues and expands until the person reaches the fullest understanding he or she ever has of his or her self and of others.

A nurse begins by observing herself.

She observes:

- Her desire for autonomy—for the power to be who she is and to become everything she can become.
- Her desire for freedom—for the power to act for herself in order to realize her own purposes.
- Her need for a true and objective understanding of her world.
- Her need to maintain her self-ownership.
- Her desire to attain good and avoid harm.

Through these observations she gains a slightly better understanding of herself. Then she observes others and discovers:

- Their desire to maintain their autonomy. She observes the pleasure they take in being who and what they are.
- The pleasure they take in the fact of their freedom.
- The actions they take to gain a true and objective understanding of their world.
- The pleasure they take in their self-ownership.
- The actions they take in order to attain good and avoid evil.

Through this process she gains a better understanding of her patient. She becomes able to act confidently and to justify her actions. The process continues and expands until she reaches her fullest ethical understanding—the widest understanding she is ever able to gain of herself and her patient.

SUMMARY

The bioethical standards serve as general guides for ethical decision making. Any rational, justifiable ethical decision must be preceded by a process of ethical decision making. Ethical decision making, in turn, must be preceeded by ethical judgment. It cannot be any better than the judgment on which it is based. Before an ethical agent can know what to do, he or she must know who is involved and why it is being done. This knowledge is gained only through judgment. Rational, justifiable judgment must be guided by the elements of individual autonomy.

These elements are principles of human nature. They are the principles that make every individual what he or she is.

A knowledge of the bioethical standards is an essential part of a nurse's context of knowledge. However, knowledge of the bioethical standards is insufficient for the nurse to effectively engage in an ethical decision-making process.

As we have seen, the individual standards can appear to come into conflict. There can be a conflict in the interpretation of an individual standard. There can, also, be conflicts between two or more standards.

Something more is needed for a nurse to apply the bioethical standards effectively and appropriately. This something more is a knowledge of the ethical elements—the elements of human autonomy.

No one can be human and be completely unfamiliar with that which makes him or her autonomous. Eveyone is familiar with the elements of human autonomy, at least, on an implicit level. It is quite advantageous for a nurse to become familiar with them explicitly.

REFERENCES

Gutman, J. (Ed.). (1949). *Spinoza's ethics*. New York: Hafner Publishing Company.

Kass, L.R. (1990). Practicing ethics: Where's the action? *Hastings Center Report, 20*(6), 6-12.

Desire and the Ethical Context

Imagine a world in which desire is not a part of human nature. This world is a tropical island floating among the clouds. On this island all the necessities of survival—fruit trees, cool water, etc.—are readily at hand. There is no motivation through discontent, no awareness that human life can be more than basic necessities. The faculty of desire has withered away, or else the inhabitants of the world never possessed a faculty of desire.

In this world there are no specifically human realities. There are no human purposes, no human choices, and no human actions. In this world every action is conducted on an animal level. Therefore nothing is good and nothing is evil. Nothing is either right or wrong.

In such a world ethics, as a study, would be inconceivable. In this world where there is no human desire, there are no vital and fundamental goals. If there are no vital and fundamental goals, there is no need for a system of principles to motivate or determine or justify vital and fundamental goals. Life itself would be unimportant. If desire were not an element of human nature, there would be no ethical realities of any sort.

Ethical realities exist in the world only because desire *is* an element of human nature.

LIFE WITHOUT DESIRE

If you recall, Rose could make no agreement with any of the peculiar people who belong to her skiing club. Therefore she could not engage in purposeful (ethical) action with them.

155

Art, if you recall, lacked autonomy. The benefit that two people can be to each other is cancelled if there is not some difference between them. Art was, in effect, identical to Rose.

Mike lacked freedom. People cannot act in cooperation with one another if they lack the capacity to take voluntary actions.

Herb had no capacity to receive and relate the truth. No agreement is possible where future events cannot be predicted. Future events cannot be predicted if they involve someone who lacks veracity. The actions of someone who lacks veracity cannot be predicted.

Fred had no capacity to exercise the virtue of privacy. He lacked self-ownership. People cannot depend upon the actions of someone who lacked self-ownership.

Bert lacked beneficence. The purpose, the very reason for being, of any agreement is the realization of some benefit. It is certainly not reasonable to make an agreement with someone from whom no benefit can be expected.

Pete lacked the ability to remain faithful to agreements. An agreement to which no one remained faithful would be no agreement at all. In a world filled with Petes there would be no agreements.

Dana, the seventh member of the skiing club, lacks all these virtues. He lacks them because he utterly lacks desire. Each of the bioethical standards depends upon desire.

During a person's lifetime he or she experiences many desires — or rather desires many things. In back of all these desires is a desire for desire itself. This is not a desire for any specific choice or decision or action. It is, rather, a desire to retain the capacity to choose, decide, and act. It is the desire for life and purpose.

A person totally without desire would not be able to understand, or to act on, the standards. The desire to retain the capacity to desire is the precondition of any exercise or understanding of the bioethical standards.

Each of the bioethical standards is either a form of desire itself or is based upon some form of desire:

- *Autonomy*, to the autonomous person, is the desire to be what and who he or she is.

Dana possesses no uniqueness in any *ethical* sense. He lacks the desire to be what and who he is, therefore, he lacks ethical autonomy.

- *Freedom* is the capacity and the desire to take action.

If someone possesses no capacity or no desire to take an action then, he is not free to take it.

Suppose that Lilly cannot fly by waving her arms. Then she is not, in any rational sense of "free," free to fly by waving her arms.

Suppose that Joe is on an ocean voyage. Joe could jump into the sea and play with the sharks, but he has no desire whatever to do this. So his "freedom" to do it is meaningless. If he absolutely lacks desire, he lacks freedom.

Dana is not free.

Dana not only lacks the desire to take actions and make agreements, he lacks all capacity for action and agreement. Since he lacks the desire and capacity for action, no ethical facts pertain to Dana in a solitary context. Since he lacks the desire and capacity to make agreements, no ethical facts pertain to him in an interpersonal context.

- Veracity is always thought of as referring to a person's telling the truth or failing to tell the truth. Veracity is much more than this. On its most basic level it is a desire to relate to some state of affairs objectively. Telling the truth to another must necessarily begin with telling the truth to oneself. A desire to communicate a state of affairs as it really is can originate only in the desire to relate to it as it really is.

Veracity as an ethical value and as a bioethical standard involves more than truth telling. It involves a nurse or patient doing what is necessary to know things as they actually are.

Dana has no desire to know things as they actually are.

Lacking all desire as he does, Dana has no desire to think of things in abstract terms. Therefore he lacks all interest in receiving or communicating truth.

In regard to matters of truth and falsity Dana lacks even curiousity. How could it be otherwise? Curiousity is a form of desire. It is the desire to know. Dana desires nothing.

- The value of privacy presupposes a desire for self-ownership. A catatonic person has no concern with privacy and cannot practice the virtue of self-ownership. This does not at all mean that the catatonic person has no right to privacy.

Dana lacks all desire for privacy. He is entirely lacking in self-interest. He has no sense of self-ownership. In order to be interested in one's self, in order to have a sense of self-ownership, a person must value things for his or her *own* sake. These are virtues that are impossible for Dana to possess.

- The case is very much the same in regard to *beneficence*. Beneficence is the doing of what is good and the avoidance of what might, forseeably, cause harm. The source of a person's beneficence is his or her benevolence — his or her feelings of good will. It is a sense of empathy with other human beings. Benevolence is the desire to see good come to others and the desire to see them suffer no harm.

Dana is entirely callous. Good and harm are equally matters of indifference to him. For Dana the standard of beneficence is an absolutely meaningless concept.

  • *Fidelity* is based upon a person's desire to make successful agreements. It is the desire to see an agreement through to its completion.

Dana is, quite obviously, incapable of fidelity. He would not want to betray a trust. Nor would he want to keep it. He is unconscious in regard to either course of action. This is because he is unconscious of and indifferent to its results.

Dana lacks all these desires. He lacks desire itself.

Dana holds no values. He makes no free choices. He takes no free actions. He has no desire to be who and what he is. In a human context there is no who and what Dana is.

DESIRE AS "THE ESSENCE OF MAN"

The great Dutch ethicist, Benedict Spinoza (1632-1677), said of desire that it is the essence of man. By "desire" Spinoza meant all of the physiological and psychological processes that constitute the life of an individual person. He defined desire as:

> [Desire is] that, which being given, [the person] itself is necessarily [given], and, being taken away, [the person] is necessarily taken [away]; or, in other words, that without which [the person] can neither be nor be conceived, and which in its turn cannot be nor be conceived without [the person]. (Gutman, 1949, p. 79)

The term "desire," insofar as it signifies an element of individual autonomy, has a specific meaning. It does not refer to any single desire for any single value. It does not even refer to the whole collection of a person's desires. It refers to, as Spinoza describes it, the defining fact of human existence. It is the nature or "essence" of every individual person.

This point is so important, and so potentially valuable to a nurse in understanding her profession, that we will examine Spinoza's definition of desire on a simpler level than he presents it and in detail:

  • There is a minor difference in the chemical composition of males and females, but basically every person has the same chemical composition.
  • Everyone's physiology is basically the same.
  • Everyone has the same world to think about.
  • Everyone's life depends on the same basic conditions.

- All people are limited, in the same ways, in the actions that they can take.
- Everyone has the same rights to life and action.

Despite all this each and every person is different in a vitally important way. There is one human attribute in which every individual person is different from every other. This attribute is human desire—especially desire as a psychological reality.

Spinoza's definition perfectly defines desire in an ethical context. A thought experiment will be helpful in gaining an understanding of the definition.

Imagine that you are just about to enter a room. One of two things might happen. The room may be unoccupied or someone may be there.

If you enter the room and there is human desire there, this is because there is a unique, individual human person there in the room. There is no human desire except the desire of a unique, individual human person.

An individual person cannot exist unless the organization of his unique desire exists. If the organization of a person's unique desire exists, then a person must exist.

An individual person cannot be known or understood unless the unique organization of his desire is understood.

If the nature of a person's desires is known and understood then that unique person is understood.

In the total absence of desire an individual person cannot exist.

Where there is human desire, a unique human person must exist.

DESIRE AND THE NURSE'S ORIENTATION TO NURSING

A professional ethic, at all odds, should be appropriate to the profession whose members it is set to guide. Every profession arises out of human purposes and desires. Nursing, and the biomedical sciences generally, arose out of the desire to regain health and well-being. Therefore a nursing ethic ought to be appropriate to this desire.

A nursing ethic needs a logical basis for sympathy with the desire to regain health and well-being. Without this basis a nursing ethic becomes dispensible. There will be no necessary and permanent connection between ethical dilemmas and ethical analysis. Ethical dilemmas will be subject to being resolved by convention and convenience.

An explicit sympathy with human desire as such is the only logical basis for sympathy with an individual. If a nurse does not have sympathy with human desire as such, she will not have sympathy with a patient's desire for health and well-being. On what basis could a nursing ethic, for instance, approve of the desire for health and well-being while disapproving the desire for autonomy, freedom, or happiness?

A nurse works to assist a patient's healing processes after surgery. These processes and the patient's desire for happiness are two expressions of the same thing—the patient's striving for autonomy and freedom. The patient's striving for autonomy and freedom is the striving to stay alive.

In order to be sympathetic with human desire a nurse need not approve of every desire that a person might hold. A nurse need not (indeed should not) approve of, for instance, a patient's desire to pursue a criminal career. But she is misguided if she disapproves of human desire as such. A nurse, at a minimum, ought to:

- Be sympathetic to the motivation of people who consult the profession.
- Be open to the propriety of human desire as such.
- Be willing to define a patient's health and well-being in terms of the patient's own desires.

A nurse who does not take this view of human desire takes a fundamentally illogical approach to her profession. Pressed to its limit her outlook on nursing simply does not make sense.

DESIRE AS THE BASIS OF THE BIOETHICAL STANDARDS

For a person to experience existence is for him or her to experience the fact that there is a world and that he or she experiences desire in relation to this world. Without desire a person's experience of his or her own existence—self-awareness— would have no biological function. Human desire should be the very center of a nurse's ethical concern. This is the only way to make a person the center of the nurse's ethical concern.

A nurse's ethical thinking should begin with desire. This is true because of the nature of ethics and the nature of desire. Ethics deals with vital and fundamental goals. The existence of vital and fundamental goals depends on the existence of someone who desires to attain them.

Autonomy

No bioethical standard is desired by a patient for its own sake. The reason for this is very simple. No bioethical standard is desirable for its own sake.

Chiang is in the hospital. His nurse, Evelyn, is quite aware of Chiang's uniqueness.

Evelyn's recognition of Chiang's uniqueness, however, is utterly valueless to Chiang. In itself uniqueness is without any ethical importance.

Uniqueness becomes autonomy when a person expresses uniqueness through unique desires. Uniqueness acquires ethical importance only when it becomes autonomy.

If Evelyn recognizes that Chiang is an accountant, a wood carver, a husband, the father of two children, and that he lives beside a river, her recognition of Chiang and his circumstances is neither evil nor good. How could it be? The census taker who talks to Chiang in his workshop recognizes this much.

Evelyn recognizes the fact that Chiang is motivated by desire. She recognizes that Chiang desires to earn a living, desires to perfect his skill at carving horses, desires to retain the love of his wife, desires the happiness of his children, and desires to return to his home beside the river. Evelyn empathizes with Chiang's desires. This fosters understanding between Evelyn and Chiang. It provides the basis for an ethical interaction between them.

Desire is the first ethical fact after which—and because of which—everything else follows. What is right or wrong, good or evil, between a nurse and her patient depends upon the obligations that their agreement places on each. Desire is the motivation out of which the agreement arises. The desires and purposes of nurse and patient determine the nature and the terms of the nurse/patient agreement.

The desire for life, well-being, and freedom from pain is the reason why there are health care settings. This desire, experienced by patients, is the reason why there are patients. The desire to assist this desire of patients is the reason why there are nurses. The interweaving of these desires is the reason for the existence of the nurse/patient agreement.

Desire brings every ethical fact that exists into existence. For any desiring being the fulfillment of desire is what is good in relation to that being. The failure to fulfill desire is what is evil in relation to that being. It is desire that brings good and evil into existence. Desire does this by bringing good into existence. Unless something were good, nothing could be evil.[1]

As you recall, Dana could experience no desire. Dana regards nothing as good and nothing as evil. Dana is truly, as the philosopher Friedrich Nietzsche described it, beyond good and evil. There are no ethical facts in Dana's world.

Nothing happens, in an ethical sense, before someone desires something and Dana desires nothing.

Freedom

Becky and June are two nurses who often care for the same patients. The patients for whom they care notice a difference in the attitudes of Becky and June. There is a pronounced difference in the experience of being cared for by one or the other. Becky seems to be in immediate contact with her patients. June seems somewhat removed from them. June's attitude seems to be: "You can do whatever you want to do. It doesn't make any difference to me." Becky's attitude, on the other hand, suggests: "I understand your desire for the things you desire. I support you in your desire for these things. I want to help you to regain your freedom to accomplish these things."

June accepts her patient's right to freedom of choice and action. Becky goes beyond this and approves of the desire that motivates these choices and actions. June accepts, but grudgingly and resentfully, her patient's right to choice and action. Becky approves of her patient's right to choose and act. She approves of this positively and benevolently.

No nurse, no patient, and no human being is concerned with freedom simply for its own sake. The value of freedom is in the fact that it allows a person to act on personal desires and pursue personal goals.

June, by simply accepting her patient's desire for freedom, misses the ethical point. In order to interact with her patient on an ethical level she would have to approve of his right to act on his desires. (By accepting without approving she may actually do nothing wrong; but she will do nothing positively right.) June embraces formalism and interacts with her patient as if he were an ethical abstraction. To interact with him on a concrete level she would have to explicitly recognize the longing, fear, and hope that motivate the exercise of his freedom.

On some level of awareness no nurse can be unaware of the importance of both desire and freedom to her patient. The fact that her patient experiences desire implies that freedom is his natural state. Human desire would be biologically unintelligible unless nature intended (so to speak) the individual person to be free.

Patients, along with people in general, desire to be free. This desire for freedom is the precondition of every other desire.

Imagine someone who had no desire for freedom—who desired in fact to give up his freedom. At the same time he desired to go skiing in Utah. The mind of this person would be in a state of impossible confusion.

Veracity

Polly was raised to always tell the truth. Therefore Polly was raised to be a poor nurse.

Frieda, Polly's patient, has had a stroke. She is paralyzed on her right side. Frieda's physician believes that the paralysis is permanent. Frieda's physical therapy is very strenuous, but she is highly motivated. She very much desires to recover, at least, the use of her arm. Frieda's therapy demands the last ounce of her motivation.

One day Frieda turns to Polly for reassurance. She asks Polly if Polly believes she will recover the use of her arm. Polly, very truthfully, replies, "No." Polly told the truth as she was raised to do. She did her patient significant harm—as a nurse should not do.

Hearing this truth, however well-intentioned it might have been, depresses Frieda's motivation for physical therapy. It interrupts the force of her desire. If Frieda had any chance to recover the use of her arm, she needed all her efforts directed toward this end. Whatever might have happened otherwise, now it is probable that Frieda will not recover.

In the context of her childhood Polly chose the right course of action. Sometimes, however, it is necessary for a nurse to abandon her childhood. There is no way to justify the course of action Polly chose, especially in a biomedical context.

Truth is, potentially, a tool by which a person creates his or her happiness and destiny. It is a tool by which a person realizes the values and purposes he or she desires. Desire cannot produce truth but without desire truth has no purpose and no value.

Nonetheless, while desire cannot shape what is or is not true, truth can, and ought to, shape desire.

In the act of recognizing her patient's right to veracity a nurse implicitly recognizes his right to desire. In recognizing any right possessed by her patient she must, to be consistent, recognize his right to desire. On the other hand, if she recognizes any of his rights, she must accept his right to veracity. Every right that a patient possesses is, directly or indirectly, a right to take an action. A person can take action only insofar as he knows the truth of the circumstances of his action.

If a human being had no capacity to know the truth, he or she would have no capacity to take action. The person would be unable to desire to take action. In order to desire a person must be able to choose from what is true. If the person could not know what is true, he or she could not make any choices.

Truth becomes a human value to people insofar as they have desires and purposes. Without desire truth has no biological value. For this reason, without desire truth has no ethical value.

Privacy

There are times when Helga, John's nurse, ought to allow John a period of isolation. There are other times when it is best that she should be there to interact with him. John is a rather withdrawn person who does not communicate easily. Helga needs a way to deal with John's privacy.

What she needs is a standard of privacy. When she is uncertain as to her best course of action, she needs the basis for a decision. When she is not sure whether a certain fact that she knows about John can be revealed or kept secret, she needs a point of reference to help her to decide. She needs a standard by which she can know what to do—by which she can resolve dilemmas before they arise—so that they do not arise.

One day, through introspection, the solution comes to Helga. The standard of privacy is John's desire. If John desires time alone she should leave him alone. If he desires to interact and it is possible, she should interact with him. To resolve a dilemma dealing with privacy Helga realizes that she should refer to John's desire. She should not try to resolve it by referring to the standard of privacy. The standard of privacy will not tell her what to do. She must deal with John's privacy from the standpoint of his desire. There is no other possible standard for privacy.

Without this tie between privacy and desire there would never be any need for ethical understanding between a nurse and her patient. Unless there was a need for ethical understanding, it is quite obvious, there would not be any understanding. There could never be an ethical intimacy between a nurse and her patient unless the patient's right to privacy has its source in his desire for privacy.

In Lana's culture people believe that things told on Halloween should be kept secret. Suppose that George tells Lana something concerning himself on Halloween. Lana holds it in the closest confidence. This has not arisen from any desire on the part of George. It has not arisen through any understanding existing between George and Lana. It does not increase whatever understanding now exists between them. This quaint practice would do nothing at all to foster ethical understanding. Only respect for privacy based on one person's understanding of the desires of another can increase understanding between them.

Privacy, the recognition of self-ownership, is a gift a nurse can give her patient. When a nurse protects her patient's privacy, she does more than prevent interruptions of his time. She protects his self-ownership.

Without a mutual respect for privacy an intimate level cannot be reached. To respect a person's privacy is simply to respect that person's desires. Not to respect a person's privacy is not to respect the person.

Beneficence

A nurse will seldom, and perhaps never, encounter an ethical dilemma that she can resolve with a ballistic accuracy. Ethical dilemmas involving beneficence lend themselves less than any other to a clear-cut resolution.

✕ DILEMMA 11-1   Wally, a 9 year old, was badly burned in a fire at his home. Iris, his nurse, comes to take him for debriding. Wally begins to cry and tells Iris he does not want to go. His face trembles and he screams, "I'll go when my Mommy comes." Wally's mother was killed in the fire. Without any further discussion Iris agrees not to take him.

The short-term benefit that Wally received by not undergoing the pain of debriding would, all things being equal, not compensate for the long-term detriment. But then, Iris must consider the possible effect on Wally if he is told, under these circumstances, that his mother is dead. Iris, has, in a sense done Wally some good — but only by doing him a great deal of harm. On the other hand it is not possible to calculate the amount of good Iris has done Wally. The harm Iris did was permanent. Perhaps the good was also permanent.

Everyone desires to give and receive that which is good. Everyone desires to avoid that which is harmful. But it is not always easy to recognize what is good and what is harmful.

Fidelity

Jose comes into the health care setting with pneumonia. Margaret is assigned to his care.

Jose desires Margaret to give him care whenever her doing this will prevent his experiencing pain or discomfort. Margaret desires Jose not to call on her when it is not necessary. A tacit agreement forms between them, as tacit agreements always form between nurse and patient.

Then Jose begins to think to himself, "I am bored. I want Margaret to overcome my boredom. This is what she is supposed to do. I will call Margaret every 20 minutes and this will overcome my boredom."

Margaret, in turn, begins to think to herself, "I want to be left alone. I want Jose to leave me alone when he does not need care. Every fourth time he rings, I won't answer."

The relationship between Margaret and Jose rapidly breaks down.

The ethical context is given birth by desire. But once the context is born, it must rule desire. The making and keeping of agreements serves to put desires in context and keep them there. It is a way to establish balance and proportion. In this way it is possible for mutual desires to be realized. Fidelity to an agreement does not limit desire. Fidelity makes it possible to accomplish things that otherwise it would not be possible to accomplish.

SUMMARY

To interact on a human level is to interact on a highly intimate level. People interact with each other on an intimate level when they share and discuss their desires. Desire is the basis of meaning in every human life. People reach intimacy when they discuss what things mean to them — when they discuss their desires.

The highest advantage of a patient is his nurse's desire to be a nurse . . . and to nurse. The appropriate ethical focus of a nurse is the desire of her patient. Her patient's desire is final. But, in any context, only his reason can tell him what he desires.

The interweaving of their desires is the ethical basis for the nurse/patient agreement. The nurse/patient agreement is seldom, and probably never, verbalized. It is an implicit agreement arising immediately between them. The ultimate basis of this agreement, therefore, is not anything the nurse or the patient says—it is what the nurse and the patient are.

NOTE

1 On evil as the absence of good where good might be expected, consult Benedict Spinoza: *Ethics*, Book IV; and Thomas Aquinas: *Summa Theologica*, 1, 48, art. 1-3; 49, art. 1; 1-II, 18 art. 1; 19, art. 5.

REFERENCES

Kass, L.R. (1990). Practicing ethics: Where's the action? *Hastings Center Report, 20*(1), 5-12.

Gutmann, J. (Ed.). (1949). *Spinoza's ethics*. New York: Hafner Publishing Company.

The Role of Reason in Ethical Decision Making

There is a folk tale that relates how one day a young man with very strange ethical ideals approached the chief rabbi of his village and expressed a desire to become a rabbi. The chief rabbi inquired of the young man what he had done to make himself worthy of becoming a rabbi. The young man, knowing that a rabbi must practice the most stringent morality, replied: "I make myself humble. I walk about with hard nails inside my shoes. Every day I have my servants beat me with a whip. I sometimes eat grass. I do not engage in frivolous conversations and I work very hard." To which the chief rabbi replied: "No one is more humble than the plow horse pulling the plow. He walks about with hard nails inside his shoes. Every day his servants beat him with a whip. He sometimes eats grass. He does not engage in frivolous conversations and he works very hard. Should the plow horse become a rabbi?"

Happily the realization dawned on the young man that, unless plow horses take ethical actions, nothing can make an action an ethical action unless it is inspired by that which is most relevant to the agent and his life—the capacity to use his mind.

THE ETHICAL STRUCTURE OF ORDINARY ACTIONS

Five days a week Tracy takes a certain action. She walks to work. Of all the actions Tracy takes, this is among the simplest. Strictly speaking Tracy's

167

walks are not ethical actions. No *single* walk she takes to work has consequences extending far enough into the future to make it an ethical action.
Still and all the walks that Tracy takes have all the elements of an ethical
action.

Let us observe Tracy on her way to work:

1. Her walk to work is the result of her desire to go to work. Tracy overrules
    all conflicting desires in favor of this desire. She does not go to work
    involuntarily.
2. She goes to work fully aware of all her alternative possibilities. This is the
    alternative she has chosen from among those available to her. Throughout
    her whole walk she remains aware of alternative possibilities as they arise.
    She will not, for instance, step off the curb into oncoming traffic. Tracy
    exercises practical reason.
3. She works in order to buy food and pay her rent. She works to finance a
    yearly vacation. She goes to to work in order to sustain and enhance
    her life.
4. Her walk is motivated by a purpose. She walks in order to attain all the
    things she is able to attain by going to work. She also walks simply in
    order to get to work—for the pleasure that she finds in working.
5. She exercises agency. Tracy is in control of her actions.
6. She is responsible for the consequences of her actions. At the same time
    no one has a right to interfere with Tracy's actions. When the streets are
    crowded, Tracy tries not to shove or bump into people. She respects the
    rights of other people. Other people try not to shove or bump into Tracy.
    They respect her rights.
7. Tracy plans her day and her evening as she walks to work. Along the way
    she is sometimes tempted to window shop. Depending on how much time
    she has, sometimes she does window shop. Tracy chooses among different
    values and different actions along her way.

DESIRE AND ETHICAL DECISION MAKING

In the nature of things desire must be at the center of the ethical decisions
which Tracy must make.

In a solitary context what any person ought to do is first determined by
what she wants to do. What action she wants to take depends on why
she is acting—the nature of her purposes. There are other principles of
ethical action to be considered. But ethical decision making *begins* in
desire.

In an interpersonal context there would never be any reason for ethical
decision making if it were not for desire. Agents form an agreement and begin
to interact. They need a way to define the purposes of their interaction. They

need a way to keep their desires in harmony. The desire that originally motivated them provides that way. Unless each was motivated by desire, there would be no reason for their interaction. There would be no way to guide their interaction. There would be no way to adjudicate disputes. That is to say, there would be no standard for them to think about in regard to their interaction. Finally, no outcome which their action might have would make any difference to them.

It is desire that brings a nurse into the nurse/patient agreement—her desire to be a nurse. The patient's desires are, so to speak, forced upon him. It is these desires that determine the decisions a nurse ought to make and the actions she ought to take. The desires that illness or injury forces upon a patient makes nursing what it is.

In one way or another whatever a person does and whatever a person is are determined, first, by desire.

The ethicist, Spinoza, tells us that "Desire is the essence of man, that is to say, [desire is] the effort by which a man strives to persevere in his being" (Spinoza cited in Gutmann, 1949, p. 201).

At one end of our existence we are programmed to fill our basic needs by desire. On the other end the highest creations of the human mind are inspired by desire.

But desire can be thought of as more than this. It can be thought of as the life-force. Even the processes that preserve the life of the organism, its physiological processes, can be thought of as a form of desire. These physiological and psychological processes have the same basic function: to preserve and/or enhance the life of the organism. Reason itself can be thought of as a form of desire. Reason, more than any other human faculty, also serves to preserve and/or enhance the life of the organism.

A person lost in a forest might feel an intense desire to create shelter for himself. He might examine all the resources about him and reason out a way to build a shelter. If he cuts his arm, the laceration will most likely heal itself. In several ways these processes—to feel, to examine, to build, and to heal—are very different. But they are alike in one very significant way. Each is a way nature has programmed the living organism to preserve its existence as a living organism. In a widened sense of "desire" each process can be thought of as a form of desire.

In the case of a patient there is the most intimate connection between these different forms of desire. A patient's rational decision to enter the health care setting is conditioned by his desire to regain his health. His decision is also an expression of desire. A patient's desire to end the pain he suffers and to regain his health is an extension of unconscious bodily processes. These physiological processes are those that the body sets in motion in the healing process.

We can view the whole process—the healing processes by which the body regenerates itself, the conscious feeling of desire and the reasoning process that produces the decision—as three expressions of one natural drive. In one way or another this whole process can be seen as the working of desire.

We can view this process mechanistically. We can look at it as three different processes, one following on another and each moving in a different direction. If we do analyze the processes in this way, we view them as billiard balls striking one another on a billiard table. Then we have carved the patient up into three parts—a body, an emotional capacity, and a mind.

To do this would be in conflict with today's bioethical thinking. Biomedicine has begun to think of the patient as a unitary being—one who is to be understood holistically. It would also be in conflict with the patient's thinking. The patient is not a mind bringing a body into the health care setting. Nor is a patient a body bringing a mind into the health care setting.

If we look at humans holistically we see their lives, as they live it, as conscious and embodied desire.

In humans reason is the instrument by which this desire preserves itself. Desire begins the process. Reason is the way that desire keeps it (keeps itself) going.

The medical arts are ways in which people preserve their lives. Medicine is the child of reason and desire.

REASON AND DESIRE

Desire is, like fire, a useful servant but a fearful master. (Author unknown)

Every person is inspired by desire to pursue the good as he sees it. The good is, as Thomas Aquinas observed, a form of the true. The true is the object of reason. The good is the object of desire.

Tomorrow morning Harriet is scheduled for a hysterectomy. Trudy, her nurse, sometimes socializes outside of the hospital with Harriet. Trudy believes that Harriet would be pleased to have a crowd of her friends visit her this evening. So she takes it on herself to make the arrangements for their visit. Trudy does this believing that what she is doing for Harriet is good, while in fact Harriet is a very private person and this is the last thing she would want.

Trudy's idea of the good, in this case, is, as the saying goes, not a good idea. It is not a good idea because it is not based on a knowledge of the facts of the situation.

That which is true is true whether or not it is good. That which can be good, however, is good only if it is true; only if it actually exists.

The pursuit of the good ought to be guided by the knowledge that it does exist, either actually or potentially. It ought to be known that that which is pursued is truly good. This is to be discovered by reason.

Ethical action is the pursuit of vital and fundamental goals. This is why the health care professions are an ethical pursuit. Its goals are vital and fundamental values. For the health care professions, as for all ethical action, it is reason which makes the pursuit of these values possible.

Socrates said of reason that it is man's means to pursue the good.

Aristotle said of reason that it is man's means to happiness.

For the American logician and philosopher of science, Charles Sanders Peirce, reason is important because it is man's means of refining his beliefs.

For the contemporary novelist-philosopher Ayn Rand, reason has ethical importance because it is man's means of survival.

Where there is good or the possibility of good in the world, where happiness is possible, where belief needs to be refined, and where survival is a problem that must be faced, there is an ethical universe. This universe calls for ethical action and practical reason.

In an ethical universe, desire is a human's source of action. Reasoning power allows a person to discover intelligible relations in his or her experience of the world. Reason allows the individual to adapt his or her actions in the pursuit of that which he or she experiences as good.

In this sense reason is the comrade-in-arms of all ethical action.

THE STANDARDS AS REASON AND DESIRE

A human is, in the classical definition, a rational animal. Imagine what a person's condition would be if he or she lacked reason. It is not necessary to create a Dana to exemplify this. Everyone's relationship to his or her reason is so intimate that one's condition if one were deprived of reason can be easily imagined. Without the use of his reason a person would have no more autonomy, freedom, nor self-ownership than an earthworm.

A nurse who totally lacked reason would not be able to understand, nor to act on, the bioethical standards. She would, in fact, not be able to act on or to understand anything at all. To the extent that a person does lack reason, or is unable to exercise it, he or she is unable to act or understand. Even minor lapses of reason, such as occur under stress, may make it temporarily impossible for a nurse to be guided by the bioethical standards.

Each of the bioethical standards is either a response to desire or is based upon some form of desire. In an ethical sense each is also a form of reason or knowledge. Each is reasoning desire.

Autonomy is, to the autonomous subject, his or her experience of personal desires. This experience is revealed through the individual's reasoning processes. Most of the things that a person experiences are experienced by perceiving them via the senses. The autonomous subject, on the contrary, experiences himself or herself, most immediately, in acts of reasoning. Even his or her desire seems to come from without. But in acts of reasoning the autonomous agent experiences himself or herself as actively expressed by action.

An ethical agent experiences freedom through awareness of his or her free actions. The agent does not think of personal freedom before acting. The agent simply thinks about acting. That the agent is free is a constant theme of his or her awareness of being in the world. The acts of thinking are the freest actions the agent takes.

The standard of veracity, as we have seen, is much broader than the issue of truth telling. It originates in and it is a part of a human need for an objective relationship to his or her world. This need is always an aspect determining the nature of awareness. In one way or another it accompanies the ethical agent's every thought and action. Every action which a person takes in order to understand, and to cope with his or her world, is taken because of a desire to attain truth.

A person's experience of self-ownership is a constant in self-awareness. It is the person's experience of the possession of his or her self as self. It is a potentiality, always right there, in the person's power to be aware—in his or her reason. Every action the individual takes, including acts of reasoning, implies a desire for self-possession. The actions an individual takes are his or her actions. Without the awareness of self-ownership there could be no such thing as *his* or *her* actions.

Beneficence, to do good or at least to do no harm, is a form of reason. This form of reason grows out of benevolence—the desire to see good come to another or to see the other avoid harm. It is reason in human interactions. Beneficence is the expression of confidence and strength realized in benefitting another. It requires the recognition of the other as a desiring being.

If there is any purpose to agreements among people then there is a purpose to fidelity to their agreements. Rational beings accomplish their purposes through the use of their reason. Fidelity is an expression of reason in human interactions and the desire that motivates these interactions.

REASON AS THE BASIS OF THE BIOETHICAL STANDARDS

All a patient's choices, values, and actions begin in desire. A nurse ought to easily understand this. All *her* choices, values, and actions begin in desire. Those choices and actions that do not begin in her autonomous desire are not her choices and actions. Not surprisingly, she experiences them as alien. She experiences them as something outside of herself. The patient's experience of his desire is precisely the same. A patient, being in a state of enforced passivity, experiences most of his choices and actions as alien and not his own. He experiences them as being forced upon him.

A nurse has a significant advantage in understanding her patient if she understands this part of his experience.

Everyone's choices, values, and actions begin in desire. Choices, values, and actions, however, should not be allowed to continue in desire alone.

A nurse's ethical thinking begins with desire. But, very early on, it should be turned over to reason. This is true because of the nature of ethics and the nature of reason. Ethical action is action toward vital and fundamental goals. Any action taken toward vital and fundamental goals must be sustained by reason. Otherwise there would be no way for a nurse to know that they were vital and fundamental goals.

Autonomy

✖ **DILEMMA 12-1**   Little Sandy is in the hospital to have his tonsils re-moved. Sandy is screaming and crying. He does not want to have the operation. The surgeon brings in the consent form for Sandy's mother to sign. Sometime later Sandy's nurse gives him the preoperative medications.

This seems to be an easy case to deal with. It seems this way only because we take so much for granted.

Sandy's tonsils are infected. It would be reasonable for them to be taken out.

On the other hand, Sandy is already an autonomous individual. Autonomous individuals have rights.

At first glance this situation seems to present no particular problems. Sandy must be operated on.

All the same ask yourself these questions:

1. Does Sandy's mother have a moral right to sign the consent form?
2. Does Sandy's nurse have a moral right to give him the preoperative medications?
3. Does the surgeon have a moral right to operate on Sandy?

Now, assuming that Sandy has no rights protecting him against this procedure (and, in our culture, we take it for granted that he has not), consider these questions:

4. When and how will Sandy acquire the rights that would protect him against this procedure?
5. Do Sandy's mother, the surgeon, and the nurse have rights that would protect *them* against undergoing this procedure involuntarily?
6. If so, when and how did Sandy's mother, the surgeon, and the nurse acquire the rights that they possess?
7. When and how will Sandy acquire the rights that his mother, the surgeon, and the nurse possess?
8. Will Sandy ever acquire the right to decide for *his* child? If so, when, why, and how?

We must assume that, at some time in his life, Sandy will acquire the right to decide for his child. If he does not, then neither did his mother ever acquire the right to decide for him. It seems as though reason is on the side of Sandy's tormenters. In reason Sandy ought to have the operation. In reason there is no reason for Sandy not to have the operation. There is no reason *except* Sandy's desire not to have it.

At the same time it is a fact that Sandy is an autonomous ethical agent. If Sandy's autonomy will not protect him, nothing ever will.

The most rational course of action to be taken is for Sandy to have his tonsils removed. Can this be the reason why the others possess the rights they do—because reason is on their side? Does Sandy lack rights, in this circumstance, because reason is against him?

Sandy's case shows the fragile interweaving of reason, autonomy, and rights.

Rights is the product of an implicit agreement among rational beings, by virtue of their rationality, not to obtain actions or the product of actions from others, except through voluntary consent objectively gained.

It seems then that a conflict between reason and autonomy is built into the nature of rights. On the one hand, people possess rights by virtue of their rationality. On the other hand, they can interact with others only if others give their voluntary consent to the interaction. This voluntary consent, in addition, must be objectively gained. People possess rights by virtue of their capacity to reason. But they can interact with others only according to the autonomy of those others.

Conflicts can arise, even among benevolent people, over the question of rights. Most of these conflicts involve:

1. One person's belief that reason demands or justifies an action.
2. Another person's belief that this action would violate his autonomy—his right to be what and who he is.

Everyone has a right not to be aggressed against, coerced, or defrauded. The implicit agreement is that no one will aggress against, coerce, or defraud another. This is the basis of ethical interaction.

In addition to the universal rights agreement a special implicit agreement is formed between nurse and patient. Special conflicts can arise here.

Conflicts sometimes arise as to what constitutes aggression, coercion, or fraud. Although one person's reason tells him the other's rights have not been violated, the other's reason will tell him they have.

Some middle ground must be found between the reasoning of one person and the autonomy of another.

✂ **DILEMMA 12-2**   Roger is an elderly man who was brought into the hospital because of dehydration as a result of the flu. While Roger is in the hospital, his physician realizes that Roger's pacemaker needs to be replaced. The physician and nurse go in to talk to Roger about the scheduling of the operation. After the physician leaves Roger tells his nurse that he has no intention of having the operation. The last time he had a pacemaker put in he suffered a stroke that left him confined to a wheelchair.

Even at his advanced age Roger has autonomous purposes for his life. When he analyzes the benefit of having the pacemaker replaced (another year of life) against the drawbacks (the possibility of having another stroke and becoming completely dependent on others, or the possibility of not surviving the operation), he decides that his most reasonable course of action is not to have his pacemaker replaced.

On the other hand when his pacemaker runs down, Roger will immediately die. This certainly seems to place reason on the side of Roger's physician.

Roger's physician feels, with a great deal of justification, that reason is on his side. The operation to replace the pacemaker would probably be a success and would give Roger another year of independent living. Whatever rights Roger has in this situation, he does not have them by virtue of any reasoning he has done. What Roger has to gain is objectively much greater than what he has to lose. It is almost beyond doubt that the course of action suggested by the physician is the course of action Roger should take. The physician believes that Roger is old and senile. He has Roger declared incompetent, and the operation is performed.

This situation places the rights that Roger has by virtue of his autonomy into conflict with the rights the physician has by virtue of his reasoning.

Ask yourself these questions:

1. Was the physician justified in the course of action he took?
2. Does a health care professional's role in society give him or her extraordinary rights?
3. What is the ethical role of a nurse in this situation?
4. The judge who declared Roger incompetent may have been legally justified; was the judge ethically justified?

One final question:

5. Is there any significant difference between Roger's situation and Sandy's?

If reason is allowed to override autonomy in conflicts among rights, this will solve a large number of problems. At the same time it will create an infinite number of problems. From then on anytime anyone feels that his or her reason justifies a course of action, he or she will have a right to violate the autonomy of another. Under these circumstances no one will have any rights at all.

If one is to have any rights, then reason cannot be allowed to override autonomy. For reason will not establish any rights. Suppose that the reasoning behind one person's argument is superior to the reasoning behind another's. Ignoring the fact that in most cases it would be difficult or impossible to prove this, there would always be a third person whose reason was superior to the second. Then there would be a fourth whose reason was superior to the third. This could go on forever. No ethical decision could ever be made.

Freedom

A person's freedom is the freedom to control personal actions. When a person is dominated by a powerful emotion or set of emotions, he or she is unable to control actions. If a person cannot control his or her actions, the person is not free. The only power a person has over his or her emotions, and, thus, over actions, is the power of his or her reason.

✖   **DILEMMA 12-3**   Alfred came into the hospital four days ago for a coronary bypass. The surgery went well, and Alfred seems on the way to recovery. A few hours ago his family was in to visit him. The room was filled with quiet conversation, and the family seemed to share a sense of intimacy.

It is now time for Alfred's first heparin injection. Lois, his nurse, has just come into his room to give him his shot. For no apparent reason Alfred refuses the medication. Lois knows that Alfred's failure to take the medicine puts his life in jeopardy. She explains to him the reason for the drug and stresses its importance.

On the one hand Lois' reason tells her that Alfred should take the heparin. There is every reason why he should take it, and no apparent reason for him not to take it. On the other hand Alfred is adamant. He absolutely refuses the shot of heparin. He also refuses to discuss the reasons why he will not let Lois give him the injection. There is no apparent reason why Alfred's freedom does not give him the right to make this decision. There seems to be here an irresolvable conflict between Lois' reason and Alfred's freedom.

Freedom is the capacity to make decisions and choices that are uncompelled by outside forces. The capacity to make decisions and choices that are not compelled by outside forces must be directed by reason. Otherwise it would not reflect the autonomy of the free person. Without reason there is no freedom.

Perhaps Alfred's decision was made under the influence of a powerful but passing emotion. If it was, then his decision was not free. In that sense the decision was not Alfred's decision. It was very much like the response of an animal to an external stimulus. It did not reflect Alfred's unique character structure or his purposes. Therefore would it not seem that Alfred had no right to refuse the injection of heparin?

Alfred has not given anyone enough information to justify the belief that his decision was coerced by some powerful emotion. Therefore it seems that Alfred does have a right to refuse the heparin.

The fact that human beings possess freedom means that ethics cannot be a type of mechanics. Humans cannot be understood mechanistically. But, as we can see above, this seems to usher self-contradiction into ethics.

We are, at least, faced with several dilemmas at the center of ethics:

1. Do justifiable ethical decisions depend, not on the facts of the ethical context, but, on a person's knowledge of those facts?
2. Are an ethical agent's reasonable beliefs sufficient to justify ethical actions?

To be free is to be free to take chosen courses of action. In the ethical sense, without reason there are no chosen courses of action. The stimulus/response behavior of an animal is very different from the deliberate and rational behavior of a person. This is why humans are ethical beings and the lower animals are not. A person's reason makes rational choice possible. It is the fact that a person's choices are rational choices—made, for better or worse, by a rational faculty—that gives him the right to freedom. A person's right to freedom is the right to make choices and to act on the choices he or she made.

Veracity

✗ **DILEMMA 12-4**   Mabel, Charlene's patient, has been diagnosed with cancer of the liver. Mabel is also 4 months pregnant with her first child. She and her husband, Mark, had been trying for a long time to have a child. Mabel's physician tells her that to treat her effectively, he will need to use chemotherapy. The chemotherapy will cause severe defects in the child, or perhaps abort the fetus. The physician recommends that treatment begin before the child's due date. He suggests aborting the fetus and starting treatment immediately. He feels that to wait until delivery would be detrimental, perhaps, fatal, to Mabel. He knows that not to wait until delivery would be detrimental and maybe fatal to the fetus.

In making her decision objectively and contextually Mabel will have to consider every relevant factor. Suppose she refuses to consider one or more factors:

- She might refuse to recognize the fact that she and the baby cannot both survive chemotherapy.
- She might refuse to consider the reasons why she ought to have an abortion and begin treatment.
- She might be unwilling to seek a second opinion and to consider the possibility of an alternative means of treatment, perhaps surgery, as a way to save herself and the baby.

In refusing to consider these factors Mabel is deceiving herself. She is, in effect, violating the standard of veracity in reference to herself.

Does the fact that Mabel is lying to herself have any ethical relevance to her nurse in the bioethical context?

What influence, if any, should this have on her nurse's choices and actions?

All reason is logical and objective. A person can be said to be reasoning only when he or she takes all the relevant factors into consideration, and follows every fact to its logical conclusion.

There are two types of reason: speculative reason and practical reason. Speculative reason has to do with such things as the reasoning a researcher goes through in an attempt to discover a cure for a disease. Practical reason has to do with such things as where a researcher ought to go to do research. It is the reasoning behind the choices a person makes based on self-interest.

Each of these types of reason depends upon truth. Logic, seeing the inner relations of things, and objectivity, seeing things as they are apart from how we want them to be, depend on truth. The purpose of each type of reason is to produce truth. The purpose is to enable the reasoner to see the inner relations of things and to see things as they are.

The purpose of speculative reason is to enable a thinker "to say of what is that it is, and of what is not that it is not." The purpose of practical reason is to enable a thinker to say of what ought to be, that it ought to be and of what ought not to be that it ought not to be. The purpose of all reason is to discover the truth.

Truth is necessary in order for one person to communicate with another. Communication is necessary for one person to understand another. Truth is also necessary for a person to communicate with and understand his or her self. When a person will not face the truth, he or she cannot effectively communicate with his or her self or with another person.

In nursing this problem arises when a patient will not face a relevant truth. It is a problem that arises when a nurse tries to communicate with her patient and fails because her patient is unwilling to communicate with himself.

How, in the case above, would it be possible for a nurse to communicate with Mabel?

Privacy

✗ DILEMMA 12-5   Dan is a 32-year-old cardiac patient. He has requested no visitors and has not had his phone connected. He wants to be left entirely alone. Rosalyn, his nurse, has taken twelve calls from Dan's friends. Other personnel on the shift have also taken several calls. Dan's right to privacy involves a right to isolation and if he has a right to privacy, then he has that right to isolation. If he has no right to isolation, then he has no right to privacy. But the way Dan chooses to exercise his privacy leaves Rosalyn without any privacy.

Here is certainly a case that needs to be adjudicated by reason. What efforts must health care personnel take to see that someone like Dan is afforded isolation?

• A person needs privacy to think, evaluate and order his or her life.
• A person needs privacy to translate thought into purposeful action.
• A person needs privacy to ensure his or her rights.

These needs are very basic and a person has a right to pursue them. No one has a right to interfere with the pursuit of these needs. Without self-ownership a person would have no right to act, no right to speak, no right to think. Indeed, without privacy, a person would have no reason to think.

Dan absolutely has a right to privacy. Rosalyn also has the same right. Neither has a right to avoid the responsibility to guide ethical actions by reason. This responsibility certainly applies to the right to privacy.

Beneficence

✂ DILEMMA 12-6   Robert, a cancer patient, comes into the hospital for evaluation. He has cancer of the bone. Radiation had been tried several months before. It proved ineffective. Robert begs his physician to end all life support measures since all he has to look forward to is more and more terrible pain. Robert's physician believes that to do this would be a form of euthanasia. He believes that euthanasia is an ethical evil. He refuses to do as Robert asks.

Robert's physician believes that he has arrived at his position through reason. He tells himself that Robert's suffering makes Robert unable to reason clearly about his situation.

Robert believes that his physician has no right to refuse. Robert's reason tells him that death would be a blessing compared with his present life and his prospects for the future. He believes that the smallest exercise of reason would lead a person to this position.

Several questions suggest themselves here:

1. Is it reasonable to believe that euthanasia, under certain circumstances, is not an evil? (Assume that any request for beneficence must be sanctioned by reason. Assume further that a person's suffering can be so terrible that he is unable to reason.)
2. Does this mean that a person in moderate pain can make a rational request for euthanasia and a person in terrible pain cannot?
3. If a person can construct a strong argument in reason not to take a beneficent action, does this invalidate beneficence as a bioethical standard?

In order that one person might act beneficently toward another, that person must have some knowledge of the other. For a nurse to act beneficently, she must identify good and evil in relation to the other person. Beneficence is an act that brings good to another or that prevents evil from befalling another. For a nurse to act beneficently, she must know where to look for good and evil. This task is far more difficult than it sounds.

Spinoza deals with the question of good and evil on its most basic level. He describes good and evil thusly:

> We call a thing good which contributes to the preservation of our being, and we call a thing evil if it is an obstacle to the preservation of our being, that is to say, a thing is called by us good or evil as it increases or diminishes, helps or restrains, our power of action. (Cited in Gutmann, 1949, p. 196)

If a patient ever examined his conception of good and evil, as a patient, he would probably describe it in precisely this way. His purpose is to live and whatever contributes to this purpose is good. Whatever tends to defeat this purpose is evil. He would find that whatever helped and increased his power of action he would have to regard as good. Whatever restrained or diminished his power to take action he would have to regard as evil.

Robert's physician took a very different view of good and evil from the view of his patient. In our pluralistic society what argument can he offer to justify his position?

In her ordinary life a nurse might have a very different attitude toward good and evil. It might have to do with dietary laws or sexual mores, political affiliations, or any number of social conventions. A nurse, however, does not deal with patients in their ordinary lives—nor in her ordinary life. She deals with patients as patients. She deals with physicians as physicians. As patients, people are concerned with "the preservation of their being" and the things that "increase or diminish [their] power of action." This is the only basis compatible with the nurse/patient agreement. In judging the actions of physicians this is the only basis for judgment in harmony with her agreement.

Reason and beneficence counsel a nurse to look at the issue of good and evil from her patient's point of view. Unless she does this, it is impossible for her to form and keep an agreement with her patient according to the purposes that brought him into the health care setting. This point of view and these purposes are the reason why there is such a thing as nursing. A nurse cannot ethically dispense with them in her ethical decision making.

Fidelity

Ken is the orderly on Karen's shift. Karen hears Ken talking "baby talk" to an elderly, senile patient, Elsie. Elsie, who is normally apathetic, responds to Ken's approach. When Ken talks to her she brightens up and smiles.

Karen, however, has been taught that this behavior is "paternalistic" and degrading to the patient. She reprimands Ken for what she sees as his ethical failure.

Karen has just graduated and is beginning work on the urology floor. As a child she was always regarded as a "good little girl." She hopes, now that she is a nurse, to be the same kind of person as she was then. She begins to plan what she will do. The first ethical decisions she makes are these:

- She will give each patient equal time.
- She will be fair. She will give each patient the same concern (regardless of the needs of the patient).
- She will do her best to charm and encourage (coerce) each patient into doing what she believes to be in the patient's best interest.
- She will behave beneficently according to general rules of behavior (rather than according to what is appropriate to her patient's context).
- She will try to do good for as many people as possible. (In a conflict between a patient and his family she will support the patient's family.)

Karen's decisions have ensured that her thinking on ethical matters concerning her profession will not objectively relate to the nature of her profession. Her approach has inspired a decision that her ethical actions will be ritualistic, noncontextual, and, therefore, purposeless.

Reason requires the reasoner to have an alert awareness of what is going on. This alert awareness is an essential precondition of any agreement. All reason is contextual. Rules imposed from without are not a substitute for reason. They are an attempt to evade the responsibility of reasoning.

Any patient who made a well-reasoned agreement with a nurse would include in the terms of that agreement:

1. Whatever can be done to preserve his life will be done—for the purpose of preserving his life.
2. Whatever can be done to save him unnecessary suffering will be done—in order to save him unnecessary suffering.
3. Whatever would violate his self-ownership will be avoided—because it would violate his self-ownership.
4. Whatever can be done to increase his freedom and well-being will be done—because it increases his freedom and well-being.

SUMMARY

That which reason demands does not change from the solitary to the interpersonal context. What is necessary to satisfy reason is the same. Only the context becomes more complex. Two people hope to bring about a certain state of affairs. They see certain interactions as bringing about that state of affairs. Each commits to these interactions. This commitment takes the form of words and ideas or concepts. Words and ideas are the instruments of reason. To perfectly fulfill her role a nurse should, whenever possible, engage the reason of her patient. This is necessary in order that their agreement can function. It is necessary in order that her patient be optimally capable of bringing reason to bear on decisions concerning the course of treatment.

Unless a nurse exercises reason, she will not find a ground on which to justify her actions. In the context of a nursing dilemma reason is attention to that context. The relevance of her justification depends on her reason, that is to say, on her attention to the context.

A nurse's exercise of reason is her greatest source of ethical confidence and strength. As the agent of her patient, confidence and strength are values that she offers him—and herself. A nurse owes it to herself to exercise reason and develop the virtues that nursing requires.

The responses of others are uncontrollable. A nurse's confidence and strength must come from within herself. They begin with reason.

REFERENCE

Gutmann, J. (Ed.). (1949). *Spinoza's ethics*. New York: Hafner Publishing Company.

Life as the Precondition of All Action

Andrew broke his leg in a skiing accident. He was put into a full leg cast about 6 hours ago and assigned to Jill. While she was assessing him, Jill noticed that Andrew's toes were cold and seemed to have a poor color.

Jill tried to get Andrew's physician on the phone, but he was not available. Since she worked in a very small community hospital, there were no interns or residents to call. When she got back to Andrew, his toes had become cyanotic.

Jill checked with her head nurse. The head nurse checked with her supervisor. Nothing was done.

Jill tried to get another physician to come, but he declined because Andrew was not his patient. Jill felt sure that Andrew was going to suffer permanent damage. Still and all she was afraid to remove the cast herself since this is not within "the role of the nurse." Because of Jill's inaction, Andrew lost his leg.

DESIRE AND THE NATURE OF A PERSON

We have already defined "desire" to include much more than the well-known psychological state. A nurse understands her patient best if, by "desire," she understands all the processes that contribute to her patient's survival and the enhancement of his life. The psychological state of desire is the best known process of this type, but every process that contributes to the survival of the organism belongs to the same family.

By including every such process under the concept of "desire" a nurse can have a well-balanced understanding of her patient. Only this understanding of his desire enables a nurse to interact with her patient in his context. This understanding of desire, as an element of autonomy, is an understanding of the entire person.

For a nurse to know her patient as a living reality is at least as important as it is for her to know any isolated psychological state or physiological process.

THE DIFFERENT ASPECTS OF LIFE

To gain an understanding of the role of life in ethics we must define "life" in the same way we define "desire." As an ethical element "life" includes the entire context of a living person. As we shall see, any narrower definition would not be adequate for an effective bioethic. Under "life" we must understand every process and action, including desire, by which an organism maintains its survival and enhances its state of being.

We have a very limited understanding of life if we look on it only as a natural curiousity. We have an adequate understanding of life only if we understand it from the perspective of the subject who is living it. In order to do this it is desirable to understand life from our own perspective.

For bioethics an adequate understanding of "life" will include such things as:

1. The body's physiological processes.
2. The integration of these processes.
3. Basic needs common to all animals: Food, water, air—the needs that are directly and immediately tied to the animal's survival.
4. Basic needs common to all human beings: Shelter, clothing, companionship, etc.
5. The life of consciousness: Perceptual experience, conceptual thought, emotion, etc.
6. The higher order needs and values of human beings: Purpose, creativity, hope, privacy, etc.—the values that are directly and immediately tied to a human level of existence.
7. The value of various activities: Walking, flying an airplane, cooking, work, etc.—conditions of physical self-expression.
8. The meaning of "aesthetic" values: Music, reading, painting, hobbies, discussion, etc.—those conditions under which a person examines and/or experiences his or her life at its best.

9. That with which a person is engaged and to which he or she is committed—the meaning, to a person, of the products of acts of choice.

A nurse can define life from the perspective of an outsider. There are,
however, a number of reasons why a nurse ought to define life from the
perspective of the living subject:

1. Medical science defines it from this perspective. If medical science thought
   of life simply as physiological survival, there would be no such thing as
   psychiatry, physical therapy, plastic surgery, etc.
2. If a nurse defines her patient's life solely in terms of its basic physiological
   processes, she will never be able to deal with ethical questions concerning
   risk, euthanasia, abortion, etc. If she defines life in terms of its basic
   physiological processes, then she will never truly experience her patient.
   She will be very much in the position of a novelist who, when she looks
   out at the characters in her novel, never really sees beyond herself.
3. If life, as an ethical concept, were defined in terms of physiological
   processes, then life as an ethical concept would pertain to all organic
   matter.

All organic matter is characterized by physiological processes. All organic
matter has basic needs that must be met if it is to survive. If a nurse made
"life," understood as physiological processes, the focus of her ethical concern, she would have to concern herself with all living matter. If she concerned herself with the freedom, privacy, and so on of all organic matter, she,
herself, could not survive. Nurses, in common with everyone else, need to
consume organic matter in order to remain alive. It would be strange indeed
if a bioethical standard logically demanded the self-destruction of the health
care professional who recognized it.

A nurse's ethical concern is not with organic matter. It is with a patient. It
must be with a patient in his entirety. This is the only kind of patients there
are, patients in their entirety.

Her ethical commitment to her patient does not arise from the fact that he
is organic matter. It arises from, and is formed by, the fact that his life is all
the things it is. A patient's life is his autonomy. In addition to his physical
needs and processes his life is his desire, his reason, his purposes, his freedom, and his power of agency.

4. If, on the other hand, a nurse defines her patient's life entirely in *abstract*
   terms, she will never be able to deal with her patient on an ethical level.
   People involved in ethical interaction are individual and concrete. Only an
   understanding of life as an element of an individual patient's autonomy
   will serve to guide ethical action. People are too different and life is too
   many things for the individual to be understood in entirely abstract
   terms.

It is not possible for a nurse to deal with her patient's life entirely on an abstract level. If this were possible, it would mean that she would hardly have to deal with her patient at all.

Only if a nurse defines the life of her patient as she defines her own life will she look at her patient as an ethical agent looks at another person in an effective ethical interaction.

A nurse's agreement is not with organic matter. Nor is the "life" that is at the center of her agreement a disconnected abstraction. Her agreement is with every aspect of an individual human being.

LIFE AS THE BASIS OF THE BIOETHICAL STANDARDS

A nursing ethic that is not appropriate to patients—and to nurses—is riddled with problems. The chief problem is that it is not an intelligible field of study. Not every ethical system is automatically intelligible. Ethics is, or ought to be, derived from a study of individual people as living, rational beings. There is no intelligible ethic of redheads or of diabetics. There is no intelligible ethic of poets or of long-distance runners. An intelligible ethic relevant only to males or only to females is an impossibility. Such an ethic would be a mistake masquerading as an ethical system.

A rational solitary ethic is one whose motivations can be justified by the benefit it brings to the person who follows it. A rational interpersonal ethic is one whose motivations can be justified by reference to the benefits and harmony it brings to the interactions of the people who are guided by it.

AN ALTERNATIVE REFERENCE POINT FOR DECISION MAKING

It is possible to make ethical decisions with the individual person, either oneself or one's beneficiary, serving as the reference point of ethical analysis. A person does this when he or she makes human purposes the center of his or her ethical system.

It is also, in a manner of speaking, possible to make ethical decisions according to rules and various social conventions.

There are drawbacks to rules and conventions that are not present in a purposeful ethic.

1. It is impossible to justify ethical actions in terms of arbitrary social conventions to a person who does not accept these social conventions. There is nothing outside of the conventions themselves to which an agent can point. There is nothing by which the agent can relate his or her decisions and actions to the context in which they arise.

   A nurse who bases her actions on social convention rather than on her patient's situation is in the position of a person who bases her actions on the flip of a coin. This is true no matter how universal, ancient, or venerable the social convention might be.

2. The ethical ideas a person adopts always depend upon that person's idea of what is and what is not good. If bioethics is to have any relevance to the biomedical situation, it must, in the case of nurses, be derived from the nurse/patient agreement. The nurse/patient agreement arises from two ideas of the good integrated and brought into harmony:

   • The benefit that a patient comes into the health care setting seeking.
   • The benefit that a nurse, implicitly, promises to her patient.

Nothing arises between a nurse and a patient from rules or conventions.

3. Happiness must be pursued. It is not something to be found out in the world ready at hand. If happiness is to be gained, it must first be desired and then it must be pursued.
   Rules and conventions are not devised to be desired. They are ways of escaping desire. They are also ways of avoiding the pursuit of happiness.
4. Belief must be refined. It is very easy to make ethical mistakes. Rules and conventions do not allow for belief being refined.

Ethical belief cannot be refined outside of the ethical context. It cannot be refined unless the nature of actual ethical agents provides the standard by which ethical truth and falsity — success and failure — are determined.

With refined beliefs a person can investigate whether an action or a value enhances life, detracts from life, or destroys life.

With rules and conventions a person cannot conduct this investigation. Rules and conventions remove an agent from the cause-and-effect aspects of the ethical situation.

5. Human survival, on every level, is contingent upon rational belief. Rules and conventions are substitutes for rational belief. They weaken the conditions of human survival.

LIFE AS THE PRECONDITION OF ALL VALUES

That which determines the nature of an ethical system and its difference from other ethical systems is the final value of the system.

Nothing can be sought or desired by anyone unless that person is alive. Life is the *precondition* of all values. As ethicist Benedict Spinoza puts it (cited in Gutmann, 1949):

> No one can desire to be happy, to act well, and live well, who does not at the same time desire to be, to act, and to live, that is to say, actually to exist. (p. 204)

In the field of ethics a nurse faces two options:

- She can choose a ritualistic ethic. This is an ethic based upon and arising out of rules and conventions.
- She can choose a purposeful ethic. For a nurse a purposeful ethic is an ethic based on her patient's purposes as codified in the nurse/patient agreement.

Nursing would be ethically unintelligible under any basis other than a purposeful ethic.

Jill, you will recall, followed the rules and did what was conventional. Her ethical actions were objectively purposeless. They were ritualistic. The final value of her ethical system was "what-a-nurse-is-supposed-to-do."

For a purposeful ethical system the final value to be gained by Jill's actions would have been Andrew's well-being. To protect the well-being of a patient is to act purposefully. This is what nursing is (or ought to be) all about. A nursing ethic ought to be all about what nursing and human life is all about.

LIFE AS THE FINAL VALUE

Life is the entire state of the living thing. As an element of human autonomy it is that state of a person which he or she experiences as his or her self.

A sense of the value of oneself and one's life is implicit in every act of valuing. In this sense life is a "pre-conscious" standard of judgment.

In the health care setting, if judgment and choice are to be determined by reference to the rights and values of a patient, then the question of the central term of the nurse/patient agreement is not problematic. The central term is the patient's life and well-being.

Consider this:

- Life is the precondition of all of a patient's other values.
- Life is the precondition of a patient's rights. To respect a patient's right to autonomy, freedom, and so on, and not to be concerned for his life and well-being is, very much, to miss the point. At the same time, to be concerned with a patient's life and well-being and not to respect his right to autonomy, freedom, and so on is to have lost one's ethical direction.
- Life is the purpose of the patient in entering the health care environment. A patient's concern for his life must be shared by his nurse, or there is no easily understood reason for her being his nurse. Life is the central term of the agreement that a nurse makes with her patient.
- A patient's motivation in entering the health care environment is the fact that his capacities and potentialities are radically circumscribed. When a patient regains his capacities and potentialities, his life is very much expanded.
- A patient, except in the most extreme circumstances, can have no rational desire before his desire for life. At the same time, in extreme circumstances, a desire for death is not an irrational desire.

DISCONTENT AND ETHICAL ACTION

Without a state of discontent there are no goals. Without goals there is no action. A person in a state of perfect contentment would desire no change. That person would have no goals and no reasons to take action.

In a state of perfect contentment a person would have no motivation at all. Since the person would have no motivation to take any action, he would, obviously, have no motivation to take ethical action.

This individual would have no motivation to take action toward vital and fundamental goals, which means that he or she would have no motivation to live on the uniquely human level.

But life is discontent. Life is an action behind every other action. Life is the first ethical action. If a person is alive, he or she has reason to be discontented and to take action. A person must take action to remain alive. Nature has programmed humans to be discontented.

The greater a person's discontent, the greater the motivation to act. The less the discontent, the less the motivation to take action. It is inconceivable that any human being would ever attain a state of perfect contentment. The processes of human life do not allow for this.

Consider a patient in a health care setting. A human being can hardly be in situation where contentment is less appropriate. He can hardly be more acutely aware of his life and desires. No one has more reason to be motivated to vital action than a patient. The action that determines all his other actions is his act of trying to stay alive and/or to regain the potentialities of his life.

The conditions that make a patient's contentment inappropriate are the conditions in which bioethics arises. A justifiable bioethic must adopt the viewpoint that his discontent forces upon a patient.

A nurse, to be an effective ethical agent, must have the same essential viewpoint as her patient. A patient is not motivated by social conventions. The rules of deontology and the evasions of utilitarianism are irrelevant to a health care setting.

A patient enters the health care setting in order to overcome the cause of his discontent. He is motivated by his most vital and fundamental goal— the preservation of his life.

The nature of human life forces particular kinds of discontent upon a person. This discontent forces vital and fundamental goals upon him. His vital goals are those that are important to him as a living being. They are the goals that make a significant difference in his life. His fundamental goals are the goals that determine what further goals he will and will not be able to choose. His life, being the precondition of all further goals, is both his most vital and his most fundamental goal.

If a nurse cannot accept the preservation of his life as her patient's ethical motivation, there will, of necessity, be an absence of ethical empathy between the nurse and her patient.

If the nurse approaches her patient believing that something other than his life and well-being are the proper goals of nursing interventions, she *begins* by betraying her agreement with him. If she rejects her powers of observation and her reasoning faculty in favor of rules, conventions, or out-of-context goals, she will never understand her patient and her patient will not understand her. They will, for all *practical* purposes, be inhabiting two different ethical worlds.

LIFE AND THE BIOETHICAL STANDARDS

Autonomy

Allison and Courtney are two nurses working in health care settings. The ethical practice of each nurse is remarkably similar.

Each nurse respects the freedom of her patient. When the patient is not being treated, or not undergoing surgery, both Allison and Courtney allow the patient to do whatever the patient wants to do.

Each nurse tells her patient the truth.

Each nurse respects the privacy of her patient. When she is not giving care, she does not disturb her patient.

Each nurse performs nursing interventions. Each does good for her patient and carefully avoids doing anything that might cause harm to her patient.

Each is perfectly true to the terms of her agreement with her patient — insofar as she understands these terms.

Neither Allison nor Courtney has ever been particularly concerned with the autonomy of her patient.

Allison's patients do not respond well under her care. Courtney's patients do very well. No nurse could have an effect on her patients significantly better than Courtney has.

Allison works in the office of a physician.

Courtney works for a veterinarian.

In so far as a person's life is more than basic physiological functioning, it is autonomous. It is, within certain limits, made to be what it is by the living agent himself.

If the autonomous aspects of a human life are ignored and only the physiological processes considered, then the person is ignored.

Suppose a person's physiological processes and the integrity of his body were demolished in a bomb blast. The person would be destroyed. This is not the only way we can imagine a person being destroyed. Suppose a magician were to change a person into a cabbage. That person would equally be destroyed. Formalistic ethical systems counsel ethical agents, in effect, to become just such a magician. They do this in the sense that they recognize no more autonomy in the people with whom they interact than that possessed by a cabbage.

A nurse who practices a ritualistic ethic—one who places something other than the life of her patient at the base of her ethical actions—embraces just such a system.

All the actions that a patient takes as a human being—all actions above the physiological level—are actions taken autonomously. Unless a nurse deals with these autonomous actions as being autonomous, she does not deal with her patient as a human being. She may as well be dealing with a cabbage.

Arguments in bioethics often imply that a person can have the right to life without a right to autonomy. A terminal patient in severe pain is kept, against his will, on life support measures. The justification for this is his "right to life." He lives for no reason other than to suffer, and the hope that a cure for his condition will be discovered. This is a possibility that no one takes seriously. His biological processes are kept intact. His love of life—everything that makes his life meaningful—is killed. He dies hating his life.

Arguments are often made in bioethics that imply that a person can have the right to autonomy without the right to life. A patient experiencing disorientation as a result of a bowel obstruction and his first preoperative medication decides to cancel his surgery. Out of respect for his autonomy and freedom the operation is cancelled and the patient dies. His fate is determined by the magical power of the words he speaks in a delirium.

A biomedical professional cannot respect a patient's right to life unless she regards him as an integrated, autonomous individual. If she thinks of him as a being whose spoken words are final she places the other aspects of his life in jeopardy.

A patient's autonomy is what he is. Not everything a patient says reflects what he is. Not everything a patient says is a reflection of his autonomy.

Freedom

Rosalyn is a nurse caring for Margaret. Margaret is a 33-year-old patient, who has had a diving accident. The accident has left Margaret a quadriplegic, dependent on a respirator. She has asked her physician to turn off the respirator and let her die.

Margaret's physician is her agent and the only way she can exercise her freedom is through him. Her physician has refused. He believes that if he were to turn off the respirator, this would be an immoral action.

Let us examine how reasonable his position is.

Suppose that Margaret were in a torture chamber. It would greatly enhance the circumstances of her life if she could escape. No one who helped Margaret to escape a torture chamber could reasonably be judged morally blameworthy.

Margaret's body, that is to say, Margaret's life, *is* a torture chamber. Margaret should not be condemned for trying to escape from the torture chamber that she is in. Why, then, should she be condemned for trying to escape from her life? Why should a physician be condemned, or condemn himself, for being willing to act to help her?

Imagine a soldier escaping from an enemy force. He has a wounded comrade-in-arms whom he cannot take with him. The enemy is notorious for torturing captured prisoners. The wounded soldier begs his comrade to shoot him. He is unable to kill himself and he wants his comrade to kill him to prevent his undergoing torture at the hands of the enemy.

Even in the context of a formalistic and ritualistic ethic it would be a difficult matter to *demonstrate* that leaving his comrade to the enemy would be a moral course of action. In the context of a purposeful ethic it would be impossible to demonstrate this.

In the context of a purposeful ethic the difference between actions taken with consent and actions taken without consent is fundamental. To borrow twenty dollars is not a wrongful moral action. To steal twenty dollars is. Rape is, rightly, regarded as an ethically unacceptable behavior. On the other hand there is nothing unacceptable about the behavior of people on a honeymoon. Assault is an evil action. Football is not. Unjustly and forcibly depriving another of his life is the interpersonal evil of murder. Voluntary euthanasia is not murder.

The physician's dilemma, if he thinks of himself as his patient's comrade-in-arms, is the same as that of the soldier. Many physicians, perhaps most, do not seem to regard themselves as the comrade-in-arms of their patient. For whether a patient like Margaret has a right to exercise her freedom through a health care professional who serves as her agent is an open question.

Veracity

✖ **DILEMMA 13-1** Chris comes into the hospital because of cholecystitis. She has been in the city only 5 or 6 weeks. She came to the city in order to get married. Her wedding is 3 days away, but it may be interrupted because of her hospitalization.

Norma, her nurse, discovers by talking to Chris that she knows Chris' fiance. She knows that he has been married before. She strongly suspects that Chris does not know this. She also knows that he abused his first wife very badly. Norma is quite certain that Chris does not know this.

So Norma faces a dilemma: Should she tell Chris the facts, as she knows them, about the man Chris is going to marry?

On the one hand, it seems that Norma would be quite callous not to tell Chris. On the other hand, this is not a health care dilemma and so it is really none of Norma's business.

This dilemma is even more complex than it seems. Whatever Norma does, she does more than simply inform Chris or withhold information. It involves more than the question of whether she should tell Chris a truth — a truth that may be very important to Chris. Whatever she does, Norma changes Chris' objective relation to her world.

Right here and now Chris must deal with her gallbladder condition. This is very unpleasant. She is looking forward to her marriage and her future, which looks very bright to her.

If Norma relates to Chris what she knows about Chris' fiance, she makes dealing with the gallbladder condition more difficult. For now Chris may not have a happy future to look forward to. Where she looked forward to joy, she now looks forward to problems. If Norma does not relate the facts concerning Chris' fiance, Chris will keep her optimistic frame of mind and enjoy the benefits that this brings to her recovery. At the same time the shock of discovering the truth will be greater because it comes so unexpectedly. And if Chris' fiance continues his practice of wife abuse, this will have very negative effects on Chris' health and well-being.

Whenever one person relates or withholds a truth from another person, in an ethical context, they change that person's objective relation to the world. The issue of truth-telling is more complex and more important than the question of whether one ought to tell the truth.

Privacy

Josie is a nurse on a trauma unit. Anthony, one of her patients, has suffered a severe head trauma that has left him brain damaged.
There are times when Anthony gets extremely agitated. He trembles so violently that it shakes his bed. Karen, his wife, has found that by getting into bed with him she can comfort him and calm him down. Josie feels a very negative reaction to this. She tells Karen that a hospital setting is not appropriate for this degree of intimacy. Josie asks Karen to stay out of Anthony's bed.

For a man and wife to get into bed together in a hospital setting is not the normal state of affairs. It is one of those things that simply is not done. Social conventions are strongly on Josie's side.

Josie evaluated the behavior of Anthony and Karen from the perspective of rules and conventions. If she had evaluated their behavior from the perspective of human life and values, her judgment might have been different. She might have gone against social convention and approved of Karen's behavior.

To respect the life of another human being is very admirable. Strangely enough, to respect his privacy is even better.

Josie can respect Anthony's right to life without respecting his privacy. Josie does respect Anthony's right to life. She wants him to live and enjoy well-being.

If Josie were to leave Karen and Anthony alone, she would show respect for Anthony's right to life and well-being. This act of respect for Anthony's privacy would enhance his life and well-being—here and now.

Self-ownership or privacy is a natural instrument through which people preserve their lives. Nature has programmed every person so that he or she experiences life as involving self-ownership. If a person did not experience the relationship between privacy and life in this way, the person could not preserve his or her life as a human being. Privacy serves biological survival. It serves the survival of the personality. If a person's privacy is taken away a part of his life is taken away—that part of his life that he or she is.

This fundamental right to privacy is very basic. The greater a person's privacy, the greater the control over his or her life. The more control a person has over his or her life, the more it is a human life and the more it is his or her own.

Beneficence

✂ DILEMMA 13-2 Donna is a nurse in the neonatal intensive care unit. Maureen, her patient, has given birth to a very premature infant. The infant does not weigh quite 2 pounds and cannot breathe spontaneously on his own. The amniocentesis reveals that the infant is suffering from Down's syndrome. A sonogram shows that the baby suffers from a severe heart defect.

Maureen asks Donna for information and advice. Her baby has only about a 5 percent chance of living. If the baby does live, he will have severe mental and physical handicaps. Maureen's physician wants to treat the baby aggressively. Maureen asks Donna if she should allow this treatment.

Considering the limited potentiality of this baby's life, the demands of beneficence are not easy to determine here. But they must be determined. Beneficence has to be a part of life for life to flourish. At the same time it is, at least, open to question whether beneficence always demands preserving life.

Life needs beneficence very much in the same way it needs justice. When a nurse diligently fulfills her part of the nurse/patient agreement, she acts beneficently. She also acts as she has agreed to act. Therefore she acts with justice.

Fidelity

When a nurse practices fidelity to the agreement, she practices fidelity to her own choice—her choice to be a nurse. In practicing fidelity to her choice she is faithful to her life. Life is the broadest context that any biomedical professional acts within. It is the most difficult context to act within. More inefficient ethical action occurs within this context than within any other. The demands of fidelity within the context of life are greater than any other ethical demands that a nurse faces.

The concept of "life" involves a person. The person is always in a world and the concept of life involves the world within which a person lives. To grasp the meaning of her patient's life a nurse must observe the world in which her patient lives and the person who lives in this world.

A person learns of the ethical meaning of human life through perceptual experience, observing the world through the senses and retaining what is learned in the form of concepts. But other people will never be more than simply *things* in the world unless a person learns of them through introspection. No one can learn the nature of other people unless the person first learns his or her own nature through introspection.

In either case—whether one is learning about the world in which one lives or about oneself and, through this, about other people living in the world—the data must be there to be observed. Every nurse, in order to learn about her patient's life and what it means to her patient, must learn about her own life and what it means to her. This is possible only if her life and its meaning is introspectively available to her. Her life and its meaning are available to her only if her life has meaning to her. If her life does not have meaning to her, as the traditional ethical theories implicitly tell her it should not, she will never understand her patient's life.

If she does not understand her patient's life, her ethical actions will be what ethical actions become under the traditional ethical theories—automatized, mechanical, untouched by reason or desire.

The suggestion is sometimes made that nurses ought to develop empathy with their patients through portrayals of suffering found in art and literature, and it is true that through art and literature a nurse can develop an emotional enthusiasm for the care she gives her patient. The emotional enthusiasm she develops is, however, like all emotional enthusiasms, transient.

A nurse cannot justify her choices, decisions, and actions—she cannot justify herself—if she does not value and respect, within herself, that which she claims to value and respect in others.

Suppose a nurse does not respect and value her own autonomy, freedom, objective relationship to the world, privacy, or rights. Suppose further that she bases her ethical choices, decisions and actions on respect for and appreciation of her patient's autonomy, freedom, objective relationship to the world, privacy, and rights. Is it not manifestly obvious that she does not believe in, and does not understand, the basis of her ethical choices, decisions, and actions?

SUMMARY

It is perfectly appropriate, ethically, that a nurse should be the beneficiary of the benefits that the bioethical standards bring to her interaction with her patient. The extent and the application of this can be determined only in the specific context. But in general:

1. If a patient accepts a nurse's respect for his autonomy, he owes the nurse a tolerance of her autonomy. If, for example, she discusses ice hockey and hunting with him, he ought to be willing to accept the fact that she is not able to be terribly bright and cheerful first thing in the morning.
2. If a patient accepts a nurse's recognition of his right to freedom, he owes her a recognition of her role as nurse and respect for her responsibilities. If, for example, she takes him to the recreation room so he can smoke, he ought to comply with her request to force fluids.
3. If a patient accepts a nurse's recognition of his right to veracity he owes her trust. If, for example, she gives him the information he needs in order to make decisions, he owes her complete information on which to base her nursing judgments.
4. If a patient accepts a nurse's respect for his right to privacy, he owes it to her not to make unreasonable demands on her time. If, for example, she protects him against interruption while he is making an important phone call, he owes it to her not to ask her to wait 45 minutes before doing his treatment.
5. If a patient accepts a nurse's beneficence, he owes her cooperation. If, for example, she gets a patient candy and a newspaper, he has a responsibility to see that his visitors do not become disruptive.
6. If a patient accepts a nurse's fidelity to their agreement, he owes her a recognition and respect for her role as a professional nurse.
7. If, for example, a patient accepts the fact that a nurse gives him attentive care and recognizes his rights under their agreement, then he owes it to her to comply with her responsible requests so that she can do what their agreement calls for.

In every case the benefits that accrue to the patient logically imply the benefits that accrue to the nurse.

REFERENCE

Gutmann, J. (Ed.). (1949). *Spinoza's ethics*. New York: Hafner Publishing Company.

The Role of Purpose

The Goals of Ethical Action

There are few consistent followers of either a ritualistic or a purposive ethical system. Most people haphazardly form the ethical system they adopt. They form it out of a combination of what they have been taught by Aunt Maude or Uncle Jeffrey and their observation of effective ethical action in real life.

A person can observe what succeeds and what fails early in life from the experience of the everydayness of family living, the give and take of playing with playmates, and the demands of school work. A person *can* observe this. Not everyone does.

Amy, a nurse on a cardiac step-down unit, is a case in point. Her ethical system is much more influenced by the ethical instruction force-fed to her by her Aunt Maude and Uncle Jeffrey than she is by her experience of successful and failing ethical interactions.

Her actions are much more ritualistic than purposive. Her actions have more in common with singing a song or reciting a poem than with cooking a meal or mowing the lawn. The goal of singing a song or reciting a poem is simply the activity itself and nothing beyond it. The goal of cooking a meal is the finished meal. The goal of mowing a lawn is having an attractive lawn. Amy's ethical actions have no purpose beyond the actions themselves. Her ethical actions, like singing and reciting, are their own reason for being.

In the context of a person's everyday life there is certainly nothing wrong with singing a song or reciting a poem. These can be enjoyable activities. But nonpurposive activity is very inappropriate to a bioethical context.

In the minor, everyday ethical dilemmas that arise in the life of a nurse, Amy experiences inner conflicts. Her ritualistic ethical system is entirely out of harmony with the bioethical standards. The ethical demands of nursing cannot be met without observation of the bioethical standards.

Amy's patients come into the health care system because certain of their values are in jeopardy. Her orientation toward her patients is appropriate to their physical or psychological condition. She interacts with them according to the narrow purpose that brought them into the health care system. But in the "human" and ethical aspects of their interaction Amy reverts back to the ritualistic rules that Aunt Maude and Uncle Jeffrey taught her.

Amy has trouble dealing with normal everyday ethical dilemmas. She is entirely incapable of dealing with the dramatic dilemmas of medicine. Her stand on the most complex and challenging ethical dilemmas of bio-medicine — abortion, euthanasia, organ transplants, genetic engineering, use of fetal tissue, restricted treatment of the elderly, treatment of infants delivered in the second trimester, etc. — is set once and for all by the rules she has adopted. She has no desire to analyze and enter into the ongoing discussions of these complex issues, except insofar as she can defend her prejudices.

Bernice, Amy's co-worker, is not intimidated by ethical matters. Consequently she can take purposeful ethical action much more seriously. Her ethical system is very heavily influenced by her observation and evaluation of the purposeful ethical actions she has observed. When she thinks deeply about bioethical questions she does not take the instruction given to her by her Aunt Susan and Uncle Fred seriously.

The ethical aspects of Bernice's interactions are much more purposeful than ritualistic. Her ethical actions are goal oriented. In the minor, everyday ethical dilemmas that occur in the life of a nurse, Bernice is guided, almost entirely, by the purposes of her patient and the nature of the health care system. She experiences little or no internal discord.

Bernice looks upon the complex and interesting ethical dilemmas of bio-medicine as the most stimulating and challenging part of being a member of the health care professions. For Bernice these dilemmas are not a threat to ritualistic beliefs. They are an exciting challenge to her to develop her understanding.

Ethics arose from the necessity of making decisions in the face of adversity. The face of adversity that confronts Amy and Bernice as nurses is very different from the face of adversity that would confront them as family members, playmates, or students. It is also very different from anything that ever confronted Aunt Maude and Uncle Jeffrey or Aunt Susan and Uncle Fred.

A ritualistic (traditional, post-Cartesian) ethic is one that holds along with the "Father of Modern Philosophy," Rene Descartes (1596-1650), that a human person is constituted of two different and antagonistic principles— mind and body. It holds, implicitly or explicitly, that the mind is spiritual, pure, and moral. It holds, implicitly or explicitly, that the body is carnal, corrupt, and evil.

This Cartesian dualism has dominated ethics since the time of Descartes.

A purposive ethic (an ethic in the Aristotelian tradition) is one which holds, along with Aristotle and Aristotelians, that a human person is a unitary being—that there is no moral opposition between a person's consciousness and the physical body. Modern biomedicine is much more Aristotelian than Cartesian. Biomedicine is in the process of change, and it is becoming more Aristotelian every year.

The Aristotelian, life-centered ethic has been under attack ever since the time of Descartes and especially since the systematic deontology of the German philosopher, Immanuel Kant (1724-1804).

After the time of Descartes and Kant the ethic of "the man in the street" became more and more formal and ritualistic. Modern man has come to take formal and ritualistic ethic less and less seriously. Modern man has not become noticeably less moral.

A ritualistic ethic is one that, implicitly or explicitly, holds that:

1. Ethical principles are what they are apart from the desires, choices, and purposes of ethical agents.
2. The reason for being of an ethical principle is to direct an ethical agent in the control of innate evil impulses.
3. The desires, choices, and purposes of ethical agents are either ethically irrelevant or ethically undesirable.

In the case of bioethics a traditionalist, by the logic of his or her position, must hold that ethics is prior to and of greater importance than the biomedical context. The traditionalist will hold, consequently, that ethics should shape the biomedical context.

A purposive (Aristotelian) ethic, on the other hand, is one which, implicitly or explicitly, holds that:

1. Ethical principles are what they are because humans are what they are and reality is what it is. The nature of appropriate ethical principles is formed by the desires, choices, and purposes of ethical agents in their interaction with reality.

2. The desires, choices, and purposes of ethical agents are not determined by innate evil impulses. In consequence the goal of ethical principles is to direct ethical agents to successful ethical action.
3. Ethical principles have their reason for being in the desires, choices, and purposes of ethical agents in their pursuit of the good. Thus, for Aristotle the goal of ethical action is happiness; for Thomas Aquinas the good is that which is naturally satisfying to the appetites; for Spinoza man's life and well-being are the goal of ethical action. Even for Plato the goal of ethical action is that which, without being unjust, benefits the individual.

In the case of bioethics a purposive ethic would hold that the biomedical context determines the ethical principles relevant to the biomedical context—that the biomedical context must determine the nature of bioethics.

Although many biomedical professionals give lip service to a ritualistic ethic, very few practice such an ethic in a biomedical context. Even the legal system consistently refuses to sanction the effects of out-of-context, ritualistic action. For a biomedical professional to approach his or her practice from a ritualistic perspective would be disastrous.

A great deal of effort has been put into various attempts to harmonize biomedicine and ritualistic or traditional ethical systems. None have yet succeeded. None will ever succeed. The traditional ethic is based on, and does not make sense without, an assumption of the mind-body antagonism. If a biomedical professional, standing on the hospital steps, looks upon the incoming patient as a pure spirit trapped in an evil body, there is no way he or she can effectively treat the patient. There is no way the professional could even communicate with the patient. No patient entering the health care system is, in that situation, willing to think of himself as a consciousness whose existence is desirable trapped in a physical body whose existence is undesirable.

Hippocrates' outlook on bioethics was thoroughly purposive. A purposive ethic also determines the ethical outlook of modern medicine. If modern medicine embraced a ritualistic ethic, then biomedical professionals would have to hold ridiculous positions. They would have to hold, for instance, that it is not ethical to cut someone. The ethical system of "the man on the street" would tell the professional that cutting someone is not ethical.

Patients enter into the health care setting motivated by their desires, choices, and purposes. It should be unnecessary to point out that the action of a patient, in entering the health care system, even though it be a purposeful action, cannot rationally be regarded as an action taken with an evil intent. But if this is not the attitude of a health care professional who embraces a ritualistic ethic, then his or her ethical attitudes and ethical actions are in a state of conflict. The ethical system that this professional embraces, is unrelated to his or her profession. It is pointless. It is, above all, purposeless.

PURPOSE AS THE BASIS OF THE BIOETHICAL STANDARDS

Purpose is the mental set of a desiring being. It is action directed toward vital concerns, toward needs and values. Purpose is the central element of a purposeful ethical decision-making model. In any action that a person takes, success or failure depends upon whether or not the person accomplishes his or her purpose. In an ethical context whether an aspect of the context is good or evil depends upon whether it assists or hinders the purposeful actions that the context calls for.

On the simplest possible level it is quite obvious that a screw driver is right for the purpose of screwing a screw into a piece of wood. It is wrong for the purpose of hammering a nail. A hammer is right for hammering a nail but wrong for screwing a screw.

If a person's purpose is to gain happiness, then those actions that will bring about conditions which produce happiness are right and good. Those actions that bring about conditions which undermine happiness are wrong and evil.

For purposes of returning a patient to a state of agency, those actions that bring about the physical and psychological conditions of agency in a patient are right and good. Those actions that undercut the physical or psychological conditions of his agency are wrong and evil.

David is in the hospital with perpherial vascular disease. His nurse, Joy, is educating him on how he must care for himself when he gets out of the hospital.

In order to do this, Joy:

- Tries to find out all she can about David so she can advise him according to his specific situation.
- Gives him all the information he needs so that he can enjoy the maximum freedom of action.
- Tells him whatever he needs to know in order to enable him to gain and retain his power of agency. She tells him nothing that he does not need to know or that might hinder his gaining and retaining his power of purposeful action.
- Allows David the isolation he needs in order to make autonomous decisions. She reveals nothing to anyone that might interfere with David's privacy when he leaves the hospital.
- Does whatever she can in order to promote David's welfare. She does nothing which might hinder David's welfare, nothing that might hinder his power to take autonomous actions.

The standard of any action, including ethical actions, is the purpose that the agent means to accomplish by the action.

QUESTION: "Why did the chicken cross the street?"
ANSWER: "To get to the other side."

If a chicken or a person wants to walk across the street, then getting to the other side is the standard of success. If a person wants to learn to use a computer, then his or her standard of success is the ability to use a computer. If a person wants to become a nurse, then the standard of success is passing the state boards. If a nurse wants to recognize the self-ownership of her patient, then that patient acting on his self-ownership is the standard of the nurse's success.

Every event that fulfills an agent's purpose is an event that signals the success of an ethical agent. The reason for being of an ethical decision-making model is to guide the action of an ethical agent to just such events. An effective ethical decision-making model for nurses is an instrument to guide a nurse in the accomplishment of ethical purposes appropriate to nursing.

THE FACETS OF PURPOSE

The world presents various alternatives to an ethical agent. An agent chooses from among alternatives according to his or her desires. When an agent chooses from among alternatives, this act of choice forms a purposeful state of mind. A purpose is the object of a desire that a person brings to the forefront or retains in his or her attention.

A choice is an objective relationship between a state of desire and an alternative that a person perceives in the world. A choice is a mental action which inspires physical action. All action is purposeful behavior.

Any purposeful ethic involves choice. An ethical system not based on purpose and choice is ritualistic and formalistic. It is like reading poetry to oneself. In relation to nursing a ritualistic or formalistic ethic cannot motivate actions appropriate to nursing. It cannot guide a nurse's actions appropriately. It cannot enable her to justify the actions she takes. It can no more be a professional ethic than tea leaf reading can be a technology.

A nurse armed with a formalistic ethic would not know what questions to ask of a context. Nor would she know what would constitute the answer to a contextual ethical question. A process of ethical justification has to do with these questions and answers. Such a process is simply an explanation of the questions a person has asked and the answers that he has acted upon.

REASON AND PURPOSE AS THE BASIS FOR ETHICAL DECISION MAKING

Purpose as an element of autonomy, in and of itself, is usually sufficient to resolve an ethical dilemma. Each of the other elements of autonomy is important only as it relates to purpose.

In order to act purposefully and ethically a nurse must always act according to the evidence she has of the array of values held by a patient. Let us examine this process through a thought-experiment:

Suppose a nurse, Sylvia, stranded on a desert island, had to make an ethical decision concerning a stranger who washed up on shore. The stranger is both naked and comatose. He has a traumatic wound to the head. Sylvia has no way of discovering the name of the stranger, let alone his specific desires, purposes, or values.

Nonetheless, it is quite possible for Sylvia's actions in regard to this stranger to be determined according to a proper nursing ethic. In this situation she can utilize the element of purpose to arrive at perfectly justifiable decisions and actions. Every nurse, in every situation of this type, with a greater or lesser amount of difficulty, can come up with an answer to these interrelated questions:

- "What would the maximum number of persons most desire in this circumstance?"
- "What would be the purpose of the maximum number of persons in this circumstance if they could act for themselves?"

Any decision that a nurse would make on the basis of a reasoned answer to these questions is ethically justifiable. There would, in fact, be no other ethically justifiable way of arriving at a decision. If a health care professional has virtually no evidence to go on, he or she must go on what little evidence there is.

Sylvia has evidence of the sex and approximate age of the stranger. This tells her almost nothing.

She can see that the stranger is a person. This tells her all that she needs to know.

It is perfectly reasonable for Sylvia to form her conclusion according to the purposes that most people would hold. Whatever purposes the maximum number of persons would hold in this circumstance, this stranger would *probably* hold.

A fireman leaving a burning house might see a packet of letters and a scrapbook on a table. If he can only save one, he has a perplexing problem. He has no way of knowing which the homeowners would prefer he save. Sylvia has no such problem.

Suppose that the stranger in our thought-experiment were conscious. Sylvia can see that he is bleeding from a cut on his head. Under these circumstances Sylvia would probably act automatically and without stopping to ask permission. But Sylvia might ask him if he wants her to stop the bleeding. The odds are overwhelming that the stranger would reply that he did. Then she would know exactly what the context calls for.

Sylvia does not have all this evidence. She does, however, have all the evidence that she needs. She has enough evidence on which to make a reasoned judgment. In a circumstance of this type, the fact that a judgment is reasoned is sufficient to justify the judgment.

In an emergency, a health care professional will almost automatically act for the purpose of saving lives. What other justification could the health care professional have for this except that the maximum number of people in the maximum number of circumstances would want their lives to be saved? Sylvia is justified by the fact that any individual person in the emergency would almost certainly want to be saved.

It is not necessary to be a mind reader to be an effective ethical agent.

That she will act according to her best judgment forms part of a nurse's implicit agreement with her patient. It forms part of a nurse's relationship to the rest of the world. It is a fundamental part of a nurse's role.

However some people are very strange.

Suppose that the stranger for whom Sylvia acted were to claim that the decision she made was a wrong decision. Suppose, for want of a better supposition, that he believes that by touching his head on a Tuesday Sylvia defiled him. He declares that he would have preferred bleeding to death to being defiled.

Let us examine the implications of this:

Under the circumstances Sylvia made her decision on the basis of all the evidence available to her — the evidence she had of the stranger being a person.

If the decision she made and the action she took, based on her analysis of the evidence, was a wrong decision and a wrong action, then either:

A. It is a fact that the majority of people washed onto the shore of a desert island, with a scalp laceration, would want to bleed to death and Sylvia should have known this,

or

B. Sylvia made a mistake in reasoning from the evidence that was presented to her. An ethical agent should not make decisions by reasoning from evidence.

If the stranger attempts to justify his claim on alternative A, he attempts to justify it on an absurdity. Imagine a group of people with profusely bleeding scalp wounds sitting on a beach and replying to offers of help with: "No thanks, don't bother. I would just as soon bleed to death."

If the stranger attempts to justify his claim by alternative B, that Sylvia should not have acted on a reasoned conclusion based on her evidence, then his position is even more absurd.

If she should *not* have decided according to her recognition of the evidence, then she *should* have acted without thinking. But, if she should have acted without thinking, then anything she did would be right. If a person *should* act without thinking, then there is no way that what he does can be *wrong*. In this case his claim that she should not have taken the actions she did contradicts itself.

Let us assume that Sylvia should have decided on what to do without thinking, without reasoning according to the evidence avaliable to her. If a person's action is based on thinking then, within limits, that action will be predictable. Thinking will limit the number of actions that might be taken. If a person acts without thinking, then the ensuing action will be unpredictable. There will be nothing to limit the number of actions that might be taken.

If Sylvia should have acted without thinking, she might have done anything at all. If she would have been right to do anything at all, then any action she took would be justified. If any action she took would be justified, then the decision and action that she actually did take could not rationally be condemned.

In the nature of things a nurse *can* justify her ethical decisions and actions through the element of purpose. Purpose is, or ought to be, directly or indirectly, the standard of *all* ethical decision making.

PURPOSE AND THE ETHICAL CONTEXT

The effects of some actions are entirely predictable. If you jump into a swimming pool, it is predictable that you will get wet. If you drop a light bulb on a sidewalk it is predictable that the bulb will break. If a patient is hemorrhaging and a nurse fails to take action, the patient will die.

The effects of other actions are very unpredictable. The course of a patient's recovery is unpredictable. A patient's notion of and need for privacy is unpredictable. The degree of independence a patient wants is unpredictable.

Ethical actions are very much of the second kind. Ethical actions cannot be taken with ballistic accuracy. The greater a nurse's knowledge of her patient's context, the greater the chance of her decision being the best one. All the same a nurse must sometimes act on very limited knowledge. She can seldom, and perhaps never, act with perfect certainty.

The first effect of an action does not justify an action. Any effect might, in its turn, become a cause of further effects. Thelma, a nurse in a rehabilitation center for children, is caring for Larry, a 10-year-old child. Larry has heard that something happened to his dog. Thelma reassures him and tells him that his mother is going to bring the dog in to see him that afternoon. This reassures Larry and makes him very happy. When the afternoon comes and Larry's mother has to tell Larry that his dog has died, the grief that Larry experiences is much worse because of the reassurance Thelma had given him.

In the same way the comfort a patient derives from false hope that is given him concerning his prognosis often increases his distress when he learns the truth.

In order to execute optimally effective ethical actions a nurse must, of course, intend good effects. But, good intentions are not enough. She must analyze the context to see what probable effects her actions will have. In order for an ethical action to be justified, it must be appropriate to the context. In order for the purpose and probable effects of an action to be understood, there must be an interweaving of the ethical context and the nurse's awareness.

The justification of ethical actions cannot be based on an infallible knowledge of what is called for and what the effects of one's actions will be. It must come through good intentions and the nurse's dedicated efforts to knowing what she is doing — and why.

PURPOSE AND THE BIOETHICAL STANDARDS

Autonomy

Audrey is 18 years old. She is a member of a very radical religious sect. The sect has been founded within the past 10 years by an extremely charismatic leader. Audrey has adopted a number of ideas from the sect that are entirely opposed to modern medical practice.
All the same Audrey believes that she would like to become a nurse. She discusses this with her friend, Marsha. Marsha, who is a nurse, is aware of Audrey's beliefs. Marsha faces the problem of whether or not she should encourage Audrey to join the profession. Audrey's purpose and her autonomy seem at odds.

A person's autonomy always determines the nature of his or her purpose. At the same time the nature of a person's purpose reveals his or her autonomy. It may be that Audrey does not perceive the conflict between her present beliefs and her desire to be a nurse. Marsha, however, has no right to assume this. This complicates Marsha's dilemma.

Every purpose is chosen. If a person holds a purpose, he or she has chosen that purpose. If that person has chosen a purpose, he or she has chosen it because of his or her beliefs in relation to that purpose. A person's beliefs form that person's autonomy. Every choice a person makes and, consequently, every purpose a person holds, is an expression of his or her autonomy.

In Audrey's case her beliefs and her purposes conflict. This is evidence that Audrey's autonomy is not fully formed. The famous rabbi, Hillel the Elder (1st century B.C.) remarked, "He who would be everything will be nothing." So it will be with Audrey, until she discovers who she is.

Nurses often face the problem of trying to resolve an ethical dilemma in harmony with the autonomy of their patient and according to his purposes. This is very difficult when there is a conflict between the patient's autonomy and his purposes.

Every conflict between autonomy and purpose is, ultimately, a conflict between two opposed purposes. In an ethical context a person's autonomy is simply those purposes that are fundamental, vital, and unique to that person—those purposes through which the person makes himself who he is. Audrey's task is to discover whether it is her religious beliefs or her desire to be a nurse that produces her more fundamental and vital purpose.

The autonomy of the people involved is the basis for the nurse/patient agreement. The fact that a person's purposes constitute his or her autonomy makes it necessary to form the agreement. The fact that the person's autonomy lies in his or her fundamental and vital purposes makes it unnecessary for the agreement to be an explicit agreement.

Freedom

✂ DILEMMA 14-1   Keith is suffering from a bleeding ulcer. He and his nurse, Jenna, have developed a very close and trusting relationship. Keith has been talking for days about wanting to get to his son's wedding in two weeks. His physician tells Keith that he cannot get the bleeding of Keith's ulcer stopped. The physician wants to operate the next day. Keith refuses to undergo the operation. Should Jenna use her influence with Keith in order to persuade him to change his mind? The line between persuasion and coercion is very thin in this context.

Human purposes are long range. They require freedom. A person's freedom is the freedom to act, or not to act, on a purpose. A person's freedom is the freedom to form, or not to form, a purpose.

If a billiard ball were free, if it could move about the billiard table whenever it choose, its behavior would be unpredictable and inexplicable. Human freedom is biologically intelligible and predictable because people have purposes.

A person possesses volition. Nature does not compel a person to think every thought he or she thinks. Nor does nature compel a person to take every action that is taken. A being's volition is the basis of human freedom. A person experiences pleasure in exercising that volition. Yet it is not volition that makes a person's freedom valuable. It is the possibility of realizing his or her purposes that makes a person's freedom valuable.

A value is the goal of an action. A person's freedom is the freedom to decide on values and to pursue them. If a person had no values, freedom would be of no value. Purpose imparts value to the freedom to pursue values.

The rights of every individual comes into being because all people have purposes. A right is an agreement. It is an agreement that everyone shall have freedom of action. Every right is a person's right to freedom to pursue purposes. A person's rights increase the range of his or her freedom and the freedom of everyone in a society.

Freedom is the standard by which individual rights can be weighed and measured.

Veracity

✖ **DILEMMA 14-2**   Russell is in the emergency room following a motorcycle accident. He is bleeding profusely from his foot and leg and has observable trauma to the head. It looks as though his foot might need to be amputated. His vital signs are very unstable. In his partial delirium he tells Selma, the nurse who is attending him, that he has been training to enter the Olympic boxing competition. He asks her whether or not his injuries will interfere with his boxing career. Suddenly Selma faces a dilemma.

Truth is a necessary precondition of purpose. Ethical agents could not act on purposes unless they had access to the objective facts of a situation. Still it seems, as in Russell's case, there are times when it may be better not to know the truth. But this seems to suggest that there are times when it is better not to have purposes. It is very difficult to see how a person would be better off without purposes.

Without purpose there would be no reason for a person to take actions. If there is no reason for a person to take actions, there is no value whatever to truth.

If, however, a person desires to act — has purposes — he or she needs truth. Truth can be, and ought to be, the best friend of purpose.

Privacy

✖ **DILEMMA 14-3**   Nina motivates her patients to follow their regimen of treatment by constantly reminding them of things they have told her they want to do. It might seem that this is taking advantage of her patients' purposes in order to violate their self-ownership. However, it may be that the benefit of following the regimen of treatment justifies Nina's gentle bantering.

A person's thinking determines what he or she will regard as central to self-ownership, as private.

If a person does not have privacy, does not enjoy self-ownership, then all the value of purpose is lost. The fact that people have and act on purposes shows the value of privacy. Every purpose is a private purpose.

If a person could not act on private purposes without interference, he or she could not maintain the effort spent on purposes. The noninterference with self-ownership that the standard of privacy counsels is the precondition of an agent's purpose.

If a person has no right to self-ownership, then he or she has no right to any purpose. If a person has no right to pursue purposes, then he or she has no right to life. Life requires privacy.

Beneficence

✖   **DILEMMA 14-4**   Larry is a 33-year-old patient who suffers from epilepsy. Larry's condition has not responded well to drugs. He had a seizure six weeks ago and fell down a flight of cement steps. As a result of his accident he sustained permanent brain damage. He is unable to perform most activities of daily living, and the brain damage has left him with severe speech difficulties. Larry was a heavy smoker before the accident and, now that he is stabilized, he has taken up this habit again. His only pleasures since his accident are watching television and smoking.

Larry has developed a chronic cough which is aggravated when he smokes. His nurse, Louise, has decided that for his own benefit it would be better if he limits and finally quits smoking. Is Louise's course of action, over the long run, beneficent or is she unjustifiably interfering with Larry's pursuit of his purposes?

Is there any plausibility to Louise's claim that she is exercising beneficence toward Larry? Or does beneficence necessarily consist in helping a person attain his purposes and not hindering him?

Fidelity

✖   **DILEMMA 14-5**   Marilu is caring for an 82-year-old woman, Lillian. Lillian has been quite active in charitable affairs. One day, while shopping, she slipped on a patch of ice. Lillian fractured her clavicle in the fall. She was taken to surgery and the fracture was repaired. Part of her post operative orders consisted in 10 mg of valium and 75 mg of demerol as needed.

Lillian became very confused and within two days did not know her name. Her physician diagnosed her as senile. He began making plans for her to be transferred to a nursing home. He contacted her daughter, who lived in a distant city. Lillian's daughter decided not to visit until her mother was transferred to the nursing home.

Marilu is convinced that Lillian is not senile, but the physician refuses to consider her reasoning. Marilu believes that if Lillian is taken to the nursing home she will never again return to her normal life. She has every reason to believe that Lillian would not want to go to the nursing home.

Under these circumstances Marilu faces a conflict between the purposes of the health care system and what she believes to be Lillian's purposes. She also faces a conflict between the demands of fidelity to her agreement with Lillian and her agreement with the health care system.

Fidelity, like purpose, has an inside and an outside. Each depends upon a state of mind in the agent and the action he takes in the outside world.

Fidelity and purpose are related in another important way. Fidelity is an instrument whereby people accomplish purposes. Cooperation assists purpose.

Fidelity makes cooperation possible. If it were not for its relationship to purpose, fidelity would have no ethical importance. It has no ethical importance in itself. Fidelity to an agreement to perform an unethical action is not an ethical value. Fidelity is only important insofar as it serves the moral purpose of an ethical agent.

SUMMARY

If there is one activity more central to human life than any other, it is the discovery and pursuit of autonomous purposes. This is the activity that relates an individual's abstract aspirations and the biological functions necessary to the organism's continued survival.

An individual person defines what is important and what is not by the purposes he or she chooses to pursue. This is the basis of a purposive ethic.

For a ritualistic ethic, on the contrary, that which is important is irrelevant. Nothing is important, but some things are necessary. A person must do his or her duty, not because something is important but because duty is necessary for its own sake.

There is a claim that a certain school of ethicists never tire of repeating: "You can't get an 'ought' from an 'is'." By this they mean that from any fact true of people or of reality it is not possible to perceive one course of action as superior to another in an ethical sense. You cannot get an ethical motivation from a fact. If a person starts from a ritualistic basis—if what a person ought to do is cut off from human purposes—then, indeed, "You can't get an ought from an is." But ethics can be purposeful and you can get *every* ethical motivation from a fact. In fact you cannot get ethical motivations from anywhere else.

REFERENCE

Gutmann, J. (Ed.). (1949). *Spinoza's ethics*. New York: Hafner Publishing Company.

CHAPTER

15

The Role of Agency

The Nature of Ethical Action

Imagine, if you will, that you are taking a stroll over a very large lawn by a woodside. As you walk, you pass one by one, a rock, a tree, and then a horse. Finally you pass a young woman and a young man.

From the "viewpoint" of the rock nothing is either good or evil. Whatever happens, it is a matter of perfect indifference. But, in order to experience the "ethical aspects" of what you see during your stroll, imagine that one thing, if only this one thing, is good in relation to the rock. There is a *very* weak sense in which the (only) good for the rock is to retain its structural integrity, to retain its "rockhood." Obviously the rock has no desire to remain in existence. That is not important. What is important is this: There is nothing morally outrageous in the fact that the rock exists and remains in existence.

Now you pass a tree. This is a very different kind of thing. The rock is inert and inanimate; the tree is alive. To stay alive the tree must sink its roots into the earth in order to draw stability and sustenance from the ground. So you encounter a sort of progression, a change in the way of being. Even so there is nothing here, in the living and acting of the tree, that is morally undesirable. Life is not, in itself, an ethical disaster.

Now you come to the horse. The horse is also alive. It is alive in an even stronger sense than the tree. The horse is conscious of its environment. It moves about from place to place in a manner that follows from its nature. The horse eats grass from the ground and apples from the tree. Yet even in this behavior of the horse there is no basis for a rational moral indignation. The existence of the horse is not a moral calamity.

So it is also with the man and woman. Here again one comes to a different kind of being—the man and woman are not only conscious, they are conscious on an abstract and conceptual level. Yet there is nothing any more intrinsically immoral in the existence of reason in the man and woman than there is in the animality of the horse. There is nothing more morally undesirable in the animality of the horse than there is in the "treeness" of the tree. There is nothing more morally undesirable in the "treeness" of the tree than there is in the "rockness" of the rock.

In a nursing context an ethical system that would seek to work around the disaster of a patient being human and being alive would be a tragic mistake. It would probably be a mistake that would lead to litigation.

ACTION

The term "action" in ethics has a very specific and technical meaning. It can be most easily understood in relation to its correlative "passion." Action and passion are both forms of behavior.

A *passion* is any behavior that an entity undergoes through a force external to itself and not as an outcome of any act of self-determination. An *action* is a behavior that an agent initiates from the self. The agent determines the execution of the action, the occurrence and the nature of the behavior. Scratching an intolerable itch or behavior exhibited under the influence of an overwhelming emotion such as fear are instances of passion. The falling of a leaf, the careening of a billiard ball, the behavior of a nail in the vicinity of a magnet are also examples of passion.

Making and completing long-range plans, meeting an inconvenient ethical responsibility, engaging in a difficult, unfamiliar thought process, lifting a heavy weight are various types of action. These, of course, are things that leaves, billiard balls, and nails cannot do.

In relation to a force that precludes volitional choice and compels behavior a (potential) agent is passive. This meaning of the term "passive" is retained in the adjective and in the noun "patient"; indeed, both terms have the same root. A patient is a person who is passive—a person who is incapable of actions according to normal capabilities.

Action, on the other hand, involves these preconditions:

1. An agent's awareness of the situation in which he or she is to act.
2. An agent's awareness of self in general plus his or her specific awareness of self in relation to the situation in which he or she is to act.

3. An agent's implicit awareness of his capacity for self-determined behavior.

All these capabilities can be possessed by a patient. What the patient lacks, to a greater or lesser extent, is the fourth capability.

4. The capability to translate his awareness into an action intended to bring about a desired result.

These preconditions of agency belong to every agent and are not inherently problematic. However, these potential assets of an agent can become problematic under the influence of a dilemma, when an agent may forget possession of these preconditions, distort his or her relationship to them, or be unable to estimate what he or she can accomplish through them.

A nurse may find the physical or mental condition of her patient functioning as a kind of dilemma, causing him to lose his awareness of, or even his interest in, his powers of agency. The demands of effective nursing, under these circumstances, call upon a nurse to rekindle this awareness if possible. This requires that she recognize the difference between her patient's passive acceptance of various states of affairs and his actual exercise of agency. An action actually expresses the nature and intention of the agent, whereas passive acceptance may not.

AGENCY AS THE BASIS OF THE BIOETHICAL STANDARDS

A person's agency is the power to act on autonomous desires that spring from his or her own reasoning. Agency is what human life is all about.

Agency requires autonomous desire. Without autonomous desire behavior is involuntary (or nonvoluntary). Involuntary behavior does not arise from agency. For instance, if a person is jostled in the street and bumps into a wall, that behavior does not arise from agency. His behavior, as we have discussed, is a passion — it arises from a force outside of agency.

Agency requires reason or autonomous thought. Behaviors that arise from the emotions as well as reflex behaviors are not actions. Actions express the specific nature of the agent who acts. Only rational beings possess agency. Only reason in action expresses the specific nature of a rational being.

If ethical action does not, in fact, properly begin with agency, with actions that arise in an agent's autonomous desire and reason, then all of bioethics is misdirected. Every bioethical standard is geared to promote agency in the service of individual purposes:

- The standard of *autonomy* is designed to protect those actions of a patient that express his unique character structure.
- The standard of *freedom* is designed to protect actions arising from the individual agency of the patient.
- The standard of truth (*veracity*) is designed to support the actions which

arise from the individual agency of a patient. It does this by allowing him to act on knowledge.
- The standard of *privacy* is designed to protect the self-ownership of a patient insofar as that self-ownership is expressed in the patient's present or future actions.
- The standard of *beneficence* is designed to protect the actions of an agent—to support his actions and to see that no harm comes to his power of agency.
- The standard of *fidelity* is designed to protect the interactions of several agents as they act toward mutual purposes.

Try to imagine applying the bioethical standards to a machine and you will see the essential relationship between the standards and the patient's agency.

AGENCY, RIGHTS AND ETHICAL INTERACTION

Imagine a desert island with one inhabitant, Jane. Jane is the island's only inhabitant. With no possibility of a division of labor and none of the tools of civilization available to her, survival is a pressing problem for Jane. Under these circumstances, what does Jane have a right to do and what does she have no right to do—what would it be wrong for her to do?

In these highly unusual circumstances it is obvious that Jane has the right to do whatever she has the power to do.

She has the right to pursue any value that she has reason to believe will bring her the maximum benefit and the right to shun whatever would tend to her detriment. She has as much right to pursue her values as she has to exist—and each for the same reason.

How could it be wrong for Jane to act to sustain her existence? Why would it be wrong for her to act toward the realization of her values? There is no logical reason why Jane should negate any aspect of her being, neither the fact *that* she is nor the fact of *what* she is.

The fact that Jane, a thinking, valuing person, actually exists is exhaustive evidence that it is right that she should exist. The fact that Jane is, by nature, a being to whom the pursuit of values is appropriate is conclusive evidence that it is right that she pursue whatever she values. Against the fact that Jane does exist, no rational evidence can be adduced to show that it would be ethically better if she did not exist. The proposition that Jane ought to renounce her life or the pursuit of her values cannot be logically or, therefore, ethically justified. It simply does not make sense.

Jane has the right to be what she is. Any alternative to this principle is incoherent. As a natural corollary to this principle we must conclude that Jane has a right to do whatever she has the power to do. Nothing Jane does can violate the rights of another. There is no other on the island.

Now, let us change the scenario somewhat.

One day Michelle is washed ashore. Holding strictly to the context of our problem, how has Jane's situation changed? How is the principle that Jane has the right to do whatever she has the power to do been modified?

Ethically the principle is unimpaired, although two significant changes have come into Jane's life:

1. As rational beings Michelle and Jane have an obligation not to violate each other's rights. Whether or not they do violate each other's rights, the obligation remains. The obligation is there not by virtue of any arbitrary decision either might make but by virtue of their defining characteristics, by virtue of what Jane and Michelle have in common—their rational nature. As a corollary of this each has an obligation to honor the agreements that she makes with the other.
2. Jane's existential position is enormously enhanced, as is Michelle's for having found Jane there.

> There are many things outside us which are useful to us and which, therefore, are to be sought. Of all these, none more excellent can be discovered than those which exactly agree with our nature. If, for example, two individuals of exactly the same nature are joined together, they make up a single individual, doubly stronger than each alone. Nothing, therefore, is more useful to man than man. (Spinoza, in Gutmann, 1949, pp. 202-203)

If the inhabitants of the island number two or number in the millions, nothing is essentially changed. Moreover, allow yourself a little thought-experiment by placing yourself in the picture. If *you* were Michelle or Jane, the ethical principles governing the situation would remain exactly the same.

If any ethical state of affairs that might apply to a particular individual is, all things being equal, right or wrong, it can only be because it is right or wrong universally, for *every* ethical agent.

TRADITIONAL PREJUDICES AGAINST AGENCY

Modern medicine can allow itself many compromises with the prejudices of popular culture. One compromise that it cannot allow is the prejudice that individual agency is evil.

If individual agency is evil, then the biomedical professions are evil. For the reason for being of the biomedical professions is to return individual patients to a more perfect state of agency.

The Greek philosopher Epicurus (341-270 B.C.) said of the origin of the prejudice against agency that: "Most men want to do good. But, even more than they want to do good, they want to do those things to which their lusts impel them. So they make themselves good by criticizing the evil they are able to perceive in others. They perfect this art by perceiving evil in *every* action which others take."

It is no accident that the ethical system that has arisen in modern biomedicine (the bioethical standards) is incompatible with contemporary views of good. Biomedicine is entirely oriented toward the increased agency of those who seek its services. Nothing opposed to agency can be compatible with the bioethical standards.

Deontology is intrinsically opposed to agency. If human actions and human agency were not evil, it would make no sense to replace the desires that motivate them with moral duties. If human agency were not evil, it would not be appropriate for utilitarianism to try to channel it into the hopeless pursuit of "the greatest good for the greatest number."

AGENCY AND PRESUPPOSITIONALISM

Most modern ethicists are, implicitly or explicitly, presuppositionalists. A presuppositionalist is a person who believes in the necessity of presuppositions, that ethical values cannot be discovered through the human experience of reality alone. A presuppositionalist believes that an ethicist must approach the experience of reality with presuppositions that arise from somewhere other than experience. Why he or she believes this and where the presuppositions arise from the presuppositionalist does not say. If he or she did, of course, it would have to be based on another presupposition. This presupposition would have to be justified in terms of another. This process would be infinite — a possibility that logic does not allow for.

It is also a possibility that medicine does not allow for. From the Hippocratic Oath to the American Medical Association's Principles of Medical Ethics biomedical professionals, or at least physicians, are called on to derive their ethical practice from the nature of their profession. If nurses are to be professionals in the same sense as physicians are professionals, and all other professionals are professionals, they must do likewise. The contemporary bioethical standards are a repudiatiation of presuppositionalism.

According to all that is given to experience without the presupposition of evil, human agency is not evil. The self maintenance of a rock is not evil. The action of a tree in maintaining its existence is not evil. The efforts of a horse to maintain its life are not evil. A visitor from another planet would be hard put to discover the intrinsic evil in men and women acting to preserve their existence.

To live, think and desire, to choose and act are not wrong. The agency of a patient is not an evil to be deplored. The agency of a nurse — her living, thinking, desiring, choosing, and acting — are not evils to be overcome.

The health care setting makes sense if and only if existence and action are good.

THE BIOLOGICAL FUNCTION OF AGENCY

Agency is the agent's interaction with his own life.

It is the instrument of reason and desire.

It is the servant of an agent's purpose.

The function of purpose is to move an agent from a lesser to a greater state of autonomy, freedom, objective connection to reality, and self-ownership.

The function of agency is to move an agent from a less refined reason and a less complete knowledge to a more refined reason and a more complete knowledge.

Agency guides reason in its vision of rational desires and in actions leading to the fulfillment of desire.

Agency enables an agent to attain a more desirable state of life.

Finally, agency serves to increase its own competency and strength. In taking physical actions a person increases the strength of his or her body. In taking the actions necessary to increase understanding, a person increases the strength of his or her mind.

AGENCY AND RIGHTS

Rights pertain to an individual's freedom of action. An individual has a right to make free choices among alternatives based on desires, purposes, and values.

In a state of solitude a person has a right to do whatever he or she is capable of doing. An individual has this right in the sense that no one else is relevantly involved and there is no possibility of violating the rights of others.

In the life of every (noncriminal) individual and in the history of the race it becomes evident that the range and effectiveness of the individual person's activities are greatly augmented if people do not have to devote time and effort to guarding themselves against aggression, coercion, and fraud. So, as a sort of evolutionary instrument, an implicit agreement arises among rational beings, an agreement not to aggress against, not to coerce, and not to defraud each other. The benefit of this agreement is so great and so obvious, the detriment of not having this agreement is so manifestly ruinous, that the agreement *literally* "goes without saying." This agreement is, in various ways, the basis of all benevolence and cooperation among people.

It is also the essential basis of the existence of laws. Laws arise because there is a need for laws. But the need arose long before the laws. This implicit agreement arose before the laws were possible. It arose with the human ability to make agreements.

To the extent that a society is free, the laws that it recognizes as most fundamental are reflections of individual rights. These laws are an explicit statement of the implicit agreement on nonaggression.

Where laws have no rational justification, where they serve no evident need, where they have no moral basis, they are resented and notoriously difficult to enforce. Not so with laws based on the implicit agreement — perhaps not even a criminal can *resent* such laws.

This preexisting agreement against aggression arises from the human condition. Without it there would be no basis for honoring any inconvenient explicit agreements. No legal system could possibly be effective. There would be no basis for agreement on a legal system. The only check on people's criminality would be the limits of their imagination and the range of their daring.

Making an agreement is not at all synonymous with having reason to believe that an agreement will be kept. Where there is no reason to believe that an agreement will be kept, there is no reason to make an agreement, any agreement. Dependable explicit agreements are made possible by this implicit agreement.

Rights can be defined as the product of an implicit agreement among rational beings, by virtue of their rationality, not to obtain actions nor the product of actions from others except through voluntary consent objectively gained.

This implicit agreement gives fiber to explicit agreements and to laws. It gives moral force to every explicit agreement and every other implicit agreement. This holds true of the unspoken but traditional agreement between nurse and patient. The nurse/patient agreement is, in effect, guaranteed by the implicit agreement that constitutes rights. The nurse/patient agreement is an agreement that nurse and patient have a right to expect that each will fulfill his or her role according to the purposes that motivate their interaction. It is an agreement that there will be fidelity and benevolence on each side.

The English philospher, John Stuart Mill (1806-1873), said that one person cannot advance the interests of another by compulsion. One person cannot *rightfully* compel another person to do something because it is better for that other person to do it, because it will make the other person happier, or because, in the opinion of the first person, it would be wise for the second person to do it.

Rights determine the actions an agent can take. Everyone has the right to be free from the coercion of others. Everyone constantly relies on the species-wide implicit agreement that people will not deal with each other coercively. A person can act freely in any social context as long as he or she does not coerce another. In coercing another a person gives up the right to exercise freedom.

> [The right to] self determination is an individual's exercise of the capacity to form, revise, and pursue personal plans for life . . . free from outside control . . . In the context of health care, self determination overrides practitioner determination. (President's Commission, 1982)

A nurse, because she is the agent of her patient, and through the implicit agreement she has with him, has agreed to protect the rights of her patient.

She has an ethical obligation to protect her patient from anyone who would violate his rights. Above all she cannot, herself, break the rights agreement.

It has been observed that rights is to a society what reason is to an individual. The health care setting is a small society.

THE QUALITY OF ETHICAL ACTIONS

The quality of an ethical action for deontology is determined by whether or not it was taken dutifully. If it is taken as the result of a duty, it is good. If it is taken against the agent's duty, it is evil.

The quality of an ethical action for utilitarianism is determined by whether it has produced "the greatest good for the greatest number." Every ethical action taken by an agent sets up a chain of further actions. What might have a good result immediately might have a disastrous result over the long term. The quality of a utilitarian's actions, theoretically, could be known only at the end of time.

The quality of an ethical action for a purposive ethic is determined by whether it can be justified in terms of justifiable intentions and reasonably predictable benefits.

The quality of an action taken according to bioethics is justifiable if that action sets up an increased agency in its beneficiary.

An ethical judgment, for a ritualistic ethic, is essentially like an aesthetic judgment. It has no reference to events occurring in the real world. The judgment of a deontologist or a utilitarian cannot be judged by the effects it brings about in the external world. It can be judged only by a subjective feeling of pleasure or approval experienced by the viewer. In this way it is identical to an aesthetic judgment. If there is no essential difference between a nurse's ethical and aesthetic judgment, then, in both cases, she is not an ethical agent. She is a mere spectator.

In her nonprofessional life a nurse can perfectly well approach her own life as a spectator. She can refrain from taking actions to influence the course of her life according to her desires. She can abandon the course of her life entirely to accidental circumstances. But she may not do this, in her professional life, for her patient.

LIFE AND AGENCY

A purposive ethic is possible only because reason is possible. For a purposive ethic to come into play reason is necessary.

A purposive ethic has its reason for being in human desire.

Life is the precondition of both reason and desire. Therefore it is entirely reasonable for a nursing ethic to hold the patient's reason and desire as its standard of judgment and the patient's life as its final good.

In order to know her patient a nurse must know herself.

A nurse must know what her life is all about in order for her to:

- Reason about that which she desires.
- Desire that which she reasons about.
- Understand her patient's reasoning about that which he desires.
- Understand her patient's desire for that about which he reasons.

The best resource a nurse can offer her patient is not her interest in his life, his reasoning, and his desires. It is her interest in her own life, her own reasoning, and her own desires. If she lacks interest in herself, she cannot understand how to be interested in her patient.

AGENCY AND THE BIOETHICAL STANDARDS

Autonomy

DILEMMA 15-1   Gwen is a nurse on the same unit as Carrie. One evening Gwen accidentally gave seconal to a patient for whom the drug was not ordered. Seconal is an addictive substance. A close count of the medication on hand and that which is dispensed is always kept at the hospital where Gwen works. If a nurse makes a medication error, this becomes part of her permanent record. When she makes three medication errors, she is suspended for three days. If she receives three suspensions, she is fired.

Carrie, the nurse who took the next night shift after Gwen, discovered the mistake. Carrie knows that Gwen is a good nurse. She does not want Gwen to get into trouble. She also knows that the patient to whom Gwen gave the seconal was not harmed by it. Carrie believes that no one will be benefited by Gwen's mistake being revealed. She fixes the records so that the mistake will not be discovered.

The next time Carrie sees Gwen, she tells her what she has done.

If you were Gwen what would you do in this context, and why? What do you think you ought to do in this context, and why?

Let us consider another, similar case:

Roseanne, a nurse, started working on the labor and delivery unit of a large women's hospital about a year ago. So far Rosanne has managed to keep the fact that she is addicted to cocaine a secret from her co-workers at the hospital.

It is Thursday night and Rosanne is scheduled to work the 3 to 11 shift. When 3:20 rolls around, Rosanne has not yet arrived. She finally arrives at 3:40 obviously under the influence of some substance.

Carolyn, the nurse who is being relieved by Rosanne, has ethical responsibilities in these circumstances. What these responsibilities are does not seem particularly problematic. *Why* she has the responsibilities she has, in this context, is more problematic than would appear on the surface.

Under these circumstances if you were Carolyn what would you do, and why?

What do you think you ought to do, and why?

There is very often a difference between what a nurse would do and what she believes she ought to do. This reveals that she does not emotionally accept the ethical system that she has adopted. This shows that there is something wrong with the nurse or with her ethical system. If a nurse and an ethical system come together and the result is discord, this is not necessarily the fault of the nurse.

Freedom

✄ **DILEMMA 15-2**   Naomi is a 46-year-old patient in the hospital for the fourth time this past year. She has undergone surgery twice for cancer of the liver. The cancer metastasized, and she was admitted a third time for chemotherapy.

Her present admission is for dehydration and pain. Naomi has asked her physician to allow her to die as painlessly as possible. She has refused her permission to continue with chemotherapy.

Naomi is the mother of three children ages 14, 16, and 17. Her physician feels that with chemotherapy Naomi could live at least long enough to get her 17-year-old to the age of 18. The physician believes that when her son is 18, he could take care of the other two children. He is putting considerable pressure on Naomi to consent to yet another treatment. He has even discussed with Jennifer, Naomi's primary care nurse, the possibility of going to court over this matter.

As Naomi's primary care nurse, what should Jennifer do in order to protect Naomi's freedom?

In order to initiate action a person must be free. The right to freedom, which the bioethical standard of freedom provides, is the right to act on one's agency. Being able to act on his agency is a person's way of being alive.

Life is action. A person's life belongs to whomever controls his or her freedom of action. If Naomi's physician is able to determine her choice of life and death, then Naomi's life belongs to him. It seems that this state of affairs surely cannot be right.

But what of court decisions forbidding the removal of life support systems? Does this mean that, in the final analysis, a person's life belongs to the courts? If an individual person's life does not belong to the person, how does a nurse work this fact into the bioethical standards?

A recognition of a person's right to freedom precedes a recognition of any further right. If a person does not have a right to act freely, then his life does not belong to him. If he does not have the right to freedom then, in the final analysis, he does not have any rights.

Veracity

✄ **DILEMMA 15-3**   Jason is a patient in a psychiatric hospital. He was admitted nonvoluntarily. He has been diagnosed as a paranoid schizophrenic. His physician has prescribed 5 mg Haldol and 2 mg Cogentin. Jason refuses to take the medication. He tells his nurse, Jessica, that the physician is trying to poison him.

Aside from what he tells her Jessica has no reason to believe that Jason's physician is trying to poison him. Would she be justified in giving Jason an injection of the medication against his will so that he would get the benefit of it? Does the standard of veracity relate to Jason at all? If so, how?

If a person could not ascertain the truth, agency would be useless to him or her. On the other hand, it is through agency that truth possesses its value for a person. Everyone implicitly values agency more than he or she values truth.

The relationship between truth and agency is the relationship between belief and action. A person cannot act unless he or she acts on beliefs. Beliefs are important to a person only insofar as they assist or hinder purposeful actions.

Privacy

✗ DILEMMA 15-4 Barnaby is a 42-year-old outpatient scheduled for a vasectomy. Barnaby had his driver's license suspended because of drunk driving. His wife, Phyllis, has driven him to the hospital.

Barnaby has not told Phyllis the truth about what he is having done. He has misled her as to why he had to be admitted to the hospital as an outpatient.

Phyllis has strong beliefs against any form of birth control. Barnaby feels that it would hurt her if she knew the nature of the operation he is having.

However, he feels that he cannot support another child on his salary. Because of his ill health he has not been able to do as many odd jobs as he once was in order to make ends meet.

Barnaby has asked his nurse and physician to keep his confidence.

After the operation, Janine, Barnaby's nurse, comes out to reassure Phyllis about his condition and to tell her when Barnaby will be able to be discharged. Phyllis asks Janine what was done to her husband.

Barnaby has set up the worst possible circumstances here. With the arrangements he made, it was impossible that Phyllis' curiousity would not be aroused. At the same time he made Janine a buffer between himself and Phyllis.

Did Barnaby have a right to do this?

If a person had no right to privacy then, of course, he or she would have no right to agency. There is no agency without private goals. In order to exercise one's agency, a person must enjoy self-ownership (as it seems Naomi did not in the case under Freedom). In addition to this a person must be able to act without being unjustly hindered.

If a person does have a right to privacy, then, by that very fact, he or she has a right to agency. If a person is left alone, there is nothing and no one to prevent acting; that person has perfect freedom.

This does not resolve the dilemma that Barnaby set up. Janine's dilemma is this: What are the limitations on the right of a patient to involve a nurse in the actions he wishes to take?

Beneficence

✗ **DILEMMA 15-5**   Rodney is one of Julia's patients in the intensive care unit. He is dying from cirrhosis of the liver. Rodney asks Julia for a small drink of water. The order left by the physician placed Rodney on NPO because of the actively bleeding ulcers in his stomach and intestine.

Despite all of his medical problems Rodney is alert and he is thirsty. He knows the probable consequences of a sip of water and yet continues to want it.

Rodney's physician is called in the hope that he will change the order. He will not. He says that he wants to be conservative and is afraid that the water would trigger more bleeding.

Despite this Rodney still continues to plead for a drink of water.

What can Rodney's nurse do?

All beneficence is beneficence in regard to agency. If one person does good for another, he or she either:

- Increases the agency of that other person in some way

or

- Bestows a value on that other person which the other person could not have acquired.

If one person does harm to another person, he or she either:

- Decreases the agency of that other person

or

- Takes a value from that other person which the other person already possesses

or

- Prevents that other person from acquiring a value which that other person could have acquired.

"What is the nature of beneficence?" This question has many aspects. It is one of the most difficult in all of ethics. It is one of the most important questions facing a nurse.

Here it is in its most dreadful aspect:

Sometimes it is better to give up a small good that a person can enjoy at present in favor of a greater good that a person can enjoy in the future.

Sometimes it is better to endure a small evil that a person can suffer at present in order to obtain a greater good in the future.

Sometimes it is better to endure a small evil in the present in order to escape a greater future evil.

Sometimes it is better to give up a small present good in order to escape a greater future evil (Spinoza cited in Gutmann, 1949).

When it is necessary for a nurse to choose for a patient or to counsel a patient, how does she weigh and measure the small present good or the small present evil in contrast to the greater future good? How does she weigh and measure the small present good or the small present evil in contrast to the greater future evil?

Fidelity

DILEMMA 15-6 Conrad is a young adult admitted for the fourth time this year with acute leukemia. This time he brought a living will into the hospital with him. His living will states that in the event that he arrests, he does not want to be resuscitated.

Conrad does arrest. A new intern happens to be in the room at the time. He asks the nurse, Amelia, to get the crash cart. Amelia explains to the intern about Conrad's living will. The intern's response is that living wills are not legal in their state.

What can Amelia do?

A nurse can never justify breaking the agreement she has with her patient. At the same time there must be a limitation to her responsibilities. These limitations are never completely clear. They can be determined only by reference to the elements of the patient's autonomy interacting with the elements of the nurse's autonomy.

According to ritualistic ethical systems agency has an ethical purpose different from the agent's purpose. The purpose of agency is to serve fidelity.

In the scheme of things agency comes before fidelity. Agency cannot exist to serve fidelity. Fidelity exists to serve agency.

If two people make an agreement between them and their sole purpose is to be able to exercise fidelity to the agreement, it would reveal a bizarre disorientation on their part. Every agreement is made for some purpose involving agency, some purpose outside of the agreement itself.

SUMMARY

Every action in a bioethical context is taken for a purpose. The purpose of an action taken in a bioethical context is some biomedical good. Every biomedical good is specific to the welfare of one or more individual patients.

The view of good held by a ritualistic ethical system is not specific to individual welfare. Therefore, it cannot be appropriate to the nursing context. In the view of ritualistic ethical systems good and evil are not functions of effects but of the agent's intention—to do his or her duty or to bring about "the greatest good for the greatest number."

If any action in any ethical system is not well intentioned, then it is not justifiable. Every action in any ethical context is taken with a view to good or evil. In a purposive ethical system the effects of an action are fully as important as the intention behind the action. The quality of the ethical action, that is to say, whether it is good or evil, is determined by the intention behind it *and* by its predictable effects.

REFERENCES

Gutmann, J. (Ed.). (1949). *Spinoza's Ethics*. New York: Hafner Publishing Company.

President's Commission for the Study of Ethical Problems and Medicine and Biomedical and Behavioral Research.

(1982). *Making health care decisions: The ethical and legal implication of informed consent in the patient-practitioner relationship*. (Vol. I). Washington, DC: US Government Printing Office.

Postscript to Parts
One and Two

In the objective relationship between the mind of a person and the reality known by the person there are three kinds of "things."

- There are "things" in the mind that have no counterpart in the world outside of the mind.
- There are "things" in the world outside of the mind that exist whether any mind is aware of them or not.
- There are "things" in the mind that do not exist outside of the mind, but, there is still something in the world outside the mind that serves as a foundation to that which is in the mind.

The first kind of "thing" exists only in the mind. This includes such "things" as leprechauns, the tooth fairy, square circles, unicorns, and so on. These "things" exist in the mind in the sense that they can be imagined. But there are no leprechauns, unicorns, tooth fairies or square circles in the real world outside of the mind.

The second kind of "thing" really exists in the world. This includes such "things" as this chair, that tree, the gust of wind blowing that newspaper, those false eyelashes, and so on. Whether or not anyone is seeing them or touching them, these "things" actually exist in the world outside of consciousness.

The third kind of "thing" does not exist out in reality. But something exists out in reality that serves as the basis of this "thing" existing in the mind.

For instance, furniture exists in the mind. Outside of the mind there is no such "thing" as furniture. But for its own use the mind observes these four chairs, this table, that sofa, this bookcase and groups them all together, according to what they have in common, under the concept "furniture." The chairs, table, sofa, and bookcase all exist in the real world apart from the mind. But in addition to the chairs, table, sofa and bookcase, there is no eighth "thing"—furniture—existing out in the real world.

Furniture does not exist in reality apart from the mind as do chairs, trees, wind gusts, and false eyelashes. But, unlike leprechauns, tooth fairies, square circles, and unicorns, furniture does not exist in the mind without a reference to reality.

The existence of furniture in the mind has a foundation in the chairs, tables, sofas, bookcases, etc., that exist in the real world.

The bioethical standards are much more like the third kind of reality, more like furniture than either of the first two kinds of reality.

There is no such thing as autonomy out in the world; there are only autonomous agents. Agents have this in common—they are all unique.

There is no such thing as freedom out in the world; there are only agents who possess or lack freedom.

There is no such thing as veracity out in the world apart from knowers who know what is true.

There is no such thing as privacy out in the world; there are only agents who possess self-ownership.

There is no such thing as beneficence out in the world; there are only agents who do good and do harm.

There is no such thing as fidelity out in the world; there are only agents who uphold or fail to uphold the terms of their agreements.

The bioethical standards are "things" that exist in the mind and not in reality. But people possess very abstract properties in common. People are autonomous. They act freely. They have a need for veracity, privacy, and beneficence. They make agreements, and they are faithful to these agreements. It is these properties of people that keep a biomedical professional's awareness of the bioethical standards tied to reality out in the world—the reality of her patients.

The hardest thing in all of reality for a person's mind to be "tied to" is people. For a biomedical professional to function on an ethical level, there must be something tying her awareness to the people of whom she is aware. This something is the bioethical standards.

Everyone is autonomous. Everyone is free. The standards pertain to every-one—to humans as human.

But, for a biomedical professional to function on an ethical level there must be something tying her awareness to more than "people." There must be something tying her awareness to her individual patients.

Those things that serve as a foundation in reality, to tie a biomedical professional's awareness to her individual patients, are the elements of autonomy.

That which determines the nature of an individual person is:

1. The collection of a person's desires.
2. The way a person uses his reason in interacting with the context of his life.
3. The vision that one has of what one's life is and what one wants it to be.
4. The hopes and purposes that motivate a person.
5. One's agency—one's mental, emotional, and physical capacities.

In order to know what is right for a person in any given context, it is very desirable to know the person. It is much easier to know a person through knowing the elements of his autonomy than through knowing that, by right, all men are autonomous, free, and so on.

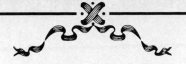

PART THREE

CASE STUDY
ANALYSIS

CHAPTER
16

Resolutions to Dilemmas

Rights can be defined as: The product of an implicit agreement among rational beings, by virtue of their rationality, not to obtain actions nor the product of actions from others except through voluntary consent, objectively gained.

Rights is a product in this sense: Valerie desires to take a particular action at a certain time. At the same time Barbara refrains from interfering with Valerie and from attempting to obtain actions or the product of actions from her. (It must be assumed that Valerie's desire is strong enough that she would not voluntarily consent to interact with Barbara.) Barbara's refraining from interfering with Valerie's action gives Valerie perfect freedom to take the action.

Responsibilities can be defined as: The product of the restrictions a person accepts on freedom of action when he or she enters into an agreement.

Responsibilities are a product in this sense: Valerie and Barbara have an implicit agreement between them that they will respect each other's rights. Every being who possesses the power of reason has this implicit agreement with every other such being. This agreement exists between them by virtue of the fact that they are rational beings. That a person is a rational being means that he or she is a being who approaches the world through reason.

Valerie, then, since she is acting on independent purposes, does not wish to interact, at this time, with Barbara. Barbara, according to their agreement, has no right to interfere with Valerie's action. This noninterference is a product of the restrictions the rights agreement places on Barbara's freedom of action.

Thus, it can be said that Valerie has a right to take the action she desires. This right, as can be seen, is the product of the implicit agreement between Valerie and Barbara.

REFINING THE CONTEXT

The one major mistake an ethical agent can make in analyzing a dilemma according to the elements or the standards is to apply the elements or standards to someone to whom they do not pertain. For instance, a surgeon is operating on a patient for a liver dysfunction. He decides that it would be convenient, while he is at it, to take out the patient's appendix. He suggests this to the nurse. She agrees that he has made an excellent point. The surgeon relates his idea to the patient's husband. He replies that they are going on vacation and this might well prevent an inconvenience from arising.

It can be argued that:

- The patient has a certain autonomy but then so do the other three people involved.
- The patient has not forbidden this action, therefore the surgeon is free to take it.
- If the surgeon operates, no deception has been involved — unless the patient's husband lied about them going on vacation.
- No invasion of the patient's privacy is involved since she is going to be operated on anyway.
- This may be a beneficent action. It may save her the necessity of having to undergo an appendectomy at some future date.
- It does not violate fidelity since the surgeon is doing everything he agreed to do, and more.

The action that the surgeon proposes to initiate involves another person, his patient. The only rights he can enjoy in this context is the rights to which his patient agrees.

The action which he proposes he would take voluntarily. He has no right to compel his patient to cooperate involuntarily. He has no right to obtain actions or the product of actions from his patient except through her voluntary consent.

In this totally silly context the actions the surgeon proposes he cannot take by right. He has no right to take the action despite the agreement of the nurse and the patient's husband. He would have no right to take this action if he had the agreement of the entire world, but not the patient's agreement.

No one ever has a right to violate the rights of anyone. Such a right would be the end of all rights. No patient ever has a right to violate the rights of a biomedical professional. Aside from this, in a biomedical context, all rights belong to the patient. No rights belong to the surgeon or the nurse. Since there is no question of the situation being an emergency and the patient is not incompetent, no rights belong to the patient's husband. The surgeon, the nurse, and the patient's husband have nothing but responsibilities in relation to the patient's rights. Their autonomy, freedom, desires, purposes, and the rest are not ethically relevant in this context.

The elements and standards must be applied to the people in an ethical context *according to their rights and their responsibilities.*

- The right to *autonomy* is the right to be oneself and to value that which one desires. It is a right not to obey the demand that a person be what he or she is not.
- The right to *freedom* is the right to act to pursue one's own purposes without interference.
- The right to *veracity* is the right to act on an objective view of reality and one's life without being victimized by deception.
- The right to *privacy* is the right to use one's reason to make one's own decisions. It is the right to enjoy independent self-ownership. It is a right not to be "taken over" by another.
- The right to *beneficence* is the right not to be harmed and to increase one's agency through agreements.
- The right to *fidelity* is the right to expect agreements to be kept. As we have seen, the right to fidelity is necessary to the existence of agreements.

Take any context where, for instance, Barbara has a responsibility to respect Valerie's rights. The fact that Barbara has a responsibility to respect Valerie's rights, in that context, does not give Barbara any rights in that context.

If one person desires to obtain a dress from another, she cannot induce the other to make or to give her a dress unless the other person agrees to make or to part with a dress. This consent must not be gained through coercion or fraud.

If one person agrees to purchase a dress from another person then: The first person has a responsibility to pay for the dress; this person has a right to receive it; the second person has a right to be paid for the dress; this person has a responsibility to give over the dress.

If one person agrees to respect the autonomy of another then, in interacting with that other person, he or she has a responsibility not to interfere with that other person's pursuit of his or her unique values.

If one person agrees to respect the freedom of another, he or she has a responsibility not to interfere with the action of that other.

If one person agrees to interact with another person on the basis of veracity, then that person has a responsibility not to harm that other person through fraud or deceit.

If one person agrees to respect the privacy of another, then that person has a responsibility not to attempt to control the actions of that other person. If one person agrees to protect the privacy of another person, then he or she has a responsibility not to permit third parties to try to control that second person's self-ownership.

If one person agrees to interact with another on the basis of beneficence, then he or she has a responsibility to do some good for that other, if possible, and to do no harm to that other person.

If Valerie takes some action toward Barbara, then the elements and the standards cannot be applied to an analysis of what Valerie's rights consist in, because, in this context, Valerie, as yet, has no rights. Barbara has not yet made an agreement with Valerie to take some positive action.

Valerie has acted to obtain actions or the product of actions from Barbara. Barbara has not acted to obtain actions or the product of actions from Valerie.

Suppose that Valerie acts toward Barbara. If Barbara agrees to interact, she responds to Valerie's action. Her response initiates further action on the part of Valerie. This process proceeds into a chain of interactions, each based on the agreement implied by the prior action.

Valerie and Barbara need the elements and standards as analytic tools since each is responsible for the forseeable consequences of the actions that she takes. By the same token each is responsible for nothing *but* the ethical actions she takes. Valerie has responsibilities but no rights when she initiates an ethical/causal chain. Barbara has no responsibilities when she does not initiate an ethical/causal chain unless she responds to Valerie's action. Her response would involve an implicit or explicit agreement.

If Barbara refuses to interact with Valerie, then she is responsible for nothing. Otherwise Barbara would, conceivably, be responsible for any event anywhere in the world. She would be responsible for events that she has not caused, that she could not have forseen, and over which she has no control.

But, in an ethical context, this is impossible. If Barbara could be held responsible for events which she did not initiate, and to which she did not agree, there would be no definable ethical reality such as "responsibility."

THE RIGHTS OF A NURSE

Once a nurse takes on the treatment of a patient, she cannot thereafter refuse to engage in legitimate interactions according to the nurse/patient agreement. The nurse/patient agreement governs every subsequent agreement or refusal.

If rights is as we have defined it, then certainly patients have rights.

A nurse also has rights. She has the right not to take actions which, as a nurse, she has not agreed to take. She has a right not to take actions except those actions to which she has given voluntary consent — and that voluntary consent must be objectively gained.

In becoming a nurse in a pluralistic society a person agrees to provide certain actions — giving treatments, giving comfort to a patient, counseling a patient, monitoring a patient's progress, and so on. She does not agree to provide more than that which is called for according to the role of a nurse. Therefore she is not responsible for providing more than this.

No one has a right to expect her to provide more than this. A nurse has a right not to have the limitations of the nurse/patient agreement exceeded.

THE FOUNDATION OF THE AGREEMENT IN THE ELEMENTS AND STANDARDS

When an agreement, such as the nurse/patient agreement, arises between Valerie and Barbara, then the rights of each is determined by the terms of that agreement.

The standards define the terms of the agreement.

The elements define the standards.

The terms of the agreement are determined by the nature — the skills — of a nurse and the purposes of a patient. Where the terms of the agreement are not clearly spelled out, as they often are not in a pluralistic society, dilemmas can arise. When dilemmas arise, the elements and the standards can help to clarify the terms of the agreement.

A NOTE TO THE READER

In going over these dilemmas the reader should recall that they are abstract case studies. In abstract case studies, of course, it sounds as though the nature of the case is very clear and the responsibility of a nurse is equally clear — and rigid. In the context of a real-life situation, however, a nurse seldom enjoys this clarity.

We would ask the reader not to think of these dilemmas and resolutions as establishing rules to be followed. Blindly following rules can be ruinous. A nurse has no ethical responsibility to ruin herself at the first opportunity.

In ethical matters there is a difference between right and wrong. It does matter what an ethical agent does. All the same it is not an ethical agent's responsibility to do everything right everytime. To do everything right every time would be absolutely impossible. No ethical agent has a responsibility to do the impossible.

There is a very large difference between a real-life context and a case study. Nothing that follows should instill a feeling of ethical incompetence in the reader.

The purpose of these analyses is to make the reader stronger and more knowledgeable. Many ethical agents do not allow themselves to know when their response to an ethical situation has been inadequate. Without knowledge there is no growth. Without growth there is no possibility of consistently appropriate ethical decision making. It is a nurse's responsibility to know. The purpose of these resolutions is to enable the reader to orient her thinking about bioethical matters and to develop, *over time*, competence at ethical decision making.

In this Part we will discuss the numbered dilemmas from Parts One and Two.

3-1, p. 30   The dilemma of whether a nurse should "declare war" on a patient's bad habits.

3-2, p. 32   A dilemma involving a physician's desire to prevent a patient from doing "what no one could possibly want to do."

3-3, p. 32   A dilemma involving the use of heroic measures to keep a dying patient alive.

5-1, p. 57   The dilemma of whether a nurse should cooperate when she disagrees with policies.

5-2, p. 57   The dilemma of a conflict between action and passion.

5-3, p. 61   The dilemma of a conflict between a patient's right to know and his unique desire not to know.

5-4, p. 62   The dilemma of whether a patient should be informed about a condition concerning which very few patients would want to be informed.

5-5, p. 64   The dilemma of a conflict between a patient's freedom of action and hospital scheduling.

5-6, p. 64   Whether a nurse ought to accept Kant's belief that apathy is an ethical strength.

5-7, p. 65   Whether a nurse ought to accept Kant's belief that it is never right to tell lies from benevolent motives.

5-8, p. 66   The dilemma of whether a nurse ought to give a patient information that his physician does not want him to have.

5-9, p. 67   A dilemma concerning whether a nurse ought to vary routine where there is no apparent reason to take action.

5-10, p. 73   The dilemma of whether a dying patient's desire for confidentiality should override his family's plans for a pleasant surprise.

7-1, p. 93   A dilemma concerning whether honesty is the best policy when honesty may be harmful to the patient.

7-2, p. 95   The dilemma of how a nurse might counsel a patient who must decide on whether to gamble on a "long shot."

7-3, p. 101   A dilemma involving a nurse's promise of secrecy.

7-4, p. 102   A dilemma involving a conflict between the standard of fidelity and optimal medical practice.

8-1, p. 109   The dilemma of whether a nurse has the right to use force to prevent a disoriented patient from ambulating.

8-2, p. 109   A dilemma involving the right of a patient to refuse to make decisions regarding his treatment.

8-3, p. 110   A dilemma involving a conflict between autonomy and veracity.

8-4, p. 113   The dilemma of whether a comatose Jehovah's Witness should be given a blood transfusion.

8-5, p. 113   The dilemma of whether the nature of a rational benefi- cence is compatible with the exercise of "gentle coercion."

8-6, p. 113   A dilemma involving the right of a terminally ill patient to die.

8-7, p. 114   The dilemma of how to deal with a demanding patient who interferes with the nurse's attention to her other patients.

8-8, p. 115   A dilemma involving a parent's right to know versus the right of a child to have his parents not know.

8-9, p. 116   A dilemma involving a nurse giving information about a patient over the phone.

8-10, p. 116   The dilemma of whether a nurse ought to feed a stroke patient or insist on the patient learning to feed himself.

8-11, p. 117   The dilemma of whether a feeble and elderly patient should be let out of restraints to freely walk around.

8-12, p. 117   The dilemma of whether a nurse ought to interfere with a patient's activities if these activities threaten his health.

8-13, p. 118   The dilemma of whether a nurse should give sensitive information to a family member before she has discussed this with her pa- tient.

8-14, p. 119   The dilemma of whether a nurse should tell a patient's wife that she did not fulfill a symbolic agreement she had with her husband.

8-15, p. 119   The dilemma of a conflict between what a family needs to know and what a patient does not want his family to know.

8-16, p. 119   A dilemma involving a conflict of whether a nurse ought to report a case of suspected child abuse.

8-17, p. 120   The dilemma of a conflict between loyalty to a patient and loyalty to the employing institution when a nurse suspects her patient is acting fraudulently.

11-1, p. 164   The dilemma of a nurse caring for a young person in exceedingly difficult circumstances.

12-1, p. 173   The dilemma of whether a child's rights protect him against a procedure he does not desire.

12-2, p. 174   The dilemma of whether a physician has a right to compel a patient to undergo a procedure which he believes the patient ought to undergo.

12-3, p. 176   A dilemma dealing with what a nurse ought to do when she has an obviously inadequate knowledge of a situation.

12-4, p. 177   The dilemma of how a nurse communicates when a patient violates the standard of veracity.

12-5, p. 178   The dilemma of whether a patient has a right to ask a nurse to take on extraordinary responsibilities.

12-6, p. 179   A dilemma involving a patient's right to seek euthanasia.

13-1, p. 191   The dilemma of whether a nurse's responsibility extends to the details of a patient's personal life.

13-2, p. 193   A dilemma involving a retarded infant with a severe heart defect.

The following dilemmas are all highly context dependent. In addition, they are quite difficult. Several are dilemmas nurses meet in their interactions with physicians. These usually are more difficult to resolve than dilemmas that only involve patients.

Several of these dilemmas do not directly involve nurses. They involve only physicians. An ethically effective nurse ought to be able to evaluate a physician's actions as well as her own actions. For this reason these dilemmas are included.

The final resolutions of most of these dilemmas can be discovered only in the actual context in which they arise. All that can be done in a case study analysis is to make the nature of the dilemmas clearer. We will offer only broad suggestions as to the direction the resolutions might take.

14-1, p. 206   A dilemma concerning how a nurse might interact with a patient who is motivated by two conflicting purposes.

14-2, p. 207   The dilemma of whether a nurse, in protecting her patient against knowing the severity of his condition, violates the element of purpose.

14-3, p. 207   The dilemma of whether a nurse's badgering her patients about their expressed desires violates their privacy.

14-4, p. 208   The dilemma of whether there is a limit on the value of a nurse badgering a patient about a bad habit.

14-5, p. 208   The dilemma of whether a nurse ought to intervene on behalf of her patient against a physician's decision.

15-1, p. 219   A dilemma involving a conflict between hospital policy and trust between nurses.

15-2, p. 220   The dilemma of whether a physician is justified in demanding that a patient live for the sake of her children.

15-3, p. 220   The dilemma of whether a psychiatric patient who is brought into the hospital against his will should be forcibly medicated.

15-4, p. 221   A dilemma concerning the responsibility a nurse has to give information to a family member who has a right to know.

15-5, p. 222   The dilemma of whether a terminally ill patient has a right to ask a nurse for something that might be injurious to his health.

15-6, p. 223   A dilemma involving the ethical status of a patient's living will if a living will is not legally recognized.

RESOLUTIONS

❖ DILEMMA 3 - 1   Why a nurse should not "declare war" on a patient's bad habits.

Autonomy: Joyce's action is an attack on Ralph's autonomy. It is, in principle, an attempt to force a change in Ralph's nature. There cannot be anything in a rational nurse/patient agreement to justify Joyce's action. To be coerced into a forcible change in his nature is not the reason why a patient comes into the hospital. Joyce has no responsibility to do this, and she has no right to do it.

It may be that if Ralph gave up his smoking habit, this would increase his long-term welfare. This is a legitimate concern of a nurse. The way to go about ensuring a patient's long-term welfare, however, is softly and gently, not by "declaring war." The way to go about ensuring a patient's long-term welfare is efficiently, not inefficiently.

Freedom: Joyce's action is an attack on Ralph's right to freedom and self-determination. If Ralph has no intention of giving up his smoking habit, Joyce has no ethical right to attempt coercion as a way of caring for him.

Veracity: No doubt it is true that bad habits are contrary to the long-term welfare of patients. But this truth delivered to Ralph frequently, vigorously, and coercively may do him more harm than good.

Privacy: If a patient, as an autonomous individual, enjoys self-ownership, then a nurse who denies his self-ownership cannot be justified in that denial. When one person coerces another, this action implies that the person is taking over the ownership of the other.

Beneficence: In a certain (subjective) sense a nurse who is attempting to, coercively, help her patient overcome a bad habit is showing beneficence. It feels like beneficence to her. Beneficence, however, is not an inner state of feeling. It is the quality of an action by which that action benefits its beneficiary. In an objective sense an attack on a patient is never beneficent.

Fidelity: The nurse/patient agreement is an agreement between nurse and patient that they will cooperate. Coercion is not cooperation. In exerting coercion the nurse violates her agreement.

Analysis of this dilemma through the elements merely confirms what analysis through the standards show.

❖ DILEMMA 3 - 2   Why a physician preventing a patient from doing "what no one could possibly want to do" is not practicing beneficence.

Autonomy: Harold is unique. His motivations for refusing the amputation of his gangrenous leg must certainly be unique. But they are his motivations; it is his leg and it is his life.

The physician, apparently, did not ask Harold why he was refusing the operation. Or, if he did, Harold's answer did not satisfy him.

Harold's motivations and values are unique. So are the motivations and values of the physician unique. In order for Harold's answer to satisfy the physician, their motivations and values would have to be harmonious. If Harold's answer *must* satisfy his physician, then Harold's physician has the same rights in relation to Harold's life as Harold has. In fact, this would give the physician not only the same rights, but greater rights than Harold.

If Harold has a right to be an autonomous individual, then he has no ethical responsibility to satisfy his physician on a decision concerning an operation that he does not want his physician to perform.

Freedom: The physician's action is an attack on Harold's freedom of choice in the matter of his own life. If this freedom is taken away, Harold has no freedom left.

Veracity: This dilemma does not involve the standard of veracity:

1. It does not involve Harold's physician attempting to deceive him.
2. Harold has no ethical responsibility, in this context, to tell his physician any truth. Harold's physician has no right to expect Harold to tell him any truth.

Privacy: A health care professional does not protect a patient's right to privacy by destroying it.

Beneficence: To destroy a patient's individual sovereignty is not to act beneficently toward him. There is no such thing as acting beneficently toward a person by giving him a benefit he does not want.

H. G. Welles wrote a story called "The Richest Man in Bogata." This is the story of a man whose airplane crashes in a valley among the mountains of Columbia. In the crash the man loses the sight of one of his eyes. The valley where he crashes is filled with diamonds. The brilliance of these diamonds has made everyone who lives in the valley blind. When the inhabitants of the valley discover what has happened to the airplane pilot, they decide that they must put out his other eye. They are all very happy not being sighted. They do not suffer the glare of the diamonds. They believe that anyone who can look out upon the valley must suffer from the glare. So they decide they will blind the pilot, out of beneficence, for his own benefit.

Coercive beneficence cannot be beneficence.

Fidelity: Ask yourself if you would enter into an agreement with a physician if one of the terms of that agreement allowed the physician unlimited freedom to do anything he wanted.

Analysis through the bioethical standards does not justify the physician's actions.

Analysis through the elements will confirm what analysis through the standards revealed.

DILEMMA 3-3 Whether, in a strictly nursing context, heroic measures should be used to keep a dying patient who is in excruciating pain alive.

Autonomy: If heroic measures are not taken and Martha is allowed to die then, certainly, her uniqueness will be lost along with her life. Her uniqueness will pass out of existence.

This fact, however, has no ethical relevance. The ethical concept of "autonomy" is not the uniqueness of a person that the outside world gazes upon. It is the uniqueness of a person as the person lives and experiences it. It is the person's self-identity as he or she experiences it. Not to allow Martha to die would not preserve her autonomy. It would violate her autonomy.

Not to allow Martha to die is not the same as forcing her to live. It is forcing her to continue dying.

Freedom: If it is Martha's desire to die and health care professionals have agreed to act as her agent, then in applying heroic measures they violate their agreement. They take an action for her that she would not take for herself.

Any claim that they violate her right to freedom in not applying heroic measures is one of the extreme points of ethical absurdity.

Veracity: As far as making her decision is concerned, Martha has all the information she needs. Her excruciating pain and the fact that she is terminal provide this. The standard of veracity does not enter into the picture beyond this.

Privacy: When a person makes an agreement with a health care professional, he or she makes it from the perspective of self-ownership. Martha made her agreement on this basis.

If someone has a right to force Martha to live in these circumstances (for instance a legislator who passes a law), then this person has taken over the ownership of Martha. This is true despite the fact that Martha has never given up her self-ownership.

It is absurd to say that Martha's self-ownership is not violated under these circumstances. If another person takes over control of Martha's actions, this person certainly violates her privacy.

Beneficence: In dilemmas involving passive euthanasia different people have widely differing views as to what constitutes beneficence. It is, finally, up to every individual to decide on what constitutes "doing good or at least doing no harm." What a person believes and what a person can justify are often very different things. Staying in the bioethical context, let us try to clarify the question of justification through a thought-experiment:

Try to imagine, in your mind's eye, that to end Martha's life and suffering would be to harm her.

Imagine that to keep her alive and suffering would be to bestow some good upon her.

Now that you have seen this, in your mind's eye, let us take it one step further.

Imagine a patient, Marian, who is dying a peaceful and painless death. The technology to keep Marian alive is available. But this technology is excruciatingly painful.

Assume that Marian ought not be kept alive under these circumstances, and then try to devise some justification for keeping Martha alive.

Is it not absurd to keep a patient in unendurable pain alive while permitting a patient who is not in pain to die?

Suppose that ethics demands that patients such as Marian, as well as patients such as Martha, be kept alive. This supposition implies that every "health care setting" ought to become a combination cemetery and torture chamber.

If a person can believe this, nothing more can be said. If a person can justify it bioethically, he or she will have transformed the nature of biomedicine.

Fidelity: The demands of fidelity, of course, depend upon the agreement.

If health care professionals agree to act as Martha's agents and they agree to act toward her with beneficence, then they agree to act toward Martha as she would act toward herself. Martha would not act to keep herself alive. If health care professionals keep her alive in these circumstances, they break their agreement with her.

Virtually no one in Martha's condition would enter a health care setting if she knew that the agreement gave health care professionals a right to force her to suffer against her will.

Euthanasia, even passive euthanasia as discussed in Martha's case, is a very complex and a very controversial subject. In order to illuminate the analysis we have made through the bioethical standards, we will analyze it through the elements.

Desire: It is inconceivable that the desire of a terminal patient in unbearable pain to continue living as long as possible could be a rational desire. The element of rational desire calls for Martha being allowed to die.

Reason: To paraphrase the great Dutch ethicist, Benedict Spinoza: Reason demands nothing contrary to nature and nature demands nothing contrary to reason.

If a person wages a war on his existence—a war that he cannot win—if he denies everything that he knows to be true, he turns his back on reason. Reason demands that a person accept the facts of his existence and the reality of his world. If reason demands anything then it demands that a person accept that which he knows to be true.

For a person to accept that which he knows to be true is for him to act in harmony with his own nature. It is for him to act in harmony with the reality of the world around him. Reason and nature demand nothing less than this.

The reality of Martha's existence calls for the exercise of reason. It calls for the biomedical professionals who are her agents to exercise reason and beneficence.

Life: Martha is alive only in the sense that an irrational animal is alive. Martha is not an irrational animal. The best promise life offers her is death. If Martha's life is allowed to speak for itself, then Martha ought to be allowed to die.

Purpose: Analyzing Martha's situation from the vantage point of purpose shows that Martha ought to be allowed to die. This is not surprising. In the context of the bioethical standards it is an ethical purpose. It is a rational purpose. And, not least, it is Martha's purpose for herself.

Agency: Every ethical agent in exercising agency should exercise it with courage and clarity of vision. If biomedical professionals are given the power to decide Martha's fate, they should decide with courage and clarity of vision. For they are her agents.

Both the bioethical standards and the elements suggest the ethical propriety of allowing Martha to die.

❀ **DILEMMA 5-1**   Whether a nurse should cooperate when she disagrees with policies.

In this case the physician is calling upon Nancy to take actions with which she disagrees. Her problem is to decide whether this is a violation of her rights and, if it is, whether she should refuse to cooperate with the physician.

In this case, Nancy is affected because of the effects of her actions on her patients. So the case must be analyzed with this in mind.

Autonomy: Nancy must decide whether she is willing to follow routine. She may believe there is no reason why a woman past the child-bearing years should not have her uterus removed. But if she does not believe this and if she is concerned with the effects of following routine on her patient, she should take some action such as whistleblowing or even quitting.

If she is not concerned with the physician's routine, then it is difficult to see how her relationship to her patients and her responsibility as their agent can be regarded as ethically proper. If this is her attitude, then she would probably not find the situation problematic to begin with. Therefore she probably would not bother to analyze it.

Freedom: It is not in Nancy's control to establish procedures. If any of her rights is being violated, it cannot be her right to freedom of action. Nor is her patient's right to freedom of action being directly violated. It is their right to veracity that is being violated. The standard of freedom is not directly relevant.

Veracity: It is virtually certain that, if this physician's patients were aware of his policies, they would not employ him as their physician. They would not undergo a hysterectomy unless they had adequate information and knew that the operation was necessary.

Nancy is surely violating the standard of veracity if she does not tell a patient that even though the patient is past child-bearing years and suffers from endometriosis, this does not in itself mean that she needs a hysterectomy.

Privacy: The rights of this physician's patients are certainly being violated, but not their right to privacy—except in the sense that the physician's invasion of their body is an invasion of their privacy. Neither is the physician violating Nancy's right to privacy. Therefore the right to privacy is not a relevant consideration here.

Beneficence: In order to meet the standard of beneficence Nancy must take some action. If she does not, she is surely violating this standard.

Fidelity: It is unimaginable that Nancy's patient has no right to expect Nancy to inform her of what she (Nancy) knows to be true. It is inconceivable that a patient would believe that her agreement with Nancy does not call for Nancy to inform her of the facts of this situation.

A patient who would believe this would have to believe that a nurse has no ethical responsibility whatever.

The elements would, quite predictably, agree with the analysis that is made through the bioethical standards.

Whistleblowing

Sometimes there are cases over which a nurse has very little control. These are cases such as:

- A physician desires to prevent a patient from "doing what no one could possibly want to do," which means that the physician desires to compel the patient to do what the physician believes the patient should want to do.
- A physician desires to inform a patient about some aspect of a condition which the patient would not want to be informed about.

- There is certain information that a patient would be benefited by having but the physician does not want him to have it.

Because of her role in the health care setting there is often relatively little a nurse can do. If she quits and turns her job over to someone who does not care, she accomplishes nothing.

The one major thing she can do is to recognize that what is being done is wrong—to recognize who is doing wrong and why it is wrong.

In cases like this the very first responsibility a nurse has is to be absolutely certain that what is being done *is* wrong. Until she has a clear vision of the context, she ought to do nothing. When she meets these responsibilities, perhaps, she cannot accomplish much by herself. But if she can accomplish anything, she has an ethical responsibility to do what she can.

Each nurse must decide for herself what she is willing to risk.

A word has been coined for risk-taking activity. It is called *whistleblowing.* "Whistleblowers sound an alarm from within the very organization in which they work, aiming to spotlight neglect or abuses that threaten the . . . [individual patient]" (Callahan and Bok, 1982, p. 277). The person who chooses to be a whistleblower hopes to stop the destructive process. Since the person does not fill the role of referee, this success is often not forthcoming.

A potential whistleblower should consider the following five questions before deciding to actually go public. The first four are from Callahan and Bok (1982, p. 278). The authors have added the fifth which is, perhaps, of even greater importance in a biomedical context.

1. Is speaking out really in the patient's interest?
2. What is the likelihood of change?
3. Is the whistleblower's responsibility to serve the interests of his patient greater than the responsibility he owes to his colleagues or his employing institution?
4. How great is the risk of retaliation and what type of retaliation might be expected?
5. What harm will occur to the patient or patients if action is not taken?

Legislation being introduced in many states will reduce the risk of being a whistleblower. The intent of the legislation is to decrease the risk and severity of retaliation. If this legislation is successful, it will decrease a nurse's risk. Therefore it will increase a nurse's ethical obligation to act for the benefit of her patient. It will place on her a stronger responsibility to try to actively promote an end to the abuses she finds in the health care system.

❧ **DILEMMA 5-2**   How a nurse can analyze the context of her decision when she is caught between an action and a passion.

Autonomy: If Sally takes action and gives Fred the dose of medication, she does not violate Fred's autonomy. If Sally remains passive and fails to give the dose of medication, she does not violate Fred's autonomy. In neither case is Fred's *autonomy* directly involved.

Freedom: For Sally to give Fred the dose of morphine would be perfectly in keeping with the agreement between Fred and his physician. For Sally to refuse, under these circumstances, would be for her to bring it about that Fred's right to free decision, choice, and action will be violated.

It is possible that a mistake has been made. It is possible that there has been a failure of communication and understanding. If there has been this mistake or this failure, it must be corrected. Otherwise the bioethical standard of freedom calls on Sally to give Fred the medication.

Veracity: When Sally took on the care of Fred, she made an agreement with Fred that she would not violate his freedom. She also had an agreement with the physician that she would follow his orders. If Sally's belief that to hasten a patient's death is never justifiable, then she should never permit herself to be in a situation such as this. The standard of veracity requires Sally to give Fred the medication.

Sally's belief is not a bioethical standard.

Privacy: It is very evident that Sally does not have the right to control Fred's actions and take over the ownership of Fred's life. It is also evident that Sally does not have the right to control the physician's decisions and actions.

The standard of privacy requires that Sally give Fred the medication.

Beneficence: For Sally to refuse to give Fred the medication because she believes it is not ethically justifiable to hasten a patient's death is not the same as for her to refuse to give Fred the medication out of motives of beneficence. For Sally to create static over this does Fred no good whatever. By prolonging his suffering it does him harm. To have placed herself in this situation is, already, to have violated the standard of beneficence.

Fidelity: It is quite obvious that in failing to give Fred the medication Sally betrays the nurse/patient agreement.

Analysis through the elements further clarifies this:

Desire: Fred desires the medication and he has a right to it.

Reason: In this situation it is not part of Sally's proper function to do Fred's reasoning for him. It is not part of Sally's proper function to do the physician's reasoning for him. It is certainly not part of Sally's proper function to demonstrate for her beliefs at Fred's death bed.

Life: It is Fred's, not Sally's, life to sustain or to bring to a close.

Purpose: Within the confines of beneficence Sally has a right to discuss Fred's decision with him. But the final purpose belongs to Fred. If Sally interferes, she violates Fred's purpose.

Agency: As a nurse Sally is an agent. She is, however, not the agent of her own desires and values. She is Fred's agent. Therefore her actions ought to be taken as Fred's agent.

Whatever she does, one ethical responsibility rests on Sally. She has a responsibility never to insert herself into this kind of situation again.

❦ DILEMMA 5-3 What to do when a patient's right to know conflicts with his desire not to know.

It is a rule that a patient has a right to know the details of his condition. When

Zelda relates all this to Mr. Wu she obeys the rule and satisfies Mr. Wu. No one can fault her for this. There are times when a patient must be told the details of his condition. This is necessary in order that he can understand and make decisions concerning his course of treatment. Mr. Goldfarb's case is not in this category.

Let us see if we can find a bioethical standard to justify Zelda's relating this information to Mr. Goldfarb:

Autonomy: Mr. Goldfarb's nature is such that he does not desire this detailed information. Having this information does not do him any good. At the same time it does him some harm.

If a patient's primary reason for entering the health care system is to receive information, then, perhaps, Mr. Goldfarb's autonomy would have a lessened relevance. In entering the health care system, it might be said, he consents to receive the information. If a patient's primary reason for entering the health care system was to receive information, however, the majority of patients who come into the hospital would discover the details of their condition and leave. Such is not the case. The primary reason for a patient entering the health care system is to regain his physical or psychological well-being.

Zelda violated Mr. Goldfarb's autonomy.

Freedom: Mr. Goldfarb has a right to know. A patient has the right to know because knowing enables him to take informed action. If knowing does not enable him to take informed action, then knowing has no value. Knowing has no value for Mr. Goldfarb.

His right to take action is prior to and logically more important than his right to know. His purpose (health and well-being) is more important than information for its own sake.

In addition to his right to know Mr. Goldfarb has a right not to know. This right ought to especially be respected when his not knowing assists his freedom of action and his well-being better than his being informed.

Veracity: Every truth which a nurse relates to a patient should be treated like a wild horse. It should always be controlled by beneficence.

The detailed truths that Zelda related to Mr. Goldfarb were not motivated by maleficence. However, Zelda should have been guided by beneficence and she was not.

The standard of veracity offers her no justification.

Privacy: In order that people, in their interactions, do not aggress against each other there must be an agreement between them to respect each other's self-ownership. Ethically, no one can be involved in an interaction unless he has given his consent. One person cannot influence the action of another person without the consent of that other person unless he takes over the ownership of that other person.

Try to imagine someone controlling the action of a pair of scissors without controlling the pair of scissors.

Between Zelda and Mr. Goldfarb, as between every nurse and patient, there is an implicit agreement that each will respect the self-ownership of the other. Zelda violated that agreement.

Beneficence: Zelda did Mr. Goldfarb harm for the sake of doing that which did him no good. Perhaps Zelda did not know the effect that her action would have on Mr. Goldfarb. If she did not know, she should have known. She cannot appeal to the standard of beneficence.

Fidelity: Zelda was faithful to the standard of fidelity just in case the nurse/patient agreement involves a nurse taking particular actions regardless of their consequences. The nurse/patient agreement, of course, does not involve this. Zelda can find no support in the standard of fidelity.

An examination of the elements of Mr. Goldfarb's autonomy will show nothing different.

DILEMMA 5-4   Whether a young girl should be informed that her physician has discovered the condition of testicular feminization.

Autonomy: There is no question but that informing Amelia of her condition will be an assault on her self-image. There is no question but that it will have a negative effect on her (developing) autonomy. An analysis of the effects of being told on Amelia's autonomy reveal these reasons why she should not be told. It reveals no reasons why she should be told.

Freedom: It is certainly the case that Amelia will enjoy less freedom by knowing of her condition. Thus, at best, the standard of freedom does not support informing her of her condition.

Veracity: It is hard to see how Amelia would be better off knowing of her condition. Benevolence does not call for her to be informed. The effect that being informed will have on her autonomy is an excellent reason for her not to be informed. The standard of veracity does not justify informing her.

Privacy: The act of informing her would surely be an invasion of Amelia's privacy. She has not invited, and it is probable that she would not invite, Dr. Richmond to inform her.

Beneficence: There is no question but that not informing her is the more beneficent course of action.

Fidelity: The agreement between a patient and a health care professional is an agreement that the health care professional will try to make a patient's state of well-being better and not make it worse.

What Dr. Richmond can do immediately will make Amelia's state of well-being better, although Dr. Richmond is not the only surgeon in the world who can do this.

On the other hand, the long-term detriment of being informed will vastly outweigh the benefit that Dr. Richmond will bestow on Amelia through his immediate action. Once Dr. Richmond does this harm to Amelia, there will be no one who can undo it.

Despite the bioethical standards, many contemporary ethicists would call for Amelia to be told of her condition. Because of the complexity of this situation let us examine it in terms of the elements of Amelia's autonomy:

Desire: Most 17-year-olds would not want to be informed. It cannot be known with certainty whether or not Amelia would want to be informed, but it can be known with certainty that she *probably* would not.

Reason: Knowing of her condition will make it more difficult for Amelia to think positively of herself and her life. The element of reason calls for Amelia not to be told.

Knowing would do Amelia more harm than good. There is, at least, a slight suggestion, in reason, that she not be told. If reason is to be beneficent, then there is a powerful demand that she not be told.

Life: No part of her life is threatened by not knowing. No part of her life is enhanced by knowing. Therefore, there is nothing at all in the element of life to suggest that she should be told.

Purpose: None of Amelia's purposes would be served by her being informed. At the same time it cannot be doubted that some of her purposes would be hindered by her knowing. The element of purpose counsels that she not be told.

Agency: Amelia's agency would be hindered by her knowing. Her self-image would be damaged. Her approach to the world would change.

Amelia has a right to know. She also has a right *not* to know. And, she has a right not to be harmed.

Contemporary ethicists offer two arguments as to why Amelia should be told:

1. Amelia will probably find out anyway.

   This is a contextual factor that must be taken into consideration in an actual context. It is, however, a factor that can be taken into consideration only in an actual, real-life context. It is a logistical factor and as such it is not one of the *ethical* aspects of the context. If there is any way that it can be brought about that Amelia will not find out about her condition, then this way should be discovered.

   That Amelia will find out anyway is a rationalization. It is a health care professional's excuse for doing his duty when he knows he should not.

2. It is suggested that Dr. Richmond has a responsibility to Amelia's relatives. Amelia must be informed in order that she can discuss this condition with them. It might be advantageous to them to be aware of the recessive disorder that may run in their family.

   Let us examine the ethical strength of this argument:
   Dr. Richmond may feel that he has a duty to inform Amelia's relatives. As we have seen, duty is an entirely inappropriate bioethical standard. So he cannot justifiably act on this feeling.

   Perhaps, however, Dr. Richmond reasons that *Amelia* has a duty to inform the members of her family.

   There is no reason to believe that Amelia has any such duty. Claiming that Amelia has a brother (and she may or may not have a brother) does not prove that she has a brother. Claiming that Amelia has a duty does not, logically or ethically, establish the fact that indeed she does have a duty. Every bioethical standard implies that she does not.

   It is probable that Dr. Richmond's reasoning, strictly speaking, is not deontological. It is not based on a declaration that either he or Amelia has a duty. His reasoning, probably, is, at least partly, utilitarian. He is probably motivated by the belief that by informing Amelia "the greatest good for the greatest number" will be served. But it can be seen that this too involves a duty.

We have also seen that utilitarianism is as inappropriate to a biomedical context as is deontology. The utilitarian standard will also fail to justify Dr. Richmond's action.

The difference, in this context, between a purposive ethic and utilitarianism is this: According to a purposive ethic Amelia is at the center of the ethical context. Dr. Richmond must expect nothing of Amelia but that she pursue her own welfare and the welfare of those whom she values.

Utilitarianism, on the other hand, allows Dr. Richmond to expect Amelia to pursue the welfare of the larger number of people whether or not she values them. This simply because they are the larger number. Her well-being must be sacrificed to their benefit.

If Dr. Richmond were motivated by a purposive ethic, he would choose among contextual alternatives. Then he would decide according to rights and responsibilities. He would try to make his decision intelligible in relation to cause and effect. He would try to bring about ethical proportion and balance.

Such a decision would call for Amelia to take on the burden of knowing about her condition only if she chose to do this. If Amelia knew all the facts, she might, out of beneficence, wish to inform her relatives. Let us subject Dr. Richmond's position, under a purposive ethic, to a rational ethical analysis:

Amelia should value her relatives only if she has some rational reason to value them. For instance, if they are abusive or contemptuous of her, she lacks a rational reason to value them. If she values them in spite of this she has no ethical reward to offer those who are not abusive or contemptuous of her.

Amelia should choose in favor of her relatives only if she has a rational and objective reason to value them. This reason would have to be sufficient to make her willing to bear the burden of knowing of her condition.

She has this objective reason only if her relatives, in turn, place a high value on her.

Let us see where this leaves us:

If Amelia's relatives place a high value on her they will be concerned with the effect of knowing about her condition on Amelia.

If her relatives would be unconcerned with the effect of her knowing of her condition, then Amelia has no objective reason to value them.

If Amelia does not have an objective reason to value her relatives, then to inform her of her condition so that she can inform them is simply to sacrifice her to the greater number. To inform her, Dr. Richmond would have to assume that Amelia is, or ought to be, motivated by self-contempt.

If her relatives place a high value on Amelia, they would not want her to undergo the trauma of knowing of her condition. They would regard the detriment to Amelia as out of proportion to the benefit to themselves.

In the context of a purposive ethic Dr. Richmond would have to conclude that:

If Amelia has no objective reason to value her relatives, then, in the context of a purposive ethic, beneficence will not be a rational motivation for her to be informed.

If Amelia does have objective reasons to value her relatives, then, her relatives will not want Amelia to know of her condition. Their balanced and proportioned desire would be to place Amelia's benefit above theirs. Rather, they would consider Amelia's benefit to be of greater benefit to them.

Amelia's relatives have reason to value Amelia only if Amelia respects their desires. If Amelia respects their desires then she ought to accede to their desire for her welfare to be protected.

It is not difficult to understand that Amelia's increased happiness and self confidence thoughout her life would be more prized by her relatives than their increased convenience.

Suppose that one of Amelia's relatives is a nurse. Should a nurse placed this high a value on her convenience? How would she relate to her patients? Could you, as a nurse, place a high value on this nurse?

In the context of a purposive ethic, there are no ethical circumstances calling for Amelia to be informed of her condition.

Nurses and the Physician's Dilemma

This is a dilemma that falls on a physician to resolve and not on a nurse. However, in the health care system, very often a physician resolves a dilemma but a nurse must deal with his resolution. Quite often it is a nurse who must explain his resolution to the patient and, perhaps, spend an entire day with the patient and/or the patient's family answering questions. These situations can be very frustrating for nurses.

Nurses should be able to analyze even the most difficult dilemmas. Knowing how to analyze difficult ethical dilemmas makes it easier to analyze simple dilemmas. It might also enable a nurse to win the respect of her colleagues in the health care system. It might make it possible for her to negotiate with them and, one hopes, to become involved with them in the decision making process.

✌ **DILEMMA 5-5** How a nurse might negotiate a conflict between a patient's freedom of action and the hospital schedule.

When a patient enters the health care system and makes his agreement with the people in the system, they do not make an agreement to do something which might, even indirectly, injure someone else for his benefit. The health care setting has a specific nature and a specific purpose and the patient must accept this nature and purpose. A patient cannot justify a demand that the health care system become something other than a health care system.

The convenience of the people in the health care system, however, is something else again. It is unreasonable for the health care system, and it is contrary to the bioethical standards, to hinder a patient's free action when a significant value is involved simply because it is more convenient to interfere. The health care system must accept the fact that the people with whom it deals are autonomous.

Analyzing this situation in terms of the bioethical standards we find:

Autonomy: It is in the nature of nearly everyone's autonomy that they value their relationship to a son or daughter. If conditions are such that nothing but convenience stands in the way of Mr. Morris seeing his son, then it would violate his autonomy not to reschedule things so that he can see his son.

If more than convenience (for instance, safety) would be hindered by the rescheduling, then, however painful it might be to Mr. Morris, the schedule should not be changed.

Freedom: Certainly it would violate the bioethical standard of freedom if Mr. Morris were kept from seeing his son for a reason involving some lesser value.

If his seeing his son were to undermine another person's greater value, then he should not see his son.*

Veracity: The importance of veracity in this dilemma is either remote or nonexistent.

Privacy: If the requirements of Mr. Morris' privacy do not violate the requirements of anyone else's privacy, then Mr. Morris has a right to do what he desires to do because he enjoys self-ownership and because, in this circumstance, he has no obligation to any other person.

Beneficence: If Mr. Morris is barred from seeing his son for an unjustifiable reason, this is a failure of beneficence.

Fidelity: If Mr. Morris is prevented from seeing his son for a less than adequate reason, then there is a violation of fidelity to the agreement.

If the reason why the schedule is not rearranged is justifiable, then to rearrange it would not be according to the terms of the agreement.

The health care system makes no agreement with a patient that it will not be a health care system. Biomedical professionals make no agreement with a patient that they will not be biomedical professionals.

Triage

Mr. Morris' case calls for ethical balance and proportion. Although Mr. Morris' case is not, strictly speaking, as complex or demanding, it is similar to a triage situation. The nature of ethical balance and proportion can be seen in an analysis of the "triage" situation.

We can conduct our analysis in a small thought-experiment:

Suppose that there is a situation in which two people each have a stake. The benefit that Barbara might retain is one she would much rather have than lose. The benefit that Valerie might retain is one which, if she lost it, would cause her extreme grief. Suppose further that there is a third party, Helen, who has a responsibility to exercise beneficence in this situation.

---

* The greater value must be a value to another person. Only Mr. Morris can decide on the rank of his values. Therefore a health care professional cannot prevent Mr. Morris from seeing his son for the sake of Mr. Morris' greater value.

Unless there are very compelling reasons to the contrary, arrangements ought to be made to allow Mr. Morris to see his son.

Helen can act to assist only one person—either Valerie or Barbara but not both.

In and of themselves neither Barbara nor Valerie is intrinsically more deserving than the other.

Helen faces a dilemma. Should she assist Barbara, or should she assist Valerie? How can she, without empty rationalizations, *justify* the decision she makes? There is no one individual who is the center of the ethical context.

There is no doubt that some benefits are more important than others. So all possible benefits can be, in effect, evaluated and numbered by Helen. She can rate them from 1 to 10 according to their importance. Class 1 benefits, for instance, are those that are least in importance; class 10 benefits those that are most important. A class 3 benefit will not motivate the person who holds it as much as a class 8 benefit would motivate him.

In a triage situation the benefactor (in our case Helen), in effect, analyzes the situation in this way:

First Helen asks herself: "If Barbara and Valerie were not two people but only one person, what would be the best thing for me to do?" She knows very well that Barbara and Valerie are not one person. But, in this situation, in order for her to make a justifiable decision, she must think of them as if they were. She must act as if they were one person. She must act to bring about the benefit that would be rated highest by this person.

If Helen could bring just one thing from a burning building, she would bring out this person's dog rather than this person's wedding dress. She would judge that this person would rate her dog at least an 8 while she would rate her wedding dress perhaps a 3.

If it were Valerie's dog and Barbara's wedding dress, she would rescue Valerie's dog, for the same reason. She judges Valerie's dog to be an 8 to Valerie; she judges Barbara's wedding dress to be a 3 to Barbara.

She would rescue Valerie's dog because this is what the (triage) situation calls for. The triage situation is an ethical situation where all the potential beneficiaries become one person.

We have been assuming that there is an equal probability of Helen's being able to salvage either Valerie's dog or Barbara's dress. We have assumed that the risk to Helen is equal in both cases. The odds for and against a benefactor being able to bring about different benefits and the risks involved must also be factored in. If Helen could easily salvage Barbara's wedding dress but the probability of her salvaging Valerie's dog was very low and/or the peril to her (Helen) were very high, then it might be more reasonable for her to salvage Barbara's wedding dress.

In a triage situation a health care professional must sort out all the possible benefits to everyone involved in the situation—wounded soldiers on a battle-

field, people injured in an airline disaster, people trapped in a burning building—regardless of whose benefits they are. She cannot make her decision
according to an agreement with an individual beneficiary. Therefore she must
make it according to the benefits that she can bring about.

If a nurse on a battlefield finds a soldier with a broken leg and a sprained
ankle, she will fix the broken leg.

If she finds two soldiers, one with a broken leg and one with a sprained
ankle, she will attend to the one with the broken leg, for the same reason.
This is the greatest benefit she can bring about.

After an airline disaster a nurse might treat the severe bleeding of a person
with a broken back before immobilizing him. There is something she can do
for his bleeding and little she can do for his back. At the same time his
bleeding presents a greater threat to his life than does his back.

If she found two survivors, one with severe bleeding and the other with a
broken back, she would attend to the one with the severe bleeding, for the
same reason that she would attend to an individual person's bleeding before
attending to his back.

According to the triage analysis Helen ought to choose her beneficiary
according to:

1. The importance of the benefit, its ranking on the scale.
2. The probability of her being able to bring about the benefit.
3. The risks she will encounter.

In a triage situation Helen ought to regard every possible beneficiary as
one person. Then she ought to direct her actions according to the most
rational desires of this one person.

She ought to do this in a situation where only one person is involved
because, in this situation, this is the greatest benefit she could bring about.
This is what the rational desire of her beneficiary would call for her to do.

She ought to do this in a triage situation, where more than one person is
involved, because this is what the situation calls for.

For purposes of analysis, ethical decision making, and ethical action a
triage situation makes everyone one person. In the context of a triage situation she ought to bring about the greatest benefit. She ought to do this
because this is, so to speak, what the rational desire of *this* one person would
want her to do.

The analogy between the triage situation and Mr. Morris' situation is obvious. So is the reasonableness of analyzing them in the same way. If the benefit
of seeing his son to Mr. Morris is a 6 and no one can receive—or lose—a benefit
of 7 or greater, then Mr. Morris should see his son. If Mr. Morris' seeing his son
would interfere with another patient's benefit that would be rated 7 or greater,
then the benefit should be given to the other patient.

A nurse should be extremely careful not to apply triage reasoning where it is not appropriate. It is only appropriate where there is an objective conflict between the values of two equally deserving beneficiaries. It is never appropriate when its application would violate the terms of an agreement or violate someone's rights.

✿ **DILEMMA 5-6**   Whether apathy is an ethical strength or an ethical evil.

Autonomy: Mrs. Narda's autonomy is never allowed to come into play. If she knew all the facts she might still opt to undergo the treatment for the sake of her children. On the other hand, if Jane informed her of the facts, she might decide not to undergo this treatment. Since the standard of autonomy calls on a biomedical professional to respect and support her patient's unique character structure, Jane should have given Mrs. Narda this information and she did not.

Freedom: People are free if they determine their actions voluntarily on the basis of the information they have. The standard of freedom calls on a nurse to support the ability of a patient to engage in free action. If this requires a nurse to give a patient information of which the patient is unaware, and the nurse does not do this, she violates the patient's right to freedom.

Veracity: If a nurse is aware of a certain body of information that would benefit her patient and she does not give this information to her patient, she violates the standard of veracity.

Privacy: In failing to give Mrs. Narda complete information, Jane has taken over Mrs. Narda's self-ownership. The standard of privacy calls for Jane to give Mrs. Narda complete information.

Beneficence: To allow Mrs. Narda to undergo experimental treatment for the sake of her children may, in some sense, be beneficent in relation to her children, although this would be difficult to show. It is not beneficent in relation to Mrs. Narda. Jane's responsibility is to her patient, not to her patient's children.

Fidelity: If everyone who entered the health care system expected to be treated as Mrs. Narda was treated—if they assumed that the agreement between a patient and the health care system depended upon the personal values of the people in the health care system—there would be an outcry that would shake the halls of many courthouses. The biomedical professions, in fact, have already been through this.

Jane surely violated the standard of fidelity.

The error of Jane's course of action can be seen even more clearly in terms of the elements:

Desire: The desire that determined Mrs. Narda's decision was not her desire but Jane's desire and the physician's desire. The evil of this is, in a grisly sense, comic.

Reason: The reason that determined Mrs. Narda's decision was not her reason but Jane's and the physician's. No one's reasoning can be replaced by the reasoning of another person.

No reasoning, in any relevant sense, went into Mrs. Narda's course of action.

Life: The only life for which Jane had an ethical responsibility was Mrs. Narda's life. Jane did not concern herself with Mrs. Narda's life. She failed the ethical element of life.

Purpose: Mrs. Narda had a right to decide, choose, and act on her autonomous purposes. This right was taken from her.

Agency: Mrs. Narda had a right to exercise her agency to whatever extent she was able. Had Jane given her the information to which she was entitled, she would have been able to exercise her agency considerably more than she did.

If the difference between good and evil, in a bioethical context, is determined by the bioethical standards and by the elements of a patient's autonomy, then Jane's apathy and failure to give Mrs. Narda complete contextual information is an evil.

❧ **DILEMMA 5-7**   Whether it is ever right to tell lies from benevolent motives.

This is a unique and interesting case in this respect. The nurse is not dealing with a patient. The patient is entirely unaffected by her nurse's actions. The nurse is dealing with the parents of a deceased patient.

The bioethical standards are the most relevant guides to ethical action that biomedicine has yet discovered. But in a case like this the relationship between the biomedical professional and the person she is dealing with is very different than her relationship to a patient. This is because there is a much stronger agreement between the biomedical professional and her patient than there is between unrelated people, even the biomedical professional and the patient's family. The nurse has no responsibility to the family's freedom, objective understanding, or privacy. There is no bioethical agreement between them.

Therefore, the best way to resolve this dilemma is by way of the elements of autonomy. Robin's parents are people, and everyone has an ethical responsibility to deal with people as people, to deal with them according to the nature of their autonomy.

Desire: It is quite obvious that no parent could have a rational desire to hear the terrible details of a child's death. The nurse inflicted an act of aggression against Robin's parents' rational desire.

Reason: When Robin's parents heard the details of their daughter's death, this did them no good and could not fail to do them harm. It harmed them emotionally. It did nothing to increase their ability to reason. Robin's nurse acted dutifully. She failed to act beneficently. She did not fail to act irrationally.

In one way or another every failure of beneficence is, at the same time, a failure of sound reasoning.

Life: The nurse's action, over a span of time, must diminish the life of Robin's parents.

Purpose: Obviously no rational purpose was served by this action. The nurse cannot justify her action by appealing to purpose.

Agency: No one's agency was increased by this. The experience they underwent at the hands of Robin's nurse will, predictably, interfere with Robin's parents getting on with their life. They will always carry this picture in their minds.

Agency does not justify the nurse's action.

Nothing justifies the nurse's action—nothing but duty. And duty is nothing.

❦ **DILEMMA 5-8**   Whether a nurse ought to give a patient information that his physician does not want him to have.

In a real-life situation this would be a very difficult case. In general these are the reasons why Verna ought to inform Mr. Rogers.

Autonomy: If Verna is right, then Mr. Rogers' most rational desire would be to go to the other hospital. If she does not give him the information, she is, at the least, failing to give support to this expression of his autonomy.

Freedom: If she does not give him the information, she restricts the actions that are open to him. In this way she restricts his freedom.

Veracity: If she does not give this information to Mr. Rogers, and their agreement calls on her to give it to him, then she fails the standard of veracity. In any ordinary context the agreement would require her to give the information.

Privacy: There is no really close relationship between this dilemma and the standard of privacy.

Beneficence: If Verna believes that this information would do Mr. Rogers some good and she has no reason to believe that it would do him harm, then beneficence calls on her to inform him.

Fidelity: If Verna is right, then not to inform Mr. Rogers is to fail to give him optimum care. This is an act of infidelity to the nurse/patient agreement.

There is not enough context to justify the need for analysis through the elements.

❦ **DILEMMA 5-9**   Whether a nurse ought to vary routine where there is no apparent reason to take an action.

This is the simplest dilemma imaginable. It will be interesting to analyze it in terms of the elements.

Desire: Put yourself in Mrs. Clay's place and ask yourself if you would want to be awakened in order to take a sleeping pill.

Reason: Awakening Mrs. Clay to give her a sleeping pill is entirely irrational. It is almost comical to think about waking her up in order to put her to sleep. It is as though someone were to pick a book up off of a table in order to put it back down on the table.

Life: No aspect of Mrs. Clay's life will be enhanced if she is awakened in order to take a sleeping pill.

Purpose: No one's rational purpose is served by awakening Mrs. Clay. Can you imagine, if Mrs. Clay could be consulted, her saying, "I wish someone would wake me up and give me a sleeping pill."

Agency: If Mrs. Clay's course of treatment calls for her to sleep, then waking her to give her a sleeping pill does not improve her agency, it interrupts it. She is already doing what her course of treatment requires.

Among other things deontology tends to deaden one's sense of humor.

❦ **DILEMMA 5-10**   Whether a dying patient's desire for confidentiality should override his family's plans for a pleasant surprise.

This dilemma was already resolved in Chapter 5. The bioethical standards are elements of the nurse/patient agreement. The standard of *privacy* requires Harry's nurse "...to reveal the fact of his son's return and let Harry decide what he desires to do." Nonetheless we will analyze the dilemma in terms of the other bioethical standards.

Autonomy: Harry's nurse must keep her agreement with her patient. If she could know that Harry's character-structure was such that he would prefer his family knowing in order that he might enjoy the surprise, then, perhaps, she should inform his family. This would not be for utilitarian reasons but for Harry's benefit and in keeping with their agreement. At all odds it is very, very unlikely that Harry's nurse could have any certain knowledge of this. Therefore it almost certainly should not determine her decision.

Freedom: Harry's freedom is involved here only remotely. The dilemma has to do with his privacy, his self-ownership. Whatever could be discovered by analyzing the dilemma in terms of his freedom could be more easily and more surely discovered by analyzing it in terms of privacy.

Veracity: If Harry believes that his nurse will not advise his family of his prognosis, and she does, then she violates the standard of veracity.

In the nature of the case she cannot ask for Harry's advice. She cannot ask him whether he wants to know that his son is coming home without letting him know that his son is coming home.

Beneficence: There is no sense in which the standard of beneficence calls for a nurse to do the greatest good for the greatest number. It calls for her to do the greatest good for her patient. Harry's nurse does this by going to Harry and discussing the situation with him.

Fidelity: The nurse can assume that Harry would desire to know that his son is safe and coming home. This knowledge would enhance the remainder of his life and, perhaps, even make the dying process easier for Harry.

A nurse's one overriding agreement is with her patient. Fidelity requires that she be true to this agreement. The nurse/patient agreement will not allow Harry's nurse to do nothing. She must discuss the situation either with Harry or with his family. She cannot discuss it with his family. She must discuss it with Harry.

❀ DILEMMA 7-1   Whether honesty is the best policy.

Autonomy: Strictly speaking Laura does not do anything that violates Adam's autonomy. Nor does she do anything that supports his autonomy. The standard of autonomy is not helpful.

Freedom: Laura, when she reveals Adam's condition to Carl, quite obviously interferes with Adam's freedom of action in dealing with Carl.

Veracity: Truth, as a bioethical standard, is more complex than a strict matter of the correspondence between idea and fact. The standard of veracity calls for truth to be purposeful and guided by concern for a patient's welfare. If veracity is not guided by purpose and beneficence, it serves no purpose as a bioethical standard. Laura has certainly violated this standard. No nurse should ever murder, rob, steal cars, assault, slander, or disobey the traffic laws. These are all excellent standards of conduct. They are not bioethical standards.

What is right and wrong action in general is determined by what human life is all about. What is right and wrong action in a biomedical context is determined by what human life is all about in a biomedical context. In her everyday existence a nurse should never stick needles into people. The situation does not call for it. In the health care setting she must often stick needles into people. The situation does call for it.

The context determines the appropriate principle. Even so, one might ponder this question: Should Laura have told Carl about Adam if Adam was not a patient but a neighbor?

Privacy: In conducting Adam's affairs without his permission Laura has taken over Adam's self-ownership. Adam's right to privacy has certainly been violated here.

It seems as if there is a conflict between the standards of veracity and privacy. There is, however, no such conflict. There has simply been a failure to apply the concept of veracity correctly. Laura did not apply it as a bioethical standard.

Beneficence: Harming her patient, in order to keep up her end of the conversation, caused Laura to violate the standard of beneficence.

Fidelity: Harming her patient is surely a breach of fidelity.

❦ **DILEMMA 7-2**   How a nurse might counsel a patient who must gamble on a "long shot."

This is a situation that Vladimir very well might want to discuss with his nurse. If he does, it is desirable that she understand the vital and fundamental factors influencing his decision. Vital and fundamental factors, in a purposive ethic, are ethical factors.

Here the bioethical standards are irrelevant. This is not, in its most important sense, a case of a nurse dealing with a patient. Nor is this a case of a nurse helping a patient deal with another person. This is a case of a nurse acting as a sounding board in order to help her patient think and make a decision for himself. Vladimir needs self-awareness. His nurse can help him to analyze his situation by reference to the elements of his autonomy.

Life: Vladimir must try to ascertain what his overall life style will be if either operation succeeds or fails. Then he must decide whether he is willing to take the risks of one course of action or be content with the results of the other course.

Purpose: In assessing all the possibilities Vladimir will have to decide on the purposes that motivate him.

Desire: Vladimir will have to decide whether his greater desire is to play again or to retain the gross motor movements of his hand. Then he must examine the strength of these desires against the probabilities of realizing each one.

Reason: Vladimir must assess the benefits and detriments of each course of action. Then he must decide on what his most reasonable course of action will be in light of his rational desires.

Agency: When Valdimir has made a decision, he ought to think about whether this decision really reflects his character and values.

There is no question of a nurse making the choice for a patient in a case like Vladimir's. Even if she is asked, it is obvious that she ought to refuse. But, if she is skilled, her consciousness can be a mirror in which her patient can see his ideas and values reflected.

DILEMMA 7-3 How strong are contextual influences on a nurse's promise of secrecy?

This is not a dilemma that a nurse is very apt to run into. However, the dilemma presented in this extreme state points up the principles involved in any dilemma of this kind.

Autonomy: The patient is unique. The nature of his desire is determined by this uniqueness. How his desire is shaped by his uniqueness in the situation cannot be known. The nurse must go on the knowledge she has. But the dilemma assumes that she has very little knowledge.

Freedom: If she reveals what her patient has told her she will, at least apparently, be taking an action against him.

If she informs the physician, she will also be taking an action for him. She will be helping him to continue acting on the purpose he had in entering the hospital.

The standard of freedom offers little help one way or the other. Or, rather, it offers too much help. It offers help in both directions.

Veracity: In order to meet the demands of the standard of veracity a nurse must be guided by beneficence. Does veracity call for her to keep her promise to the patient? Or does it call for her to inform the physician so that he can take the best possible action? In order to discover the demands of beneficence she has to know the probable outcomes of different courses of action.

There is no way the nurse can know what direction beneficence takes.

Privacy: Finally we find some assistance in the standard of privacy.

The nurse does not take over the ownership of her patient unless she does something for him that he would not do for himself. If she does something for him that he would do, then she is simply acting as his agent.

On considering the dilemma from the vantage point of privacy it is possible to see one important fact: Silence maintains the patient's privacy and self-ownership only if he would be willing to harm himself.

Perhaps he would. Perhaps his reason for wanting to keep his condition secret is important enough that he would be willing to endure this harm. The nurse must ask herself, however, why he would have told *her* if this is the case? If secrecy here is important enough for him to endanger himself in this situation, why would he have told his nurse?

Consideration of the case under the standard of privacy tends to indicate that the nurse should tell the physician what the patient told her.

Beneficence: Contextually it seems as if beneficence calls for telling. But the harm of telling is not known. Action is behavior arising from knowledge. An agent should always prefer to act on what he does know rather than on what he does not know.

The harm of not telling is known. If this harm is at all serious, then that which is known ought to override that which is not known.

Beneficence, guided by reason, suggests that the nurse break her promise of secrecy.

Fidelity: Fidelity requires the nurse to make a choice. She must exercise fidelity either toward her promise or toward her patient. Her promise, of course, was a promise to her patient. All the same she owes fidelity not to one aspect of her relationship to her patient but to the entire relationship. In the context of a purposive ethic she owes fidelity to her patient and to what she knows.

A ritualistic ethic would demand that a nurse keep her promise — but very few nurses would.

A purposive ethic would demand that a nurse keep her attention on the purpose that brought her patient into the hospital.

When a patient tells a nurse a secret, he should not forget that the first purpose of the health care system is his health and well-being. Secrecy for the sake of secrecy must give way to health and well-being.

✿ DILEMMA 7-4 Whether the standard of fidelity is capable of clashing with optimal medical practice.

The standard of fidelity is not capable of clashing with rational medical practice. The standard of fidelity binds a nurse to the overall nurse/patient agreement. It does not bind her to fulfill any minor agreement that would violate this agreement.

When the biomedical professional originally made his promise, it was perfectly in line with the agreement between a biomedical professional and a patient. When a cure for the patient's condition was discovered, this entirely changed the context. Under these altered circumstances it would be perfectly contrary to their agreement for the biomedical professional not to resuscitate the patient.

Any specific promise a biomedical professional makes to a patient or a patient makes to a biomedical professional must be taken in context. As the context changes the way the promise is kept may change.

✿ DILEMMA 8-1 Whether a nurse has the right to prevent a disoriented patient from ambulating.

Autonomy: Glenda, in recognizing Rick's context, respects his autonomy.

A patient's autonomy is expressed in his rational desires. Whatever is against Rick's rational desires is against his autonomy. His desire to ambulate, however, is not a rational desire. If he acted on this momentary desire, he could destroy his power to act on long-term desires. Glenda defended Rick's power to act on rational desires. In this way she defended his autonomy.

Freedom: A nurse who interferes with a disoriented patient's short-term efforts does not necessarily violate his freedom. She may protect his freedom. A patient's freedom is related to his reason. His freedom is the freedom to take action. Action is a behavior guided by reason.

If Rick's freedom has to do with his autonomous purposes and his life, then Glenda has defended Rick's freedom. She has not violated Rick's right to freedom of action unless the standard of freedom refers to any momentary urge that passes through a person's mind. Of course it does not. The choice a patient makes while he is in a delirium does not have the same ethical status as a choice he would make in a more lucid moment.

Veracity: The standard of veracity plays no part in this dilemma.

Privacy: Efforts that do not express the nature of the agent do not express his self-ownership. Long-term efforts, efforts guided by an agent's power of abstract reasoning, express the nature of the agent and his self-ownership.

Picture a patient scratching his knee. His nurse lifts up his wrist in order to take his pulse. This may be rude, but it does not violate her patient's privacy, his freedom, or his autonomy. Privacy, freedom, and autonomy have to do with something other than itches, reflexes, and behaviors taken in a delirium.

Beneficence: Nursing is a form of beneficence. It is beneficent for a nurse to take nursing interventions. Nursing interventions protect a patient's agency and sustain his life.

Fidelity: Nursing interventions are acts of fidelity.

It will become obvious that there are no contradictions between the bioethical standards. The bioethical standards simply must be understood in terms of the elements of autonomy. If the elements are understood, then autonomy is understood. If autonomy is understood, then the other standards will be understood. The elements force a nurse's attention onto her patient. Ethical facts come into focus when her attention is on her patient.

DILEMMA 8-2   Whether a health care professional is right in attempting to compel a patient to make decisions regarding his treatment.

- It is true that in delegating responsibility to the health care professional a patient is exercising his freedom. The health care professional is an agent acting for his patient.
- In a health care setting a patient's power of choice and decision are weakened. The knowledge he might act on is limited. The most rational exercise of his freedom might well be to delegate responsibility to a health care professional. This is constantly assumed in emergency situations. In these situations the health care professional goes about his task with no questions asked.
- A patient's relationship to a health care professional, or any type of professional, *does* always involve a delegating of reponsibility.

   On the other hand:

- In delegating his right to freedom the patient is not refusing to exercise it.
- In recognizing the nature of his autonomy the patient is not abandoning it.
- It is ethically desirable that a patient assume responsibility for himself and delegate as little as possible. But what is "as little as possible" for one person in one context will not be "as little as possible" for another person in another context.

   In some contexts a patient's best course of action may be to delegate responsibility.

DILEMMA 8-3   How a nurse resolves the dilemma of a conflict between autonomy and veracity.

Ken and Rachel are friends. This adds a complication to the dilemma. Because of this complication the best way to analyze the dilemma is through the elements rather than through the standards.

The dilemma arose because Rachel is unsure of how to interact with Ken in this situation. She must analyze the elements of his autonomy as they function in this context.

Desire: Ken would desire to get his affairs in order, but he does not want to be made aware of the seriousness of his condition.

If Rachel is noncommittal* with Ken it allows him either to deny the seriousness of his condition, or accept it internally but without having it thrust at him from the outside.

If Ken cannot be motivated in this way to get his affairs in order, then his desire is obvious: Ken, above all, does not want to know the seriousness of his condition.

Reason: A noncommittal approach on the part of Rachel can help Ken exercise his reason much better than Rachel thrusting the details of his condition at him can.

Life: Only Ken can compute the importance of his terror in the present as opposed to his desires for the future.

Purpose: Ken's purposes are in conflict. No one but Ken can tip the balance.

Agency: His agency is involved in getting his affairs in order. His condition precludes agency. As a long-term factor the element of agency cannot enter into Rachel's deliberations.

❧ DILEMMA 8-4 Whether a comatose Jehovah's Witness should be given a blood transfusion.

Autonomy: There is no way to have certain knowledge of this patient's autonomy.

Freedom: As his agent his nurse ensures his freedom by acting for him. But she has no way of knowing what actions he would take if he were free; that is, if he were conscious. The fact that this patient belongs to a particular religious sect does not necessarily mean that he accepts every practice of this religion.

If he were conscious and declared that he did not want a transfusion, then in the context of the bioethical standards that would end it. But he is not conscious, and the direction that his freedom would take if he were is not known.

Veracity: The standard of veracity offers no guidance in this case.

Privacy: The patient is unable to express his ideas and desires. Therefore there is no way to know what his privacy would consist in.

Beneficence: It is impossible to know what would be beneficent in relation to this patient.

Fidelity: This situation offers no grounds for an agreement.

This is a case a biomedical professional must decide for himself and without any help from the bioethical standards. Since the nature of this patient's autonomy also is not known the elements of autonomy offer little guidance.

The element of life offers what may be little more than a suggestion:

A person's religion is, to a greater or lesser extent, an important part of his life. But every whole is greater than any one of its parts. The patient's life is more than his religion. The best decision that can be made in this situation is that he be given the blood transfusion. This option will allow him to pursue his autonomous purposes for his life. Otherwise he will die, and all the options of his life will be closed off.

---

* By "noncommittal" we mean Rachel should say something like "If you do not recover. . . ." rather than "Ken, you are dying and therefore. . . ."

❦ **DILEMMA 8-5** Whether the nature of a rational beneficence precludes the exercise of "gentle coercion."

A rational beneficence does not violate autonomy. Neither does "gentle coercion." A person with a future is more than the sum of his present emotions. A little "gentle coercion" might be necessary to help him to reestablish his thinking processes.

❦ **DILEMMA 8-6** Whether a comatose patient with no chance to recover from his condition should be allowed to die.

All four arguments are misleading:

- The unique individual that he once was does still exist. The state of being that he once enjoyed, however, no longer exists. Even if it were true to say that, "The autonomous individual no longer exists," nothing would follow from this. If anything *ought* to be done, this can only be because an autonomous individual *does* exist. If an autonomous individual does not exist, then there is nothing that *must* be done.
- There is no way that anyone can benefit this patient. What should be done cannot be determined by beneficence. There is no way to exercise beneficence in relation to this patient.
- Life is not precious to him. Nothing is or can be of any value to him. If a tribute can be paid to him and to his life, that tribute might be his death as well as his continued existence.
- The notion of autonomy involves two other notions—uniqueness and independence.

It is true that no one has a right to terminate the life of an autonomous individual. This is not because an autonomous individual is unique. It is not because when he is observed he appears different from other people. An autonomous individual acquires the right to life through the fact that he is independent.

Every person and the context of every person is unique. Certain general principles, such as the individual person's independence, must guide every action in any context similar to this. Consideration must also be given to the actual differences that exist in the context.

In this person's context there are four relevant differences:

1. He has requested that he be allowed to die.
2. He is now permanently dependent on the efforts of others.
3. None of the elements of human autonomy now characterize him. He is conscious of no desires; he is totally out of touch with the world. He engages in no reasoning processes. His life consists in basic physiological processes; this is not autonomous. He has no purposes. He has no power to exercise agency.
4. Allowing his life to terminate is not the same as terminating his life.

The recognition of this patient's autonomy does not speak against allowing him to die. The bioethical standards do not demand that he be kept alive.

❦ **DILEMMA 8-7** How does a nurse deal with a patient who makes demands on her that interfere with her attention to her other patients?

The center of Irene's attention cannot be Henry alone; she has other patients.

She cannot make an agreement with Henry that would violate the well-being of her other patients. Therefore her dilemma cannot be resolved by analysis through the standards or the elements.

Irene must analyze this as a triage situation.

❦ **DILEMMA 8-8**   Whether a parent's right to know overrides a nurse's responsibility to her patient.

This is a very simple dilemma. It is resolved by the fact that Marilyn has an agreement with Bobby.

Marilyn, of course, also has an agreement with Bobby's parents. But Marilyn is a nurse. A nurse is a professional. As a professional Marilyn's agreement with Bobby is superior to any agreement she may have with his parents. This agreement overrides any pleasure Marilyn might derive from unguarded small talk.

Many times it will happen that Bobby's health and well-being will require that his parents be given certain information. In that case Marilyn should give them the information. But this is not because of her agreement with Bobby's parents. It is because of her agreement with Bobby.

Let us assume, for the sake of argument, that Bobby's parents have a right to know of his bedwetting. Even in this (questionable) case, they have no right to expect Marilyn to tell them.

Marilyn's only responsibility in this case is to Bobby. Their knowing will not increase Bobby's health or well-being. Bobby desires Marilyn not to tell. In most cases a nurse cannot know whether or not a patient's desire is as well-reasoned as it might be. In this context it is quite clear that Bobby's is a perfectly rational desire.

❦ **DILEMMA 8-9**   Whether a nurse should give out information on the phone if this information might help or might harm her patient's best interest.

Lotte's only responsibility is to Ray. Her only agreement is her agreement with Ray. This agreement does not include taking the word of a caller and informing the caller of Ray's condition. It might seem as if Lotte is interfering with Ray's freedom. She is not. Ethically Lotte cannot interfere with Ray's freedom unless he expresses a desire.

It is reasonable to assume that if Ray had expected the call, or regarded it as important, he would have expressed a desire to her. He would have asked her to give the caller the information he wanted. It is also reasonable to assume that, if the matter were important, the lawyer would have sent someone to the hospital. Lotte has no responsibility to assist Ray's lawyer in his failing to act as Ray's agent.

Before she gives any information to the caller, Lotte ought to talk to Ray.

Ray might be unable to talk to her. If Ray were unable to talk to Lotte, then he would be unable to talk to his lawyer.

Perhaps the caller *is* Ray's lawyer. In this case it would have been better had Lotte given him the information. But Lotte could not know this. She can only justify acting on what she does know. In this context Lotte took the only justifiable action she could.

If she gave him the information she would have done the best thing for Ray. But she would have done the best thing by accident. It is not possible to justify an accident.

❧ DILEMMA 8-10   Whether a nurse ought to feed a stroke patient who must learn to feed himself.

This dilemma calls for Yvonne to ascertain ethical balance and proportion. If the long-term physical and emotional effects of feeding himself exceed the short-term effects of his not feeding himself, then Steve should feed himself. If the short-term effects outweigh the long-term effects, then Yvonne should feed him.

Yvonne should refer to the context of the dilemma. There will be short-term demoralizing effects on Steve if he feeds himself. There will be a long-term enhancement of his life and purposes in beginning to feed himself now.

Yvonne must weigh and measure one against the other and then make her decision.

❧ DILEMMA 8-11   Whether a feeble and elderly patient should be let out of restraints so that she can walk around.

Every possible consideration should be given to Margaret. Let us grant this without argument.

There are two different facts in conflict with each other:

1. Sandra should not assist Margaret in actions that will predictably injure her. To do this would be contrary to the nature and purpose of the health care system.
2. Aside from this Margaret has a right to freedom of action.

These two facts can be brought into harmony if Margaret is allowed to walk around when she can be watched and assisted. When she cannot be, "gentle coercion" (persuasion) should be exerted to keep her in the safety of her wheelchair.

Sometimes a dilemma can be resolved by not choosing one possibility over another. An agent can meet both demands of the dilemma. He can do two things, at different times, and according to changes in the context.

❧ DILEMMA 8-12   Whether a nurse ought to interfere with a patient's activities if these activities threaten his well-being.

Autonomy: Charlie cannot leave his identity and his life situation behind.

Freedom: Ingrid deals with one aspect of Charlie's life. He deals with every aspect of his life. He has a right to be free to do this.

Veracity: The standard of veracity will extend as far as "gentle coercion" but no further. Once Ingrid has related the facts to Charlie, he has a right to do whatever he wants to do.

Privacy: Ingrid ought to warn Charlie. If it is possible she should exert "gentle coercion." But Charlie is a private individual and he has a right to decide and act for himself.

Beneficence: Strictly speaking, for Ingrid to do nothing is neither beneficence nor a failure of beneficence. If she interferes, this is against Charlie's freedom.

Actions she takes against Charlie's freedom are not acts of beneficence. Beneficence is not very relevant here.

Fidelity: Fidelity to their agreement requires Ingrid to look after Charlie's health and well-being without violating the bioethical standards. The bioethical standards are the terms of their agreement.

❖ DILEMMA 8-13 What actions should a nurse take when she is asked a question by a family member and this has not been discussed with her patient?

Karen and her nurse have an agreement. The bioethical standards are the terms of this agreement. The agreement provides Karen's nurse with no preexisting knowledge of what she ought to do in this situation.

Let us see if we can analyze the situation in terms of the elements of autonomy.

Desire: Only Karen knows what she desires. So this is no help to Karen's nurse.

Reason: It is up to Karen's reason to deal with this. Her nurse's only obligation is not to make it more difficult for Karen.

Life: It is up to Karen to integrate this situation into her life. Obviously her nurse cannot help her with this.

Purpose: Karen's nurse has no purpose to serve and no right to try to guess Karen's purpose.

Agency: Karen's nurse cannot act as her agent in this situation.

The elements of autonomy provide no more direct guidance, in this circumstance, than the bioethical standards. The elements, however, do imply a principle by which the dilemma can be resolved. This principle calls for Karen's nurse to evade the question and get away. We will now turn to that principle.

Awareness and Ethical Action

Contextual action is action taken on the basis of objective judgment.

Contextual action requires an awareness of the context of the situation. It also involves an agent's awareness of the context of his or her knowledge.

Awareness is not simply desirable for effective ethical action. It is absolutely essential to it.

In circumstances like that of Karen and Steve we would suggest to the reader this overarching ethical principle:

If you do not know why you are going to do what you are going to do, do not do it.

This principle is not always easy to apply. It must be applied in a context according to the context. But it is directly implied by the elements of an ethical agent's autonomy.

Desire. An agent can be motivated by either his or her own desire or that of a beneficiary to whom the agent is responsible. If, on the other hand, an agent is aware of no desire, then the agent has no basis for action and no responsibility to act.

Reason. Not to act when one does not know what one is doing is the essence of practical reason.

Life. When you do not know why you are doing what you are doing, you cannot effectively guide your actions. You cannot know what effect it will have on your life or the life of your beneficiary. Under these circumstances it is irresponsible to take action.

Purpose. To act without knowing what you are doing is to act purposelessly. This cannot be justified. The purpose of an action is its ethical justification.

Agency. To act without knowing what you are doing is to act without agency. It is not acting at all. It is a behavior that is not guided by awareness. It is a "violation" of your agency.

❦ **DILEMMA 8-14** Whether a nurse should tell a patient's family member that a symbolic agreement the patient and family member had was not realized.

Of course, not telling Denise does not violate the standard of veracity.

If there is any dilemma whose resolution is given right along with the context, this is it. Only a formalism utterly inappropriate to nursing would counsel Lucy to inform Denise that she had not succeeded.

We can be quite certain that Lucy would not do this.

❦ **DILEMMA 8-15** Whether a nurse should tell a family member facts the family member needs to know if her patient does not want his family told.

If this dilemma simply involved the relationship between Ike and Joan, it might be analyzed as follows:

Autonomy: It is Ike's autonomous desire that Helen should not be told. He has no responsibility to justify his autonomy to Joan.

Freedom: Joan can explain to Ike that he is putting her in the middle and try to persuade him to inform Helen. But Ike has a right to do whatever he wants to do.

Veracity: Veracity does not play an important role in this dilemma.

Privacy: Joan cannot betray Ike without betraying the standard of privacy.

Beneficence: Joan has no way of knowing whether what she is doing will or will not do Ike any good or do him any harm. She does not discover much from the standard of beneficence.

Fidelity: Joan's agreement is with Ike not with Helen.

This dilemma, however, does not involve the relationship between Ike and Joan. The resolution given above is not the resolution of the dilemma. The dilemma involved in this case involves the relationship between Joan and Helen.

There are legal entanglements to this dilemma. Joan and her colleagues might be sued by Helen if Joan does not give Helen the information she needs to get her affairs in order. This being the case Ike has no right whatever to place Joan in jeopardy.

Let us examine Joan's situation in terms of the elements.

Desire: No one would reasonably choose to pursue an occupation in which they would have no way to avoid periodic law suits. Ike has no logical right to assume that nursing is such an occupation. The law may be unclear in situations like this. This lack of clarity would not prevent Helen from suing Joan and the hospital.

Reason: If Joan were to keep Ike's confidence in this situation, it would be irrational on her part. It is irrational for Ike to expect this.

People in the biomedical professions have no implicit agreement with a patient to expose themselves to lawsuits.

Life: Joan's life would be greatly diminished if her patient's whim could place her in jeopardy.

Purpose: Joan's purpose, as a nurse, is to provide some value for her patient. She would have no motivation for this unless she had purposes for herself. If she acceded to Ike's wishes, Joan could allow herself no long-term purposes. Her future would be, at best, entirely unpredictable.

Agency: Joan's agency, as a nurse, should be devoted to the health and well-being of her patients. What Ike asks of her has nothing to do with her role as nurse.

Joan can and ought to talk to Ike and, if necessary, explain why she cannot keep his condition a secret from Helen.

❦ DILEMMA 8-16 Whether a nurse ought to report a case of suspected child abuse.

It will be seen that the elements will illuminate this dilemma best.

Desire: Shawn's desire for help is rational. Doris' desire for secrecy is not.

Reason: Shawn needs Alice to help him act on his reason. Doris is not acting on reason if Alice is right in her suspicion.

Life: Shawn has a right to a better life.

Purpose: Shawn's purpose is justifiable. Doris' is not.

Agency: Alice is Shawn's agent.

❦ DILEMMA 8-17 Whether a nurse should inform her employing institution when she suspects her patient is acting fraudulently.

Autonomy: Art is autonomous. His uniqueness in this case motivates him to act unethically. Wilma has no obligation to respect Art's autonomy.

Freedom: Art has no right to freedom to act unethically. Wilma has no responsibility to help him. Further, Wilma has no right to help him.

Veracity: The standard of veracity does not demand that Wilma remain silent in order to help Art defraud the hospital.

Privacy: No one has a right to be assisted in concealing unethical actions.

Beneficence: Wilma owes beneficence to the hospital.

Fidelity: Wilma, as a nurse, never makes an implicit ethical agreement to engage in an unethical action.

❦ DILEMMA 11-1 How a nurse deals with a young person in exceedingly difficult circumstances.

Bioethical dilemmas are among the most complex and the most difficult that any human being ever faces. Wally's case is certainly among these. It will be difficult to resolve this dilemma with optimum beneficence—in such a way that

Wally is done some good and no harm. If she handles it badly, a nurse can do Wally much more harm than good. A nurse who can handle this beneficently must be able to exercise a sort of ethical artistry.

Autonomy: Wally is in the health care system. The health care system has its own specific structures and purposes. The health care system is responsible for the health and well-being of everyone who enters it.

On the other hand Wally is young. He did not come into the health care system on his own. He was not even brought in after discussion. He is suddenly thrust into a strange environment.

Taking Wally for debriding without his consent suggests a mind/body dichotomy. It suggests that Wally's body can be taken for treatment and his consciousness can be left behind. This interaction between Iris and Wally would be truly inhuman. Iris' momentary reflection on her own nature would show her that such interaction is ethically undesirable.

Whatever its benefits, and they are obvious, compelling Wally to go for treatment at this time would violate his autonomy.

Freedom: It is part of the implicit agreement that is the basis of human rights that the young shall be protected. What are the right and wrong things for Iris to do depends on the context of her relationship with Wally. It may be necessary for her to establish a relationship very quickly.

There are overwhelming reasons why Wally ought to go for debriding. Nonetheless if Iris were to take him by coercion, this would be a violation of his freedom.

Veracity: If Iris is to deal with Wally on the basis of truth, she will have to tell him that his mother is dead. The absence of ethical value in this is obvious. For Iris to put both burdens on Wally at one time would be fiendish.

Privacy: Wally now has some self-ownership. He has a potential for full self-ownership. Badly handled, the overwhelming adversity he faces can stunt this potential. A nurse never knows how much good or how much harm in a person's life she can do. Her pride ought to compel her to do the best she can.

Beneficence: Beneficence calls for Iris to do as much good and as little harm as possible. Ideally this would consist in finding a way to get Wally to treatment without inflicting force on him. It would involve telling him of his mother's death under optimum circumstances.

Fidelity: The nurse/patient agreement begins with an exchange of values. This may be the best way for Iris to go. In order to do good and avoid harm to Wally it may be best for her to continue this exchange. Iris needs to "hang loose." She needs to begin to bargain with Wally, to find some way to trade values with him. This will avoid the trauma to Wally that a violation of his autonomy and freedom would involve.

A skillful and effective nursing intervention here calls for Iris to treat Wally, not as a "big boy," but as a human person. Even though Wally is legally a minor this is a very fine place to avoid "paternalism."

Analysis under the elements of Wally's autonomy might clarify even more what is to be done.

Desire: Wally's desire to wait for his mother is rational. Force is irrational. Force would be a psychological assault on Wally.

Suppose Wally had been treated at the scene of the fire. He probably could have been treated without a prior discussion and without psychological harm. But his hospital room takes him away from the noise and stress of the disaster. It suggests that now there is a chance to think and to discuss. The situation calls out for Iris to *bargain* with Wally.

Wally is very fortunate if Iris has the abilities of a "con man." Iris should not tell Wally that his mother is alive. Aside from this, at this moment, truth is the last thing to be considered.

Reason: In Wally's context it is perfectly reasonable for him to want the comfort of his mother's presence. Effective and skillful communication and trade will have to be carried out at this level. There is probably no way Wally can reason on a more abstract level than this.

Life: Wally ought to be treated with the highest consideration. With the loss of his mother he is at a point where he must begin to build his life again.

Purpose: In order for Iris to trade with Wally effectively she must discover the nature of Wally's most rational (practical) purposes. She must discover what she can make Wally see as his most desirable purposes under these conditions of his life.

Agency: The purpose of exchanging values with Wally is to enlist his desire for some purpose, to motivate his agency and increase his cooperation with Iris.

❦ DILEMMA 12-1 Whether a child's rights protect him against a procedure he does not desire.

The concept of rights is very difficult to deal with. Rights, as a concept, form a logical bridge between ethics and political science. Each, as a general rule, has a different outlook on the nature of rights.

For purposes of bioethical analysis rights can be seen as:

. . . the product of an implicit agreement among rational beings, by virtue of their rationality, not to obtain actions nor the product of action from others except through voluntary consent, objectively gained.

1. In the same way the rights agreement arises, to a greater or lesser extent, among all people everywhere, another agreement arises. This agreement arises by virtue of the reasoning power of a parent, the undeveloped state of the child's reasoning power, the naturally dependent state of the child and the bonds of love that exist between parent and child. It is the agreement that a parent will protect and nurture the child. It is a bond of benevolence uniting parent and child. This agreement calls for a parent to decide for a child in a situation where the child is incapable of deciding for himself.

   Sandy's mother does have a moral right to sign the consent form.
2. Sandy's nurse has a moral right to give him the preoperative medications. She is acting as the agent of Sandy's mother. She is doing what Sandy's mother would do if she were able.
3. The surgeon is also acting as her agent. He also is doing what Sandy's mother would do if she could.
4. Sandy will acquire the rights that would protect him against this procedure when there is no longer a need for the parent/child agreement.

5. Sandy's mother, the surgeon, and the nurse have rights that would protect them from undergoing this procedure involuntarily. With maturity they have acquired this right.
6. Sandy's mother, the surgeon and the nurse acquired the rights that they possess when they acquired the experience and the rational capacity to decide for themselves.
7. Sandy will acquire the rights that his mother, the surgeon, and the nurse possess when he acquires the experience and the rational capacity to take over his parent's role in making his vital and fundamental decisions.

Sandy's desire is not a rational desire. It is the short-term whimsical desire of a child. It is true, and Sandy knows it to be true, that his desire must give way before the parent/child agreement.

Sandy's uniqueness cannot protect him. It will begin to protect him only when it becomes a rational autonomy. Until then it is not sufficient for the exercise of rights. An irrational autonomy will protect Sandy's short-term whims only against his rational self-interest. He becomes ethically autonomous only when his autonomy is strong enough to protect Sandy against his whims.

DILEMMA 12-2 Whether a physician has a right to compel a patient to undergo a procedure which the patient ought to undergo.

1. Even assuming that this is a procedure that he ought to undergo, Roger's physician and the court were not justified in the course of action they took. Roger's reasoning and decision might not have been the best, but they are not entirely irrational. Sometimes the rights of others prevent us from doing that which we very much want to do. If this were not the case, there would be no reason for the existence of rights. Roger's rights should have prevented the physician from doing what he wanted to do.
2. A health care professional's role cannot give him extraordinary rights. These extraordinary rights would be a right to violate the rights of others. There cannot be such a thing as a right to violate the rights of others. If there were such a right there could not be any rights at all.
3. The nurse's role in this situation would be to counsel Roger, to apply "gentle coercion," and to offer no encouragement to Roger's physician.
4. Let us assume that the method by which the judge who declared Roger incompetent became a method common in the legal system. It is obvious that this would make the legal system an all-powerful tyranny where no one would have any rights whatever. The purpose of the judicial system would no longer be to protect rights. Its purpose would become to arbitrarily establish rights for some people and to violate the rights of others.

There are several significant differences between Roger's situation and Sandy's:

• There is no parent/child agreement between Roger and his physician. There is no basis for such an agreement between them.
• Because of the parent/child agreement Sandy's rights were not violated. Roger's rights were violated.

- Sandy does not have the rational capacity nor the experience to decide. Roger has. Sandy is immature. Roger is not immature or even senile.

At his age Sandy's situation speaks for itself. Roger's does not. Sandy's mother has a right to speak for Sandy. Roger has a right to speak for himself.

❧ DILEMMA 12-3 What a nurse ought to do when she has an obviously inadequate knowledge of the situation.

Autonomy: In the context of her present knowledge Lois will probably not be able to understand and deal with Alfred's autonomy.

Lois ought to contact Alfred's family to try to obtain the information she needs.

Lois cannot act on knowledge she does not have. Before she gives up on Alfred, she ought to try to discover why she is giving up.

Freedom: Lois cannot force him to take the heparin. This would violate Alfred's right to freedom.

Veracity: It is not known that the standard of veracity is an issue in this context.

Privacy: Alfred's right to privacy includes his right to refuse the heparin.

Beneficence: Lois cannot force Alfred to accept her beneficence.

Fidelity: After Lois has stressed the reason for and the importance of the drug, fidelity calls for and permits nothing beyond "gentle coercion."

If you think about the ethical dilemmas which Alfred's case involves, it is obvious that:

1. Justifiable ethical decisions depend, not on the facts of the ethical context, but, on a person's knowledge of those facts. Justifiable ethical decisions cannot depend on facts that are not known. No decision of any sort can be made on the basis of facts that are not known.
2. An ethical agent may often feel guilt over the results of a decision that was made when the decision was made on inadequate knowledge. The self-guilt the agent assumes may very well be worse than the unfortunate result of the decision. If the agent made the decision on a logical reading of all the knowledge that was available, the decision would be perfectly justifiable regardless of its results.
3. An ethical agent's reasonable beliefs are sufficient to justify ethical actions. There is nothing whatever that an ethical agent can act upon except his or her reasonable beliefs.

There is no need for an ethical agent to do better than he can do.

❧ DILEMMA 12-4 The results of a patient violating the standard of veracity. The fact that Mabel is lying to herself has great ethical relevance in this context.

Autonomy: By lying to herself Mabel has closed off her autonomy to Charlene. In refusing to consider one or more relevant factors Mabel takes herself out of any objective context. She has broken the connection between the context of knowledge and the context of her situation. She has broken the connection between Charlene and herself. Mabel presents no autonomy and no objective context with which Charlene can deal.

Mabel has not considered the fact that the two outcomes open to her are opposed to each other. She cannot have the child and fight her cancer. Mabel can establish an objective context only by considering all the alternative possibilities and deciding on one choice.

The fact that she is unwilling to consider every possibility makes it difficult or impossible for Charlene to communicate with her.

Freedom: Mabel is unwilling to make an objective judgment based on every alternative open to her. Under these circumstances she cannot engage in free action. She has bound herself. Charlene cannot try to influence her freedom. She has given up her freedom.

Veracity: Charlene owes Mabel the truth. A patient also has some responsibility to give truthful communications to the health care professionals caring for her. Mabel is violating this standard. This gives Charlene no basis for effective ethical action.

Privacy: Mabel is using her privacy to protect herself against the reality of her situation. She is defending herself against the value of the counsel that Charlene could give her.

Beneficence: Mabel is walled off from the influence of Charlene and other health care professionals. Under these circumstances beneficence is not possible.

In order for Charlene to benefit Mabel, Mabel will have to analyze her situation and apply some level of reason to the course of action she decides on. Mabel seems entirely unwilling or unable to do this.

Fidelity: In this narrow aspect of their relationship there is no communication between Mabel and Charlene. Since there is no communication there is no agreement other than the most basic nurse/patient agreement. In everything outside of this dilemma Charlene owes Mabel fidelity. Mabel's method of resolving this dilemma, however, is so inappropriate that Charlene has nothing to give fidelity to.

Charlene ought to help Mabel in everything she can. In the context of *this* dilemma, until Mabel becomes willing to open herself up to all the alternatives of her situation there is little Charlene can do.

The bioethical standards have been of little help in resolving this dilemma. For the bioethical standards to be significantly helpful a patient must be willing to consider all the relevant facts.

Since Mabel is not willing to exercise her autonomy the elements offer no real help.

🌼 **DILEMMA 12-5**   Whether a patient has a right to ask a nurse to take on extraordinary responsibilities.

Autonomy: Dan's autonomy gives him no justification for failing or refusing to recognize Rosalyn's privacy.

Freedom: Dan's freedom gives him no justification for violating Rosalyn's freedom. Dan will not accept his calls; he desires to be free from interruptions. At the same time, he is not willing to refuse them outright; he is unwilling to be free from interruptions.

He is not justified in making Rosalyn suffer the consequences of this absurd conflict.

Veracity: This dilemma does not involve the standard of veracity.

Privacy: The basis of this dilemma is that Dan is trying to live a peculiar contradiction. On the one hand, he desires to protect his privacy against his callers. He does not want to do this, however, by simply refusing to take their calls. He is willing to take their calls through Rosalyn. He has arbitrarily decided to surrender Rosalyn's privacy rather than his own. This is, obviously, an irrational demand on Rosalyn's time. It is a violation of Rosalyn's right to privacy.

Beneficence: Rosalyn owes Dan a balanced and proportional beneficence. Enslaving herself to the telephone for Dan's sake is not a balanced and proportional beneficence.

Fidelity: To include secretarial work as a term of the nurse/patient agreement would obviously be absurd.

❦ **DILEMMA 12-6**   Whether a patient has a right to seek euthanasia.

There is a consensus of opinion on the resolution of very few, if any, dilemmas like Robert's. There are loud voices raised on either side of the complex bioethical dilemmas that technological advances in medicine have generated.

There is vigorous opposition to letting Robert die. There is equally vigorous support for his "right to die." Either side of the question can raise ethical principles in support of their position.

There is no question that principles are important. Without principles there is no guidance. But in a pluralistic society the individual, not the principle, must be at the center of ethical decision making. Decisions must be made in the context of an agreement. They cannot be made, ethically, through principles without benefit of the agreement.

In a pluralistic society no one should interfere with voluntary agreements. No one should try to impose his ethical viewpoint universally, unless universal discord is acceptable.

A health care professional can justify her ethical decisions according to her agreement with her patient. She can do this, however, only if their right to make an agreement is recognized. If they have no right to make an agreement, then there is no way for the health care professional to justify her ethical decisions. She cannot justify decisions made according to a "principle" that amounts to a rule or a whim. There is nothing to point to beyond the rule or the whim. There is no reason for another person to accept this "principle."

Imagine this in your mind's eye:

A health care professional is called up before a judge. He must justify a decision he made, or an action he took, to this judge.

The judge is not a judge in a law court. In fact, it may be the professional judging himself. For the purposes of our thought-experiment, imagine that this is someone who will judge the professional's decision or action fairly and objectively.

The judge asks, "Why didn't you . . . (take a particular course of action). That might have had a better result."

The health care professional replies, "I see what you mean. That might have been better. I didn't think of that."

The judge says, "You can't be expected to be infallible. But next time try to do better."

Under these circumstances an agent learns from his mistakes and does not repeat them. But a health care professional who guides his actions either by whims or by rules could not say to the judge, "I didn't think of that."

It would be absurd for him to say this. It goes without saying that he did not think of it. He does not *think* of anything at all.

At the same time there is something that the judge cannot say to the health care professional who guides his actions by whims or rules. The judge cannot say, "You can't be expected to be infallible." There is no standard by which a person who accepts a whim or a rule as his final authority can be in error. The results of his actions may be tragic, but he cannot be in error. The hospital may become a bedlam of human suffering, but his ethical actions, according to the whim or the rule, are flawless.

Neither could the judge say, "Next time try to do better." In order to try to do better the follower of whims or of rules would have to admit that the method of deciding was mistaken. No one would be motivated by a whim to do better. And the rule forbids an examination by the rules-follower.

Outside of a purposive and patient-centered ethic there are many compelling arguments, based on various principles, for keeping Robert alive. There are also many compelling arguments, based on other principles, for letting Robert die. None of these arguments will justify the decisions and actions of a health care professional. In addition to whatever objective value they may lack there is no consensus of agreement on them.

It may be that one position or the other is entirely right. It may be that there is some unknown way to demonstrate that the other way is entirely wrong. If so, then guidance by ethical principle without reference to the patient is possible. But, until this is shown, biomedicine's best course of action is to remain centered on the patient.

If the right to agreement is recognized, then justification in terms of an agreement is possible. Justification in terms of an agreement means justification in terms of the rights of a patient. The bioethical standards are the terms of the agreement between health care professional and patient.

In the context of a purposive ethic:

• If a person's life is not worth living, then euthanasia is not an evil.
• If a person would, objectively, be better off dead then, under these circumstances, euthanasia is not an evil.

Perhaps another question must be answered along with the question of whether euthanasia is an evil. That question is this:

Can any one person make that judgment for anyone else?

A judgment made without evidence is entirely arbitrary and valueless. This is a truism (not always honored) of our legal system. A judgment made without evidence is not justifiable. A justifiable judgment is one that can be justified on the basis of the evidence on which it was made.

Robert has made the judgment that he wants to die. Robert's physician has made the judgment that Robert should not die. In the context of a purposive ethic who has the best evidence to go on?

Autonomy: If Robert desires to die but his right to die is not recognized, then his autonomy counts for nothing.

Freedom: Robert cannot have a right to freedom but no right to die.

Veracity: If veracity is to play a role in the decision then the decision makers will have to recognize the reality of Robert's state of being.

Privacy: It is difficult to see how Robert could be a private individual and lack the right to die.

Beneficence: If beneficence is understood in human terms, then beneficence calls for Robert to be allowed to die.

Fidelity: This is, of course, the question at hand — whether or not the bioethical standards are to be terms of the bioethical agreement. If they are then, it seems, Robert ought to be allowed to die.

It is enlightening to examine Robert's case according to the elements of autonomy.

Desire: Assuming that there is no conflict between the rational and the ethical: Robert's prospects for the future promise only more and more terrible pain.

The decision maker should ask himself this question: Under these circumstances is it rational for Robert to desire to end his life?

It is more to the point to ask the question in another way: Under these circumstances is it rational for Robert to want to continue to live?

Reason: Can anyone make a rational judgment that Robert's desire to die is not reasonable?

It is certainly possible for the conditions of life to compel one to want to die.

Does it make any sense to say that it would be more reasonable not to want to die when one is *compelled* to want to die?

Life: There are conditions under which it is reasonable to want to live. There are conditions under which it is reasonable to want to die. If this second group of conditions cannot justify a desire to die, then the first cannot justify a desire to live.

Purpose: Is it proper to become purposeless if death is the only purpose possible?

Agency: The question of euthanasia is very far from settled in our society.

There is another question, more difficult than the question of euthanasia, that must also be answered. That is the question of whether a patient can expect his physician, who is his agent, to assist him in dying. It is not at all certain whether a patient's right to agency, through his physician, extends this far.

❧ **DILEMMA 13-1** Whether a nurse's responsibility extends to the details of a patient's personal life.

Autonomy: If Norma tells Chris, this is not an attack on Chris' autonomy.

Freedom: If Norma tells Chris, she does not interfere with Chris' freedom. If she does not tell Chris, Chris' fiance may, very brutally, interfere with Chris' freedom.

Veracity: What veracity demands can only be determined by the greater benefit for Chris. Would it be better that she not know in order that she might have an easier recovery? Or would it be better that she know in order that she may avoid serious long-term problems?

Privacy: Neither alternative that Norma may choose involves a violation of Chris' privacy.

Beneficence: If Norma were to tell Chris of her suspicions, this might enable Chris to avoid the greater harm.

Fidelity: The standard of fidelity calls for an attempt to be made to meet the demands of the standard of beneficence.

This dilemma can be resolved only in the actual context of Chris and Norma's situation. Norma can understand this situation only by careful attention to it. But something can be learned from the elements of autonomy.

Desire: Chris desires to recover, get married, and live happily ever after. She does not desire to recover, get married, and become an abused wife. Unless her desire to live in a fantasy is stronger than her desire to do the best possible in the real world, she would want to know about her fiance.

Reason: Reason counsels that not knowing, over the long term, would involve the worst of both worlds. Not knowing may cause Chris to fail to find her desired happiness. At the same time it could have a very negative effect on her health.

Life: The element of life suggests that Chris ought to be told. Life is much longer than the period of time from now until her discharge.

Purpose: There is no reason to believe that the pursuit of unhappiness is Chris' purpose. There is reason to believe that ignorance of her context will not assist in her pursuit of happiness.

Agency: If Chris had full knowledge, she would probably want to investigate. If the man who Chris plans to marry is not the wife abuser, he will not resent Chris investigating. If he is the wife abuser, it does not matter that he resents Chris investigating.

DILEMMA 13-2 How a context involving a retarded child with a severe heart defect can be analyzed.

We are assuming that nonaggressive treatment in this situation is a real possibility.

The physician has asked the mother and father if this is what they desire. They have not rejected this alternative.

We also assume that nonaggressive treatment is not a question to be answered entirely at the discretion of the parents. Maureen, the infant's mother, does not approach it as a question requiring only her arbitrary decision.

Some (but very few) ethical dilemmas are not much more than questions of etiquette. Others involve the deepest values of human life. This dilemma is one of that type. It is very difficult and, outside of the actual context, it would be improper to approach it dogmatically. But analysis in terms of the elements will throw some light on it:

Desire: If meaningful answers could be evoked from people born in the condition of Maureen's baby, then the desires of these people could be known. The question cannot be asked. The answers can only be inferred.

There is a school of thought that holds that infants in this condition should never be treated aggressively. There is another school of thought that holds that infants in this condition should always be treated aggressively. In the context of a purposive ethic there would be two major ethical considerations:

- The reasonable desires of the infant's parents. What is reasonable in this context is determined by the benefit the child will bring to their lives in contrast to the detriment it will bring to their lives.

    It is very easy to make a moralistic analysis of the situation and ignore the rights and values of the parents. But the process of analysis ought to be realistic. The answers derived from analysis ought to be appropriate to the real world.

- The desires of the individual person the infant will become insofar as these desires can be inferred. The best possible estimate of this should be made and put into the analysis.

Reason: Reason demands that the decision be made in context. Analysis against the background of a purposive ethic would preclude a judgment made on the basis of preexisting beliefs. A purposive ethic would hold that the only relevant beliefs are those that are gained from an examination of the infant and his parent's context.

Life: A proper ethical decision, in the context of a purposive ethic, would depend upon an interweaving of:

- The effect the infant will have on the life of the parents. This aspect of the dilemma can be used to justify nonaggressive treatment only if caring for the infant would be significantly detrimental to the life of the parents. A matter of simple inconvenience to the parents cannot justify nonaggressive treatment.

    (It must be observed that if the parents have carried the analysis this far, they are not motivated by simple convenience or inconvenience.)

- The decision the infant would make, for or against his life, in the future, if he were capable of making such a decision.

Purpose: Purpose ought to be analyzed from two sides. The future purposes of the infant ought to be a powerful consideration. The only other consideration ought to be the purposes of the infant's parents.

Agency: A life without agency is not a full human life. It is not necessarily an undesirable life either.

An Exercise in Introspection

To introspect is to contemplate one's inner states—one's thoughts and feelings. Introspection does not, in itself, give sufficient grounds for making a decision or taking an action. The value of introspection is to enable a decision maker to refine his understanding of the evidence on the basis of which he will make a decision.

With this in mind let us try a thought-experiment:

Imagine that Audrey is standing by the neonatal intensive care unit looking at the infants. She points out Maureen's baby to a nurse standing beside her. The nurse says, "This baby is mentally retarded and has a severe heart defect. He is a very happy baby. He might have a very happy life but his parents have decided to forego aggressive treatment." Hearing this, Audrey feels a strong emotional urge to go to the infant's parents and offer to adopt him.

Picture the same scene again. This time the nurse standing beside Audrey says, "This baby is mentally retarded and has a severe heart defect. He has esophogeal atresia and several other conditions. He will need numerous operations and may never be able to eat. He has a very burdensome life to look forward to." Do you think that, under these circumstances, Audrey would have as powerful a motivation to go to Maureen and offer to adopt the baby?

You can judge that, in the second case, Audrey would have much less motivation. She might well feel an emotional drive to keep a child whose life would be more pleasant than painful alive. She would not be highly motivated to keep a child alive if the child's life would be filled with more pain than pleasure.

You can make this judgment by looking into your own thoughts and feelings.

You should never take an action based only on this judgment. To do so would be to turn your back on your patient's autonomy. This introspective judgment, however, gives you a piece of evidence that should enter into your decision-making process. It can certainly *help* you to judge what is better and what is worse in every situation of this type.

❀ **DILEMMA 14-1** How a nurse might deal with a patient who is motivated by two conflicting purposes.

If Keith has the operation and the operation goes well, he may get to his son's wedding. Then he will enjoy two benefits. If he does not have the operation, he may bleed to death and never get to anything, ever again.

Autonomy: Keith's autonomy will reveal itself when he decides that one of these two purposes is more important to him than the other. It may be that Keith, himself, is not fully aware of his autonomous desires. Hopefully his final decision will reflect his autonomy and his values. There is always the chance that it may be made in a state of confusion, or when he is not thinking clearly.

If Keith does have the operation, he may miss the wedding.

It may be that attending his son's wedding is more important to Keith than having the operation.

If his son knew the circumstances, he might be willing to postpone the wedding.

It is perfectly proper for Jenna to try to talk to him about his options. Keith cannot complain if Jenna does help him to make a decision that is consistent with his values.

Freedom: Jenna has no right to interfere with Keith's freedom. She certainly has a right to talk to him. She can try to motivate him to exercise his reason. Keith's situation calls for the exercise of reason.

Jenna also has some freedom in this context.

Every nurse has the freedom that a benevolently motivated bystander would have. In addition she has the freedom that the nurse/patient agreement gives her.

Veracity: There is one aspect of veracity that is important in this case. It is important that Keith face the truth concerning his condition and the detriments of each course of action that he might take. In the final analysis the responsibility for honoring this standard rests on Keith.

Privacy: If Jenna applies "gentle coercion" to Keith, she will not violate his self-ownership.

A patient's self-ownership does not forbid conversation. It does not forbid effective nursing care.

Beneficence: The idea that beneficence would forbid Jenna to apply "gentle coercion" to Keith involves an eccentric, short-sighted notion of beneficence.

Fidelity: Fidelity demands that Jenna try to persuade Keith. Jenna is Keith's agent while he is in the health care setting. The agreement between them does not involve, as one of its terms, that Jenna shall remain passive.

❦ DILEMMA 14-2   Whether a nurse, in protecting her patient against knowing the severity of his condition, violates the element of purpose.

This is not a simple ethical dilemma. However, the problems that it presents all circle around the demands of the standard of veracity. We can look at this:

Autonomy: Under ordinary circumstances Russell has a right to refuse an amputation. He also has a right, if he desires to exercise it, to do what is best for his health.

Russell is in an unstable condition. In addition to his leg and foot injury, Russell has suffered a trauma to the head. This makes anything he says suspect. It is possible that his autonomy will not assert itself in the choice he makes. The desires he expresses may not reflect his autonomy. They may be little more than free association.

Freedom: In a normal situation a patient has a right to choose among his alternatives. He can choose whichever alternative his autonomy inclines him to.

Generally the type of situation that Russell is in is treated as a kind of triage situation. The health care professionals involved try to do the best they can. In an emergency situation, where a patient may be disoriented, this is not at all unreasonable or unethical.

Veracity: Selma faces the problem of putting Russell in the context of his circumstances without putting stress on him. She will also want to avoid suggesting anything to him that might be injurious to his well-being.

In order to reassure him Selma can say something like, "We'll take care of you. Why don't you just let us do whatever is best?" Under the circumstances there is little chance that Russell will be boxing in the Olympics. This would not necessarily keep him from using boxing in the Olympics as a rationalization for a bad decision.

Privacy: Privacy is not a major consideration here. In the emergency room considerations of privacy do not figure significantly in ethical decisions. Provided that a patient is treated efficiently there is seldom, if ever, a real violation of privacy in the emergency room.

Beneficence: Russell's condition is unstable. At this point in time hearing the truth may put him into shock. Beneficence demands that Selma prevent stress to Russell. The saying has it that, "He who fights and runs away, will live to fight another day." Perhaps Selma ought to, so to speak, take Russell running away until the emergency is over.

Fidelity: Fidelity demands that Russell receive the best possible care. This would involve getting him through the emergency situation as easily as possible. It requires letting him make whatever decisions are possible, later, under calmer circumstances.

DILEMMA 14-3 Whether a nurse's badgering her patients about their expressed desires violates their privacy.

It is desirable to maintain a degree of privacy in any relationship. In the nurse/patient relationship some degree of privacy can be maintained. However, a certain degree of privacy, necessarily, is lost. There is a certain part of the privacy of the nurse and her patient which must be shared. The enjoyment of perfect privacy in a health care setting is not possible.

Within the confines of the nurse/patient agreement Nina's bantering does not violate the self-ownership of her patients. When truth is not harmful, it does not violate a person's self-ownership to hear it.

It is not unethical to be a "pain in the neck." Nina may be a very beneficent "pain in the neck."

DILEMMA 14-4 Whether there is a limit on the value of a nurse badgering a patient about his bad habit.

Generally speaking, a nurse should begin the resolution of an ethical dilemma by orienting herself onto the realities of the situation. This is not only true of nurses, it is true of anyone who has an ethical dilemma to resolve.

This is a dilemma that is difficult to resolve out of the context. But surely this can be said:

Larry smoked when his range of activities was much greater than it is now. The fact that his range of activities is now much less than it was is no reason, in itself, for him to stop smoking. It would not be difficult for the gentlest bantering about Larry's smoking to become an ethically unjustifiable coercion.

Autonomy: Larry's reduced range of activities lessens his opportunity for self-expression and enjoyment. He does not seem motivated to care for his health more vigorously now than he did before his accident. Perhaps this is not an unreasonable attitude on his part.

Freedom: With the loss of his agency Larry lost much of the potential for the exercise of his freedom. No doubt this loss causes him suffering. The fact that smoking is bad for his health may not be justification for causing him more suffering.

Veracity: Veracity always demands of a nurse that she face the facts. When she has faced the facts it demands that she face them again—from her patient's perspective.

Privacy: Smoking and watching television are the only exercises of his privacy that Larry has left.

Beneficence: Louise's desire for Larry to stop smoking has caused her to break him into two parts: a body and a mind. For the sake of his physical health Louise is willing to launch an assault on his mind and his emotions. This is not good nursing.

Fidelity: Louise has no agreement with Larry that would justify her treating him as though he were a puppet.

❧ **DILEMMA 14-5**   Whether a nurse ought to intervene on behalf of her patient against the physician's decision.

Every health care professional is limited in the actions he can take. Every nurse must come to terms with this fact. Nurses today practice within a pluralistic society and in the bureaucracy of the health care system. It would be unreasonable for a nurse to expect that she can remake the system in her image.

This is a dilemma where a nurse must make a judgment as to what she is willing to risk. But ethically she owes her greatest fidelity to her patient.

Marilu may decide that there is nothing that she can do. Based on this decision she *may* do nothing. Marilu has no ethical obligation to do the impossible. She does have an obligation to know the difference between the right thing to do—the thing that her agreement calls for—and the wrong thing to do. She also has an obligation to know why it is impossible to do it.

In this situation for Marilu to continue to dispute with the physician would not make sense. It would be a formalistic action that might make Marilu look very good in her own eyes. It probably would not do much to help Lillian. The best thing for Marilu to do may be to contact Lillian's daughter and explain the situation to her.

❧ **DILEMMA 15-1**   Concerning a conflict between hospital policy and trust between nurses.

Holding oneself to a high level of ethical perfection cannot be a fault. Holding oneself to a level of ethical perfection within the bounds of reason and possibility is also not a fault. There is a reason for this: The highest level of ethical perfection a person can attain is a level somewhere within the bounds of reason and possibility.

To act with ethical balance and proportion is very difficult. Sometimes that which an ethical dilemma calls for is opposed to what it would seem to call for on its surface. This may be true of Gwen's ethical dilemma. Formalism would call for Gwen to report what she did and what Carrie did. Within the framework of formalism this would certainly appear to be an exemplary ethical action.

Perhaps it would be. All the same it is possible to argue that this action would not be particularly productive:

Carrie broke the rules. There is no denying that. Nonetheless Gwen should think very carefully before returning Carrie's beneficence with an action that will be maleficent in its effects.

Gwen's action did no harm to her patient.

Gwen and Carrie ought to do what is best. There is nothing either can do that is superior to resolving to do better in the future. That is to say there is nothing that will make a difference in the lives of their patients that is superior to this action.

If Gwen reports their action, they will be punished and that will be the end of it. Because of the laws governing addictive substances Carrie's punishment might be quite severe. This fact ought to play a role in the resolution of the dilemma. It speaks against the justice of Gwen doing the conventional thing and reporting Carrie.

In principle, punishment wipes the slate clean. With the clean slate that follows punishment a person tends to become careless. The clean slate makes it easier to repeat mistakes. The "burden" of remembering a mistake is often a motivation not to repeat it. Punishment removes the burden.

If Carrie cannot "cover for" Gwen because she would be unable to trust what Gwen might do, this would make a difference in the relationship between Gwen and Carrie. If nurses cannot trust each other, this is so much the worse for the profession of nursing.

If Gwen's sees her purpose as giving the best care she can to her patients, then exposing Carrie will not further this goal. If this were the right thing to do it would have a peculiar effect. It would keep the better nurses on suspension and the worst nurses at the bedside.

Punishment makes sense when it will improve efficiency. Improved efficiency increases the welfare of patients. There is no reason to believe that punishment will improve efficiency in this case. If punishment would tend to demoralize Carrie and Gwen, it will not improve their nursing care.

Whatever she does, Gwen has an ethical responsibility to know why she is doing it. In the very narrow context of her childhood training, of course, she should report Carrie. But, as we have seen, the wider the context she examines the more reason there seems not to report Carrie.

The case with Carolyn and Roseanne is quite different. It is absurd to imagine that Carolyn best protects her patient's welfare by not reporting Roseanne.

Autonomy: Cocaine will obviously impair Roseanne's ability to deal with her patient's autonomy. It will impair Roseanne's ability to care for her patients on any level.

Freedom: Roseanne's inability to function will very probably interfere with her patients' right to self-determination. It will make it impossible for Roseanne to efficiently function as the agent of her patients.

Veracity: Beneficence and veracity call for Carolyn to report Roseanne.

Privacy: Roseanne will be unable to defend her patient's privacy. At the same time Roseanne herself has given up her right to privacy.

Beneficence: In the condition that she is in, Roseanne cannot act toward her patients with beneficence. She will not even be safe.

Fidelity: Carolyn's agreement, both with the hospital and with her patients, calls for her to report Roseanne.

There is no agreement among nurses that they will not report each other under these circumstances. If there were such an agreement it would very much change the nurse/patient agreement and the nature of nursing.

In the very narrow context of loyalty to a fellow nurse Carolyn ought to cover for Rosanne. The wider the context which Carolyn examines, however, the more it becomes obvious that she ought to report Roseanne.

The first dilemma involves the question of whether nurses have a right to protect themselves. The second involves the question of whether nurses have a right to defraud and aggress against their patients.

These are two very different questions.

What Is the Virtue of a Good Nurse?

For every ethical agent some mind set, some ethical attitude, is inevitable. No one can face the world without some orientation toward it.

For most ethical agents this mind set is very unstable. Most ethical agents do not know why they are doing what they are doing; they have no objective purpose. They simply follow their duty or their assumed responsibility to a greater number. They submit to what they assume is demanded by social conventions. They hold no final goal that their actions are oriented toward. Therefore their actions are unpredictable and vacillating. They swing from an intense ethical enthusiasm for some problems to an attitude of ethical indifference for others. At certain times they may approach every problem, however minor, with excessive ethical fervor. At other times they are unmoved by an interest in any ethical dilemma.

It is impossible to practice a traditional, ritualistic ethic and not fall into one of these mind sets. No one ever knows for certain where his or her duty lies. No one ever knows for certain how to bring about the greatest good for the greatest number.

In every ethical dilemma an agent either does well or does badly. Insofar as the agent does well he or she is virtuous. Insofar as the agent does badly, he or she is vicious.*

The fact that a nurse (agent) does well in one instance does not, in itself, make her virtuous. The fact that she does badly in another instance does not, in itself, make her vicious. A person *is* virtuous or vicious insofar as he or she has a consistent mental set.

The virtuous person has a constant ethical attitude. This attitude is a determination to do well. It is a necessary precondition of the virtuous mental set. It is not possible to hold this virtuous mental set without the preexisting ethical attitude. To attempt this is to attempt to be virtuous without effort— automatically.

This mental set does not guarantee that in every dilemma an agent will do the best thing—or even the right thing. It is a predisposition to do the right thing. If an agent who acts without this mental set does well, it is by accident. In contrast, if an agent who acts from this mental set does well, he does well purposefully.

The possession of this mental set requires that it be possible for an agent to:

1. Know the right thing to do.
2. Know why this is the right thing to do.
3. Know how to do it.

---

* "Vicious" is a technical term that does not necessarily mean motivated by an evil intention. Where virtuous means ethically efficient, vicious simply means ethically inefficient.

This is the value of a professional ethic that is purposive. If a nurse regards honoring her agreement with her patient as doing well then:

1. Knowing the right thing to do means knowing what her agreement calls for.
2. Knowing the terms of her agreement (the standards) enables her to know why this is the right thing to do.
3. If there is any question about the right thing to do, or the best way of doing it, a consultation with her patient will answer the question.

The actions of a vacillating nurse are inappropriate to the context. They are disproportionate and not well balanced.

A good nurse has an openness to her patient's values. Her patient is the focus of her attention. She has a virtuous mind set. She has a certain disposition and a tendency to behave in appropriate ways. This requires an openness to her patient's values. Her patient's values are formulated in the nurse/patient agreement.

For all these reasons a purposive ethic for nursing is very desirable.

A purposive ethic is, certainly, the ethic every patient hopes for.

❦ DILEMMA 15-2   Whether a physician is justified in demanding that a patient live for her children.

Naomi's physician is determined that she shall practice a utilitarian ethic. He assumes that she has no right to change her circumstances by her decision.

Autonomy: Naomi is autonomous and no one has a right to decide her course of action but Naomi. There is no reason why Naomi's decision *must* be determined by anything but her autonomy.

Freedom: The course of action that Naomi's physican proposes would certainly violate her freedom.

Veracity: Veracity does not play an important role in this dilemma.

Privacy: Naomi is a private person and the actions that she ought to take are determined by who she is. Who she is can be determined only by Naomi.

Beneficence: Naomi is the physician's patient. There is an agreement between Naomi and her physician. This agreement places an ethical obligation on the physician. The physician has no ethical obligation to anyone beside Naomi — unless the course of action which Naomi proposes would violate the rights of a third party. It does not. Naomi does not violate the rights of her children in refusing chemotherapy, not under any defensible definition of "rights."

Fidelity: This physician obviously has no sense of fidelity to his patient.

❦ DILEMMA 15-3   Whether a psychiatric patient who is brought into the hospital against his will should be forcibly medicated.

There is a strong tide of opinion that supports the idea that "Every human being of adult years and sound mind has a right to determine what shall be done with his own life…" (President's Commission, 1982, p. 20).

Everyone has the right to be free of outside interference. The acceptance of a person's right to determine what shall be done with his or her life ought be part of the mind set of every person involved in making ethical decisions for others.

Competency is very difficult to assess. According to the President's Commission of 1982 the assessment of competency depends upon values, goals, choices, life plans, and purposes. The assessment of competency, then, is an ethical assessment. Ethics is concerned with values, goals, choices, life plans, and purposes. It is not surprising that the issue of competency makes many ethical abuses possible. The criteria for assessment that the President's Commission has set down are ethical criteria. The criteria are ethical in the framework of a *purposive* ethic.

The President's Commission (1982, pp. 57-60) has identified three elements of competency. To establish competency a person must:

1. Possess a set of values and goals that are reasonably consistent and that remain reasonably stable so that they do not radically conflict.
2. Have the ability to understand and communicate information so that it can be known that this person can appreciate the meaning of potential alternatives.
3. Have the ability to reason and deliberate about choices in light of values so that he or she can compare the impact of alternative outcomes on personal goals and life plans.

A person's decision-making capacity is impaired if it fails to, at least, minimally promote his or her desires and purposes.

It is very difficult to determine incompetency. A patient who does not want to do what a nurse or physician wants him to do, or what they think is best for him to do, is not necessarily incompetent. It may be that this patient has a better outlook on the context of his life than the nurse or physician have. With this better outlook his judgment may be superior to that of the nurse or the physician.

On the other hand, it is not necessary to regard every statement a person makes as reflecting his desires and purposes. A child's vision is not sufficiently long range to always express his real desires and purposes. The same may be true of a patient in extreme pain, one in shock, or one with brain metatasis, mental retardation, or psychiatric problems. He may be able to act, at best, only on urges. The difference between desires and purposes, on the one hand, and urges, on the other, is that urges are short-term motivations while desires and purposes are integrated into a person's life.

The desires of the truly incompetent patient are not the result of an objective reading of the facts facing him. In this sense they are not desires at all. The expression of his desires is the product of a kind of free association.

If a person is unable to express his desires and purposes, this, in itself, does not establish that someone else has a right to do it for him. The best that another person can do is to help him establish a longer range outlook. Ideally a health care professional, when dealing with an incompetent patient, would ally himself with that patient as he is when he has a clear vision of his life purposes.

The situation of an incompetent patient is very much like the situation of a child. There is one major difference: The child is in this situation a very long time; the patient, it is hoped, will be in this situation a very short time.

For different reasons neither an incompetent patient nor a child has the rational capacity to make decisions. The relationship between a health care professional and an incompetent patient is the most delicate of all bioethical relationships. It may be that this relationship calls for an agreement very similar to the parent/child agreement.

When acting for an incompetent patient a health care professional must attempt to do for the patient what the patient would do for himself if he were able. The health care professional must try to put himself in his patient's shoes. In order to do this he must obtain some familiarity with a patient's situation and values. If he cannot obtain this understanding of the patient's context then, perhaps, he should act toward his patient as he would act toward the naked comatose stranger of Chapter 14. He should act on the strongest probabilities.

The first purpose of a health care professional ought to be to protect his incompetent patient. This requires that he protect his patient against himself—and other health care professionals. A health care professional can look upon the treatment of a psychiatric patient either from the perspective of utilitarianism or as a triage situation.

From the utilitarian perspective the professional's viewpoint will be "extensionalist." He will be interested in the effect of his action on the group—on the patient's family, the rest of the hospital staff, etc. His goal will be the greater good for the greater number, not the welfare of his patient. This cannot fail to narcotize his concern for his patient.

If he looks at the situation as though it had the same form as a triage situation, his viewpoint will be "intentionalist." He will be interested in the effect of his action on his patient. This will make the welfare of his patient the center of his attention. This is where the center of his attention belongs.

The legal and ethical positions of the incompetent patient, at present, are very much in conflict. Ideally ethical decisions would be made for the incompetent patient only within the following parameters:

- For a health care professional to assume responsibility, make ethical decisions, and take actions for a patient, there ought to be some implicit or explicit invitation for him to do so. Otherwise there is a violation of the patient's self-ownership. With the violation of the patient's self-ownership, there is coercion. Coercion is not ethically justifiable.

  The only exception to this would be in a situation strongly analogous to that of the naked comatose stranger. But, even here, there is a kind of implicit invitation.
- There are times when the psychiatric patient is in virtually the same state as the naked comatose stranger. Then the same conditions for treatment would hold.
- A radical ethical differentiation should be made between the patient who comes into the health care setting voluntarily and the patient who does not. The patient who comes in voluntarily makes an implict agreement with the people in the health care setting. The patient who does not enter voluntarily makes no such agreement. His privacy is violated. If he has a right to privacy, he has a right to refuse to make an agreement. He has a right to have this refusal accepted.*

---

* It goes without saying that this only holds when the patient has not threatened or committed any criminal action. If he has then, of course, it becomes a legal matter, and the ethics of the situation are very different.

This is the only course of ethical action consistent with the bioethical standards. This course of ethical action is very much at odds with the laws presently governing these situations. The current laws provide the patient some protection; however, they provide much more opportunity for exploitation.

There is a very old saying to the effect that, "Where there are many laws there is much tyranny." This is because where there are many laws, people do not concern themselves with ethical thinking or ethical analysis. They come to follow the letter of the law and beyond this they do whatever is convenient.

Bioethicist Morris Abram, head of the President's Commission for the Study of Ethical Problems in Medicine and Biomedical and Behavioral Research (1982), stated:

. . . [W]hile recognizing the important role that the law has played in this area, the Commission does not look to the law as the primary means of bringing about needed changes in attitudes and practices. Rather, the Commission sees "informed consent" as an ethical obligation that involves a process of shared decision making based upon the mutual respect and participation of patients and health professionals. Only through improved communication can we establish a firm footing for the trust that patients place in those who provide their health care.

Everyone, whatever his or her condition in life, possesses individual rights and ethical status. People possess rights by virtue of their rationality. This does not mean that someone who is irrational does not possess rights. The possession of rights is species wide. Everyone, regardless of physical or psychological condition, possesses the right to ethical treatment. Suppose it were possible to pick and choose which members of the human species would have their rights recognized. Obviously, under these circumstances, there could be no trust among ethical agents. Without the possibility of trust among ethical agents no one could possibly possess rights. For this reason the possession of rights must be enjoyed by every member of the species.

When making a decision for an incompetent patient, it is especially important to make the decision according to the values and goals of the patient. Otherwise the bioethical standards have been violated.

Throughout history the treatment of psychiatric patients has been the scandal of medicine. Every health care professional ought to remain fully aware of the right of an individual to make decisions for his or her own life. When it becomes necessary to force a patient to do something or to restrain the patient from doing something, a health care professional should never take the situation as the status quo.

The difficulties of dilemmas involving psychiatric patients are very complex. They cannot be captured in a case study. In Jason's case it certainly appears that his agency is impaired. In all likelihood, if he were in touch with his life, he would want to recover from his present condition. If it is justifiable to treat him against his expressed desires (or urges), the person who does treat him should not lose sight of the fact that the purpose of treatment is to return Jason's agency to him.

✿ **DILEMMA 15-4**   What responsibility does a nurse have to give information to a family member who has a right to know?

The term "rights" is abused more than the sum of all other ethical terms. That
Phyllis has "a right to know" is a figure of speech. Phyllis' "right" to know is not an
ethical right.

Janine's ethical responsibility is not to Phyllis but to her patient. Her only
recourse, under the circumstances, is to tell Phyllis, "You will have to ask
Barnaby."

✿ **DILEMMA 15-5**   Whether a terminally ill patient has a right to expect
something from a nurse that might be injurious to his health.

This is several dilemmas in one.

- Whether a patient in these circumstances has the right to something he wants if it
  may be injurious to his health is one dilemma.
- Whether a physician is justified in refusing him is another dilemma.
- Whether a nurse has a right to disobey the physician's orders is a third.
- Whether a nurse has an ethical obligation that overrides the physician's order is
  still another dilemma.

Obviously a dilemma of this complexity can be resolved only in the context. But
analysis will reveal something about it.

Autonomy: Rodney's autonomy is expressed in this desire. This desire is very
short range. But, in fact, Rodney has no long-range desires. His desire is the
expression of his autonomy in his present circumstances.

Freedom: If it is probable that the drink of water would not increase Rodney's
suffering, or if his increased suffering could be alleviated, then we must consider
the following:

When Rodney entered the health care system, he was better able to act for
himself. As time passed he sank into a more and more helpless state. To refuse
Rodney's dying request while he is in this state is to violate his right to freedom.
Had Rodney known that he would be subjected to this violation, it is, in principle,
possible that he would not have come into the health care system. In light of the
fact that Rodney cannot recover, it is an action entirely lacking ethical balance and
proportion. The physician's action was a callous violation of Rodney's freedom.

If it is probable that the drink of water would increase Rodney's suffering, and if
his increased suffering could not be alleviated, then the "violation" of Rodney's
freedom is not outside of the agreement between Rodney and the people in the
health care setting.

Veracity: Julia owes Rodney an explanation of what might happen if he does
take the water.

Privacy: Julia has a responsibility to the physician. She enjoys a position of
trust in relation to the physician. It would be understandable if she did not find the
position particularly enjoyable in this situation.

Julia has an agreement with her patient. If there is a low probability that the
water will increase Rodney's suffering, then in failing to give him water Julia would

be failing to act as her patient's agent. This would be a violation of the nurse/
patient agreement and of Rodney's self-ownership.

If there is a high probability that the water will increase Rodney's suffering, then
in not giving him the drink of water Julia would not violate his self-ownership.
Beneficence is one of the terms of the agreement. The agreement is an agreement
to spare Rodney suffering.

Beneficence: What is and what is not beneficent at every step of the way must
be determined in the context.

Fidelity: Julia is Rodney's agent. She is also an agent of Rodney's agent—the
physician. If the drink of water would increase Rodney's suffering, then Julia really
does not face a dilemma. If it would not then she must determine where her greater
loyalty ought to lie. She must also decide what she is willing to risk. On the one
hand, she risks retribution from the physician. On the other hand, she risks com-
mitting a senselessly cruel act.

❖ DILEMMA 15-6   What is the ethical status of a patient's living will if a
living will is not legally recognized?

Every agreement is an agreement to take or to refrain from taking action. The
agreement that the nurse and, for that matter, the intern, has with the patient is an
agreement to act in his place.

The intern is lead by a formalistic standard. His decision has nothing to do with
his patient, their agreement, the bioethical context, or, for that matter, the law.

His attitude is one which, we hope, is not prevalent in the health care setting. He
is willing to do evil in order to appear to be good.

REFERENCES

Callahan, D., and Bok, S. (Eds.). (1982).
Ethics teaching in higher education.
New York: Plenum Press.

Gutmann, J. (Ed.). (1949). *Spinoza's ethics.* New York: Hafner Publishing Company.

President's Commission for the Study of
Ethical Problems and Medicine and
Biomedical and Behavioral Research.
(October, 1982). *Making health care
decisions: The ethical and legal impli-
cations of informed consent in the
patient-practitioner relationship* (Vol.
I.) Washington, DC: U.S. Government
Printing Office.

Epilogue

As the old man walked the beach at dawn, he noticed a young man ahead of him picking up starfish and flinging them into the sea. Finally, catching up with the youth, he asked him why he was doing this. The answer was that the stranded starfish would die if left until the morning sun.

"But the beach goes on for miles and there are millions of starfish," countered the other. "How can your efforts make any difference?"

The young man looked at the starfish in his hand and then threw it to safety in the wave. "It makes a difference to this one," he said.

Source Unknown

If something does not make a difference, if it does not bring about a change, it is ethically irrelevant. Whatever is relevant in an ethical sense must make some difference.

A nurse can make a difference. A nurse can make a profound difference to each of his or her patients—one by one. One by one can make a very great number. But, in an ethical context, no number is greater than one.

Glossary

abstract Refers to the more general and less contextual. For instance, "A nurse has a duty to society" is more abstract (more general and less contextual) than "A nurse has a responsibility to her patients."

action A behavior arising in the volition of an agent to which the agent assigns a subjective and personal meaning. A behavior that an agent initiates from within, and that remains under the agent's control.

agent One who initiates action.

agency The power or capacity of an agent to initiate action.

analysis The process whereby one seeks to understand a whole by examining its basic parts.

apathy Lack of interest in the things that a person generally considers worthy of attention.

appropriate Whatever gives an agent a greater power of agency is appropriate for that agent, for instance, an understanding of the nature of a dilemma is appropriate for its solution. Freedom from suffering and disability are appropriate to every human being. It is for this reason that nursing is an essentially ethical occupation. Nurses join with patients in a profoundly ethical endeavor.

autonomy Uniqueness; that moral property of an agent whereby the agent has the right and power to take independent action based upon his or her unique values and desires. A person's right to be what he or she is and to be dealt with according to that uniqueness.

balance The property of an interaction whereby there is a mutual exchange of values; a satisfactory arrangement of value received for value given; reciprocity.

benefactor An agent who acts so as to bring about a benefit to a beneficiary.

beneficiary One who benefits from an action. The recipient of a benefit.

beneficence "To help or at least to do no harm" (Hippocrates).

benefit "Something that enhances or promotes well-being" (American Heritage Dictionary, 1982).

benevolence A psychological inclination to beneficence.

bioethics Ethics in relation to the health care professions.

burn-out "A syndrome of physical and emotional exhaustion involving the development of a negative self-concept, negative job attitude, and loss of concern and feeling for patients" (Pines and Maslach, 1978).

choice The intentional resolution of an alternative.

concept A mental image, held in the mind, of something existing in reality; the act by which a person knows an object in reality; the idea of that which is known.

conditions Existing circumstances. The circumstances that are necessary in order for some state-of-affairs to come about.

consequences That which follows as the result of a cause; the moral effects of an initiated cause.

context (*of the situation*) The interwoven aspects of a situation that are fundamental to understanding the situation and to acting effectively in it.

(*of the context*) An agent's awareness of the relevant aspects of a situation that are necessary to understanding the situation and to acting effectively in it.

(*solitary context*) A context involving only one person — the agent.

(*interpersonal context*) A context involving more than one person.

decision A choice made between alternative values or courses of action.

deontology "The theory that . . . actions in conformance with . . . formal rules of conduct are obligatory regardless of their results" (Angeles, 1981).

desire One's psychological orientation toward a purpose. More broadly, the capacity of an organism whereby it acts to retain its values, including the value that is its own life.

determinism The doctrine that human choices are the effects of necessitating conditions; the theory that all conscious behavior is a response to outside forces in the same way that the behavior of physical entities is always a response to external forces.

determine To bring something — a state of awareness or a state of being — into existence; to direct a course of action.

dilemma A situation in which one is faced with a conflict of purposes or with purposes whose value is not clear.

duty An ethical sanction demanding adherence to a rule without regard to consequences.

element "The fundamental, essential, or irreducible constituent of an object" (American Heritage Dictionary, 1982). Thus the roundness of a ball is an element of a ball. Its color is not.

ethics A system of principles to motivate, determine, and justify actions taken in the pursuit of vital and fundamental goals.

ethicist One engaged in the theoretical study of ethics.

evil The evil of a thing is that which negates (blocks) its efficient functioning as the kind of thing it is (failure, the violation of rights and illness are, for instance, all evils); inappropriate or disproportionate to the context.

explicit Actually spoken or agreed to — not merely understood implicitly.

freedom An agent's capacity and consequent right to take independent actions based on the agent's own evaluation of the situation.

fidelity Adherence to the terms of an agreement.

formalism The theory that ethical action is action that conforms with certain forms of behavior; an ethical formalist is one who concentrates entirely on the abstract category into which an action can be placed, without regard for the context or the effects of the action.

fundamental Essential to making a thing the kind of thing it is; the fundamental element of a thing is that which best explains its behavior (for instance, roundness is essential to the rolling of a ball; therefore, roundness is a fundamental property of a ball.)

good The good of a thing is that which assists its efficient functioning as the kind of thing it is (success, respect for rights, and health care, for instance, are all goods); appropriate or proportionate to the context.

hedonism The ethical theory that only those actions which produce pleasure in the agent are appropriate ethical actions.

implicit That which is logically suggested by the explicit but which is not made explicit (the explicit being that which is actually spoken and consciously agreed upon); understood without being openly expressed.

intelligibility That aspect of an object or state of affairs whereby it is recognizable as the kind of thing it is (if the fundamental nature of a state of affairs is easily recognizable, then the state of affairs is intelligible; if any aspect of a state of affairs makes the state of affairs recognizable, then that is its fundamental aspect).

intention The state of affairs that an agent acts to bring about; a mental act of attention to an object.

interwoven Systematic; composed of interacting, interrelated, or interdependent facts that form a complex whole (for instance, sweaters are made up of interwoven strands of yarn).

introspection The act of directing one's attention back into one's own subjectivity; the act of reflecting back onto one's own psychological processes.

justice A willingness to extricate another from a condition of adversity in which he or she was placed by another; the act of establishing proportionality on behalf of one whose rightful purposes have been interfered with by another or who has lost the product of his or her actions through the actions of another; the act of reestablishing proportionality on behalf of one whose rights have been violated; the appropriate dispensing of rewards and punishment.

justify To describe or explain in terms of, or as related to, a purpose.

justification A description in terms of how something meets a purpose—the purpose as formulated in a decision or agreement; demonstration that something is correspondent with the terms of an agreement.

life The process wherein an organism generates and sustains actions directed toward the attainment of its needs and purposes according to its potential.

logical According to the demands of understanding; intelligible (for instance, intelligible reasoning).

maleficence To do harm or to refuse to do good where good might be expected.

mercy A willingness to extricate another from a condition of adversity.

meaning That which facillitates a vital purpose; "x has meaning" means x will help an agent to attain a goal.

mores Rules or standards of behavior as related to a certain society; the ethical conventions of a society.

normative "Having to do with an established standard of behavior" (Runes, 1983); having to do with ethics.

objective Existing apart from a perceiving subject; having actual existence or reality (thought that is uninfluenced by emotion or personal prejudice is objective).

objectivity A willingness to know something as it is apart from emotion or personal prejudice.

obligation A sanction of action in terms of good and evil or right and wrong.

passion A behavior that an agent undergoes through a force external to self and not as the outcome of his or her act of self-determination.

patient One who has lost or suffered a decrease in agency.

precondition "A condition that must exist before something else can occur" (American Heritage Dictionary, 1982).

presupposition An idea that implies the truth of another idea [the first idea could not be true unless the second idea were true; for instance, the idea that people must control their natural tendency to perform evil actions presupposes the idea that people actually have a natural tendency to perform evil actions (which is a presupposition of the first idea)].

proper Appropriate to the context; meeting a requisite standard.

proportion A measure of benefit or value between one action or the product of the action in comparison with another action or the product of another action according to the standard of reciprocity.

principle A basic fact, truth, or law from which other facts, truths or laws proceed; the motivating ground of an action.

privacy Self-ownership; the right of an individual to be free of undesired or undesirable interaction.

purpose That state of affairs which is the object of an action motivated by desire; the psychological condition that accompanies an orientaion toward bringing about this state of affairs.

purposive ethic An ethic that holds that an action is to be evaluated in terms of its predictable results.

rational Tending to appropriate proportions; well reasoned; appropriate to the context.

reason The faculty of thinking; thinking being a process of awareness directed toward: (1) what is relevant, (2) what is appropriate, (3) what is balanced, and (4) what is proportional – in the demands of a context and the agent's responses to these demands.

reciprocity A balanced interchange of benefits or values; an appropriate balance between value given and value received.

relevant Serving to affect ethical proportion (something is relevant to a context if the context cannot be fully understood without it).

rights The product of an implicit agreement among rational beings by virtue of their rationality not to obtain actions or the product of actions from others except through voluntary consent objectively gained.

Rights means, in one sense, the

product (freedom from aggression) of an agreement (not to aggress). In another sense rights is the agreement itself. In either sense the generic term (freedom from aggression; agreement) is singular. Therefore, the term rights is a singular term.

It is a grave ethical mistake to regard the term rights as a political rather than a more fundamental, ethical term and to regard it as plural—an everchanging product of legislation.

ritualistic ethic An ethical system that holds that ethical principles are right or wrong without regard for the desires, choices, and purposes of the people involved.

standard That by which the ethical appropriateness of an action can be measured. Various standards that have been proposed are:

Socrates: Knowledge of that which is beneficial

Plato: The Good

Aristotle: The actions that noble and virtuous people would take

Aquinas: Happiness

Spinoza: The preservation and enhancement of the agent's life

Kant: Duty

Bentham: The greatest good for the greatest number

Rand: The preconditions of "man's life qua man"

system The interrelationships of the elements that make up a whole.

term "A condition or stipulation that

defines the nature and limits of an agreement" (American Heritage Dictionary, 1982).

triage A triage situation is a situation calling for choices to be made when the benefits that can be brought about in the situation are limited. The choices may be choices among benefits or beneficiaries or both.

utilitarianism "The theory that one should act as to promote the greatest happiness (pleasure) of the greatest number of people" (Angeles, 1981).

value The object of an action that is motivated by an autonomous desire; that which is instrumental in the realization of a purpose.

veracity (*as a bioethical standard*) The imparting of knowledge to another when this knowledge will do that other some good or at least do more good than harm.

virtue "Action according to the nature of that which acts" (Spinoza cited in Gutmann, 1949). (for instance, it is a virtue in a horse to run swiftly; it is a virtue in a boat not to sink; it is a virtue in a person to live rightly and well—according to a purposive ethic "virtue" refers to a person's ability to act to fulfill his or her rational desires).

vital Essentially related to the preservation or enhancement of life, as, for instance, a vital need or a vital desire.

volition The power to take uncompelled and purposeful actions.

REFERENCES

American heritage dictionary. (1982). (2nd college edition). Boston: Houghton Mifflin.

Angeles, P. (1981). *Dictionary of philosophy.* New York: Barnes and Noble.

Gutmann, J. (1949). *Spinoza's ethics.* New York: Hafner Publishing.

Pines, A., & Maslach, C. (1978). Characteristics of staff burn-out in mental health setting. *Hospital Community Psychiatry, 29,* 233-237.

Runes, D. D. (Ed.). (1983). *Dictionary of philosophy.* New York: Philosophical Library.

Supplemental Readings

CHAPTER 1

Gorovitz, S. (1986). Baiting bioethics. *Ethics*, *95*(3), 356-374.

Hospers, J. (1972). *Human conduct: Problem of ethics*. New York: Harcourt, Brace Jovanovich, Inc.

Loewy, E. H. (1987). The uncertainty of certainty in clinical ethics. *The Journal of Medical Humanities and Bioethics*, *8*, 26-33.

Loewy, E. H. (1988). Comparative medical ethics: An introduction. *Journal of Medicine and Philosophy*, *13*(3), 225-229.

CHAPTER 2

Ketefian, S., & Ormond, J. (1988). *Moral reasoning and ethical practice in nursing: An integrative review*. New York: National League for Nursing.

Reilly, D. E. (1989). Could an ethics committee have prevented Linare's tragedy? *Medical Ethics Advisor*, *5*(6), 69-84.

Reilly, D. E. (1990). Ethics and values in nursing: Are we opening Pandora's box? *Nursing and Health Care*, *10*(2), 91-95.

CHAPTER 3

Axelrod, R. (1984). *The evolution of cooperation*. New York: Basic Books.

Churchill, L. R. (1989). Reviving a distinctive medical ethic. *Hastings Center Report*, *19*(3), 28-34.

Gauthier, D. (1987). *Morals by agreement*. Oxford: Oxford University Press.

Kamin, F. M. (1985). Supererogation and obligation. *Journal of Philosophy*, *82*(3), 118-138.

CHAPTER 4

Andrews, L. B. (1986). My body, my property. *Hastings Center Report*, *16*(5), 28-38.

Benoliel, J. Q. (1989). Ethical perspective: In favor of autonomy. *Rehabilitative Nursing*, *14*(5), 254-255.

Davis, A. (1986). Informed dissent: The view of a disabled woman. *Journal of Medical Ethics, 12*(2), 75-76.

Donnelley, S. (1988). Human selves, chronic illness, and the ethics of medicine. *Hastings Center Report, 18*(2), 5-8.

Eckman, S., & Norberg, A. (1988). The autonomy of demented patients: Interviews with caregivers. *Journal of Medical Ethics, 19*(4), 184-187.

Engelhardt, H. T., Jr. (1989). Fashioning an ethic for life and death in a postmodern society. *Hastings Center Report, 19*(1), 7-9.

Kapp, M. B. (1989). Medical empowerment of the elderly. *Hastings Center Report, 19*(4), 5-7.

Kjervik, D. K. (1990). AIDS and the duty to warn. *Journal of Professional Nursing, 6*(1), 10, 64.

Pires, M. (1989). Ethical perspective: A nurse's reaction to Tom's story. *Rehabilitative Nursing, 14*(5), 255-256, 268.

Ridley, B. (1989). Tom's story: A quadriplegic who refused rehabilitation. *Rehabilitation Nursing, 14*(5), 250-253.

Salliday, S. A. (1990). Ethical problems: Stand up for the patient. *Nursing 90,* 26-27.

Salliday, S. A. (1990). Ethical problems: Family background. *Nursing 90,* 111.

Simms, M. (1986). Informed dissent: The views of some mothers of severely intellectually handicapped young adults. *Journal of Medical Ethics, 12*(2), 72-74.

Veatch, R. M. (1987). The ethics of promoting herd immunity. *Family and Community Health, 10*(1), 44-53.

CHAPTER 5

Brandt, R. B. (1979). *A theory of the good and the right.* Oxford: Clarendon Press.

Gorovitz, S. (Ed.). (1971). Mill's utilitarianism: *With critical essays.* Indianapolis: Bobbs-Merrill.

Hazlitt, H. (1969). *The foundation of morality.* New York: Van Nostrand.

Karin-Frank, S. (1987). Genetic engineering and the autonomous individual. *Philosophy, 22* (Suppl.), 213-229.

Blowing the whistle on incompetencies. (1989). *Nursing 90, 19,* 47-50.

Wolff, R. P. (Ed.). (1969). *Kant's foundations* of the metaphysics of morals: Text and critical passages. New York, Bobbs-Merrill.

CHAPTER 6

Stevenson, C. L. (1967). *Facts and values.* New York: Yale University press.

CHAPTER 7

Hull, R. T. (1985). Informed consent: Patient's right or patient's duty. *Journal of Medicine and Philosophy, 10*(2), 183-197.

O'Neil, R. (1983). Determining proxy consent. *Journal of Medicine and Philosophy, 8*(4), 389-404.

Schade, S. G., & Muslin, H. (1989). Do not resusciatate decisions: Discussion with patients. *Journal of Medical Ethics, 15,* 186-190.

Wierenga, E. (1983). Proxy consent and counterfactual wishes. *Journal of Medicine and Philosophy, 8*(4), 405-416.

Zurin, D. A., & Pauker, S. G. (1984). Decision analysis as a basis for medical decision making: The tree of Hippocrates. *Journal of Medicine and Philsophy, 9*(2), 181-214.

CHAPTER 8

Callahan, J. C. (1984). Liberty, beneficence and involuntary confinement. *Journal of Medicine and Philosophy, 9*(3), 261-294.

Callahan, J. C. (1985). Response to Rebecca Dresser's involuntary confinement: Legal and psychiatric perspectives. *Journal of Medicine and Philosophy, 10*(3), 199-202.

Dresser, R. (1984). Involuntary confinement: Legal and psychiatric perspectives. *Journal of Medicine and Philosophy, 9*(3), 295-299.

Strasser, M. (1986). Mill and the right to remain uninformed. *Journal of Medicine and Philosophy, 11*(3), 265-278.

CHAPTER 9

Anderson, L. (1985). Moral dilemmas, deliberation and choice. *Journal of Philosophy, 82*(3), 139-162.

CHAPTER 10

Haldane, J. (1989). Voluntarism and realism in medieval ethics. *Journal of Medical Ethics, 15*, 39-44.

Tannsjorn, T. (1985). Moral conflict and moral realism. *Journal of Philosophy, 82*(3), 113-117.

CHAPTER 11

Dagi, T. F. (1983). How can one die better? *Journal of Medicine and Philosophy, 8*(4), 431-435.

Stevens, J. C. (1984). Must the bearer of a right have the concept of that to which he has a right? *Ethics*, 68-74.

CHAPTER 12

Gatens-Robinson, E. (1984). Clinical studies and the rationality of the human sciences. *Journal of Medicine and Philosophy, 11*(3), 265-284.

Hamlyn, D. W. (1985). Self-deception. *Journal of Medical Ethics, 11*(4), 210-211.

CHAPTER 13

Doerflinger, R. (1989). Assisted suicide: Pro-choice or anti-life? *Hastings Center Report, 19*(1) (Special Suppl.), 16-19.

MacQuire, D. C. (1984). *Death by choice* (2nd ed.). Garden City, NJ: Doubleday.

Mayo, D. J. (1986). The concept of rational suicide. *Journal of Medicine and Philosophy, 11*(2), 143-155.

CHAPTER 14

Anderson, F. (1985). Human gene therapy: Scientific and ethical considerations. *Journal of Medicine and Philosophy, 10*(3), 275-292.

Fletcher, J. C. (1985). Ethical issues in and beyond prospective clinical trials of human gene therapy. *Journal of Medicine and Philosophy, 10*(3), 293-309.

Tauer, C. A. (1985). Personhood and human embryos and fetuses. *Journal of Medicine and Philosophy, 10*(3), 253-266.

CHAPTER 15

Foot, P. (1978). *Virtues and vices*. Berkeley: University of California Press.

Iserspn, K. V., & Rouse, F. (1989). Case studies: Prehospital DNR orders (commentaries). *Hastings Center Report, 19* (6) (Special Suppl.), 17-19.

Lomansky, L. (1987). *Persons, rights and the moral community*. Oxford: Oxford University Press.

Loring, L. M. (1966). *Two kinds of values*. New York: Humanities Press.

Packard, J. S., & Ferrara, B. M. (1988). In search of the moral foundation of nursing. *Advances in Nursing Science, 10*(4), 60-71.

Putnam, D. A. (1988). Virtue and the practice of modern medicine. *Journal of Medicine and Philosophy, 13*(4), 433-443.

Thomson, J. (1977). Some ruminations on rights. *Arizona Law Review, 45*, 306-315.

Veatch, H. B. (1985). *Human rights: Facts or fancy*. Baton Rouge: Louisiana State University Press.

Veatch, R. M. (1988). The danger of virtue. *Journal of Medicine and Philosophy, 13*(4), 445-446.

Yarling, R. R. & McElmurry, B. J. (1986). The moral foundation of nursing. *Advances in Nursing Science, 8*(2), 63-73.

ADDITIONAL GENERAL READINGS

American Nurses' Association (1985). *Code for nurses with interpretive statements*. Kansas City, MO: The Association.

Blanshard, B. (1961). *Reason and goodness.* London: George Allen and Unwin, Ltd.

de la Boetie, E. (1975). *The politics of obedience: The discourse of voluntary servitude.* New York: Humanities Press.

Brandt, R. B. (Ed.). (1961). *Value and obligation.* New York: Harcourt, Brace and World, Inc.

Capron, A. M. (1987). Anencephalic donors: Separate the dead from the dying. *Hastings Center Report, 17*(1), 5-19.

Coulte, D. J., Murray, T. H., & Cerreto, M. C. (1988). Practical ethics in pediatrics. *Current Problems in Pediatrics, 18*(2),142-193.

Cranford, R. E. (1988). The persistent vegetative state: The medical reality (getting the facts straight). *Hastings Center Report, 18*(1), 27-32.

Davies, J. (1988). Raping and making love are different concepts: So is killing and voluntary euthanasia. *Journal of Medical Ethics, 14*(3), 148-149.

Engelhardt, H. T., Jr., & Callahan, D. (Eds.). (1976). *The foundations of ethics and its relationship to science.* Hastings on Hudson, NY: Hastings Center.

Fenigsen, R. (1989). A case against Dutch euthanasia. *Hastings Center Report, 19*(1) (Special Suppl.), 22-30.

Ganthies, D. (1963). *Practical reasoning.* Oxford: Clarendon Press.

Gewirth, A. (1978). *Reason and morality.* Chicago: University of Chicago Press.

Gillon, R. (1988). Euthanasia: Withholding life-prolonging treatment and moral differences between killing and letting die. *Journal of Medical Ethics, 14*(3), 115-117.

Green, T. H., & Grose, T. H. (Eds.). (1964). *Hume's essays: Moral, political, and literary.* London: Scientia Verlag Aalen.

Hamilton, E., & Cairns, H. (Eds.). (1973). *The collected dialogues of Plato.* Princeton, NJ: Princeton University Press.

Haria, C. C., & Snowden, F. (Eds.). (1984). *Bioethical frontiers in perinatal intensive care.* Natchitoches, LA: Northwestern State University of Louisiana Press.

Hoppe, H. H. (1983). Is research based on causal scientific principles possible in the social sciences? *Ratio,* 173-202.

Horan, D. J., & Mall, D. (Eds.). (1977). *Death, dying and euthanasia.* Washington, DC: University Publications.

Hospers, J. (1961). *Human conduct.* New York: Harcourt, Brace and World, Inc.

Kass, L. R. (1985). *Toward a more natural science: Biology and human affairs.* New York: The Free Press.

Ketefian, S. (1989). Moral reasoning and ethical practice in nursing: Measurement issues. *The Nursing Clinics of North America, 24*(2), 509-529.

Koop, C. E. (1989). The challenge of definition. *Hastings Center Report, 19*(1) (Special Suppl.), 2-3.

Kukse, H. (1986). Death by non-feeding: Not in the baby's best interest. *Journal of Medical Humanities and Bioethics, 7,* 79-90.

MacIntyre, S. (1981). *After virtue: A study in moral theory.* Notre Dame, IN: University of Notre Dame Press.

McKeon, R. (Ed.). (1941). *The basic works of Aristotle.* New York: Random House.

Moore, G. E. (1903). *Principia ethica.* London: Cambridge University Press.

Norton, D. L. (1976). *Personal destinies.* Princeton, NJ: Princeton University Press.

Nozick, R. (1974). *Anarchy, state and utopia.* New York: Basic Books.

Olthuis, J. H. (1969). *Facts, values, and ethics* (2nd ed.). Assen, Netherlands: Royal Van Gorcum, Ltd.

Parachine, A. (1989). The California humane and dignified death initiative. *Hastings Center Report, 19*(1) (Special Suppl.), 10-12.

Pegis, A. (Ed.). (1945). *The basic works of St. Thomas Aquinas.* New York: Random House.

Polanyi, M. (1968). *The tacit dimension.* Garden City, NJ: Doubleday.

Popper, K. R. (1973). *Objective knowledge.* Oxford: Oxford University Press.

Prichard, H. A. (1972). Does moral philosophy rest on a mistake? *Mind, 21,* 487-499.

Rachels, J. (1986). *The end of life.* New York: Oxford University Press.

Ramos, M. C. (1987). Adopting an evolutionary lens: An optimistic approach to discovering strength in nursing. *Advances in Nursing Science, 10*(1), 19-26.

Rand, A. (1961). *For the new intellectual.* New York: New American Library.

Rand, A. (1964). *The virtue of selfishness.* New York: New American Library.

Rautio, K., Dean, D., & Gregg, D. (1990). Ethical guidelines for the Colorado Society of Clinical Specialists in Psychiatric Nursing. *Journal of Psychosocial Nursing, 28*(2), 38-39.

Rawls, J. (1971). *A theory of justice.* Cambridge, MA: Harvard University Press.

Reed, P. (1989). Nursing theorizing as an ethical endeavor. *Advances in Nursing Science, 11*(3), 1-10.

Rigter, H. (1989). Euthanasia in the Netherlands: Distinguishing facts from fiction. *Hastings Center Report, 19*(1) (Special Suppl.), 31-32.

Sidwick, H. (1952). *The method of ethics.* London: Macmillan.

Szasz, T. (1977). *The theology of medicine: The political and philosophical foundations of medical ethics.* New York: Colophon Books.

Van De Veer, D., & Regan, T. (Eds.). (1987). *Health care ethics.* Philadelphia, PA: Temple University Press.

Vaux, K. L. (1989). The theological ethics of euthanasia. *Hastings Center Report, 19*(1) (Special Suppl.), 19-22.

Veatch, R. M. (1981). *A theory of medical ethics.* New York: Basic Books.

Weil, W. B. (1989). Ethical issues in pediatrics. *Current Problems in Pediatrics, 14*(12), 623-698.

Weinberg, J. R., & Yandell, K. E. (1971). *Ethics.* New York: Holt, Rinehart, and Winston, Inc.

Wild, J. (1953). *Plato's modern enemies and the theory of natural law.* Chicago: University of Chicago Press.

Wolf, S. M. (1989). Holding the line on euthanasia. *Hastings Center Report, 19*(1) (Special Suppl.), 13-15.

Wolfgang, K. (1966). *The place of value in a world of facts.* New York: Liveright.

Index

4591